Sanitary and Environmental Engineering: Relevance and Concerns

Sanitary and Environmental Engineering: Relevance and Concerns

Editor

Rok Fink

MDPI • Basel • Beijing • Wuhan • Barcelona • Belgrade • Manchester • Tokyo • Cluj • Tianjin

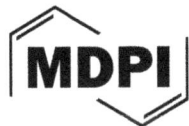

Editor
Rok Fink
Department of Sanitary Engineering
Faculty of Health Sciences
University of Ljubljana
Ljubljana
Slovenia

Editorial Office
MDPI
St. Alban-Anlage 66
4052 Basel, Switzerland

This is a reprint of articles from the Special Issue published online in the open access journal *Processes* (ISSN 2227-9717) (available at: www.mdpi.com/journal/processes/special_issues/sanitary_environmental_engineering).

For citation purposes, cite each article independently as indicated on the article page online and as indicated below:

LastName, A.A.; LastName, B.B.; LastName, C.C. Article Title. *Journal Name* **Year**, *Volume Number*, Page Range.

ISBN 978-3-0365-7753-1 (Hbk)
ISBN 978-3-0365-7752-4 (PDF)

© 2023 by the authors. Articles in this book are Open Access and distributed under the Creative Commons Attribution (CC BY) license, which allows users to download, copy and build upon published articles, as long as the author and publisher are properly credited, which ensures maximum dissemination and a wider impact of our publications.

The book as a whole is distributed by MDPI under the terms and conditions of the Creative Commons license CC BY-NC-ND.

Contents

About the Editor vii

Preface to "Sanitary and Environmental Engineering: Relevance and Concerns" ix

Rok Fink
Special Issue—"Sanitary and Environmental Engineering: Relevance and Concerns"
Reprinted from: *Processes* **2023**, *11*, 1378, doi:10.3390/pr11051378 1

Wei Yang, Peiquan Shen, Zhaoyi Ye, Zhongmin Zhu, Chuan Xu and Yi Liu et al.
Adversarial Training Collaborating Multi-Path Context Feature Aggregation Network for Maize Disease Density Prediction
Reprinted from: *Processes* **2023**, *11*, 1132, doi:10.3390/pr11041132 5

Mojca Jevšnik, Lucija Pirc, Andrej Ovca, Marina Šantić, Peter Raspor and Karmen Godič Torkar
A Multimethod Study on Kitchen Hygiene, Consumer Knowledge and Food Handling Practices at Home
Reprinted from: *Processes* **2022**, *10*, 2104, doi:10.3390/pr10102104 17

Damjan Slabe, Eva Dolenc Šparovec and Mojca Jevšnik
Hygiene and Food Safety Habits among Slovenian Mountaineers
Reprinted from: *Processes* **2022**, *10*, 1856, doi:10.3390/pr10091856 33

An Galičič, Jan Rožanec, Andreja Kukec, Tanja Carli, Sašo Medved and Ivan Eržen
Identification of Indoor Air Quality Factors in Slovenian Schools: National Cross-Sectional Study
Reprinted from: *Processes* **2023**, *11*, 841, doi:10.3390/pr11030841 49

An Galičič, Natalija Kranjec, Jan Rožanec, Ivana Obid, Eva Grilc and Branko Gabrovec et al.
Spread of SARS-CoV-2 Infections in Educational Settings by Level of Education, Taking into Account the Predominant Virus Variant
Reprinted from: *Processes* **2022**, *10*, 1947, doi:10.3390/pr10101947 65

Boyu Xia and Linchang Zheng
Ecological Environmental Effects and Their Driving Factors of Land Use/Cover Change: The Case Study of Baiyangdian Basin, China
Reprinted from: *Processes* **2022**, *10*, 2648, doi:10.3390/pr10122648 75

Yizhun Zhang and Qisheng Yan
Application of Beetle Colony Optimization Based on Improvement of Rebellious Growth Characteristics in $PM_{2.5}$ Concentration Prediction
Reprinted from: *Processes* **2022**, *10*, 2312, doi:10.3390/pr10112312 93

Qiufei Wang, Siyu Li and Ye Yang
Simulation Analysis of Implementation Effects of Construction Waste Reduction Policies
Reprinted from: *Processes* **2022**, *10*, 2279, doi:10.3390/pr10112279 111

Melani Sigler Zekanović, Gabrijela Begić, Silvestar Mežnarić, Ivana Jelovica Badovinac, Romana Krištof and Dijana Tomić Linšak et al.
Effect of UV Light and Sodium Hypochlorite on Formation and Destruction of *Pseudomonas fluorescens* Biofilm In Vitro
Reprinted from: *Processes* **2022**, *10*, 1901, doi:10.3390/pr10101901 123

Kaća Piletić, Bruno Kovač, Matej Planinić, Vanja Vasiljev, Irena Brčić Karačonji and Jure Žigon et al.
Combined Biocidal Effect of Gaseous Ozone and Citric Acid on *Acinetobacter baumannii* Biofilm Formed on Ceramic Tiles and Polystyrene as a Novel Approach for Infection Prevention and Control
Reprinted from: *Processes* **2022**, *10*, 1788, doi:10.3390/pr10091788 . . . . **139**

Rok Fink
Terpenoids as Natural Agents against Food-Borne Bacteria—Evaluation of Biofilm Biomass versus Viability Reduction
Reprinted from: *Processes* **2023**, *11*, 148, doi:10.3390/pr11010148 . . . . **155**

About the Editor

Rok Fink

Dr. Rok Fink is an associate professor at the Faculty of Health Sciences of the University of Ljubljana, Slovenia. His expertise includes sanitary engineering with a focus on biofilms, material science, bacterial adhesion, and sanitation, and has researched extensively on environmental health with the spotlight on prevention and control measures for surface hygiene.

Preface to "Sanitary and Environmental Engineering: Relevance and Concerns"

The environment consists of living and non-living elements that interact with each other and can affect their health and lives. Now more than ever, humanity is called upon to take action to protect the environment and public health. The environment in which we live is the most important factor in our health and well-being. Human activities have a significant impact on the atmosphere, lithosphere, hydrosphere, biosphere, and even outer space. Biological, chemical, physical, and social risk factors are part of our daily lives, and scientific research is constantly challenged to understand and mitigate these interactions to make life on Earth more sustainable. This reprint contains 12 articles on various filed of sanitary and environmental engineering. It provides current research on sanitary and environmental engineering with a focus on mitigation of the impact of mankind on the environment and vice versa. This reprint should be of interest to scientists, students, and engineers from practice. I hope you will find this book useful and that you will enjoy reading it as much as we enjoyed writing it. This Special Issue is a result of the collaborative work of many researchers in the field of sanitary and environmental engineering with the spotlight on food safety, indoor air quality, environmental protection, waste management, and microbial populations.

Rok Fink
Editor

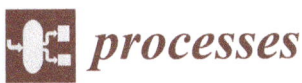

Editorial

Special Issue—"Sanitary and Environmental Engineering: Relevance and Concerns"

Rok Fink

Faculty of Health Sciences, University of Ljubljana, Zdravstvena pot 5, 1000 Ljubljana, Slovenia; rok.fink@zf.uni-lj.si

Citation: Fink, R. Special Issue—"Sanitary and Environmental Engineering: Relevance and Concerns". *Processes* **2023**, *11*, 1378. https://doi.org/10.3390/pr11051378

Received: 17 April 2023
Revised: 21 April 2023
Accepted: 29 April 2023
Published: 3 May 2023

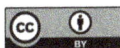

Copyright: © 2023 by the author. Licensee MDPI, Basel, Switzerland. This article is an open access article distributed under the terms and conditions of the Creative Commons Attribution (CC BY) license (https://creativecommons.org/licenses/by/4.0/).

The environment consists of living and inanimate elements that mutually interact and affect each other's health and lifespan. Anthropogenic sources of pollution are of particular concern as they are increasing exponentially, constituting a rate faster than ever before in the Earth's history. A 2016 report reported that 24% of global deaths are due to changing environmental factors [1]. In addition, since 1970, the average wildlife population size decreased by 69% [2]. These phenomena show that health and environmental sciences are key factors in terms of responding to the changing environment in order to live healthily, in coexistence, and in prosperity. Major concerns regarding health and the environment are at the heart of the Sustainable Development Goals of the United Nations Educational, Scientific, and Cultural Organization [3], which are a collection of interconnected goals intended to serve as a common blueprint for global peace and prosperity for the current period and in the future [3]. In addition, the sustainable development goals are directly or indirectly related to sanitation and environmental technology. For example, the goals of no poverty and no hunger can greatly improve public health, facilitate improved well-being, and promote healthy lifestyles at all ages, and ensuring clean water and sanitation can improve water security and facilitate access to sanitation. In addition, the realization of sustainable cities and communities can make our settlements safe, resilient, and sustainable. Responsible consumption and production will reduce pressure on the environment, reduce food waste and chemical use, and increase recycling. Climate action will strengthen the resilience of communities and increase adaptive capacity and responses to climate-related disasters. Ecosystem conservation will protect organisms from degradation and biodiversity loss. Finally, international cooperation will strengthen the implementation of these goals through the exchange of knowledge, expertise, and experience between nations. More than ever before, humanity is being called upon to take action to protect the environment and public health. The environment in which we live is the most important factor of our health and well-being. Human activities have a significant impact on the atmosphere, lithosphere, hydrosphere, biosphere, and even outer space. Biological, chemical, physical, and social risk factors are components of our daily lives, and scientific research is constantly challenged to understand and mitigate these interactions to make life on Earth more sustainable (Figure 1). The sustainability of human societies and the biodiversity that supports them requires the responsible management of natural resources, including the development of technologies and regulations.

This Special Issue, *Sanitary and Environmental Engineering: Relevance and Concerns*, addresses these issues and proposes solutions to current and future crises. Food safety is an important value in modern society, especially as we face increasing environmental changes and geopolitical tensions. For example, a study by Yang et al. [4] showed that predicting the disease density of maize through a multi-scale patch-embedding module could accurately predict maize diseases, which would thereby increase food safety. In addition, Jevšnik et al. [5] analysed food safety knowledge, practises, and hygiene statuses in a household kitchen and found inadequate hygiene in a quarter of the cases analysed. Although they found that the respondents had some knowledge about hygiene, they failed when presented with a real situation. A study by Slabe et al. [6] surveyed climbers with respect to their food safety habits and reported that food safety training should be included in general training programmes for climbers. Indoor air quality affects our health by causing sick building syndrome and other lung diseases. Galičič et al. [7] highlight macro- and micro-climatic factors and the distance of schools from pollution sources as having important influences on indoor air quality. However, indoor air quality has also influenced the spread of SARS-CoV-2. As reported by Galičič et al. [8], non-pharmacological measures such as self-testing, hygiene, and ventilation should be used if the pandemic slows down. All this shows once again how different factors and hazards in sanitation are interconnected and should not be neglected in decision making (Figure 1). Changes in the environment, especially of an anthropogenic nature, are of the most concern and have significant impacts on humans and ecosystems. The eco-environmental quality index was introduced by Xia and Zhen [9], which considers both land use and environmental quality. They found that land use is the most important factor of the quality of the ecological environment, whereas other factors do not play a significant role. In addition, Zhan and Yang [10] found that adding the PM 2.5 concentration model helps to predict impacts using the beetle swarm algorithm. In addition, Wang et al. [11] simulated an environmental policy to reduce construction waste and concluded that the policy should be implemented in relation to the phases of urban development. The simulation, prediction, and modelling of environmental factors are essential to understand causes and consequences and evaluate environmental interventions. Nevertheless, cleaning and maintaining hygiene at a sufficient level requires the application of the correct disinfection approach. For example, Zekanović et al. [12] proved that a combination of ultraviolet light and hyperchlorination is more effective against *P. aeruginosa* biofilms than either of the methods used separately. Similarly, Piletić et al. [13] analysed combined methods of gaseous ozone and citric acid against *A. baumannii* and found a 99.99% inhibition rate. In the last decade, natural detergents have attracted a great deal of attention due to their low toxicity and remarkable performance in cleaning and disinfection. A study by Fink [14] showed that natural terpenoids can be as effective as a standard antimicrobial agent chlorhexidine against *E. coli*, *P. aeruginosa* and *S. Typhimurium*.

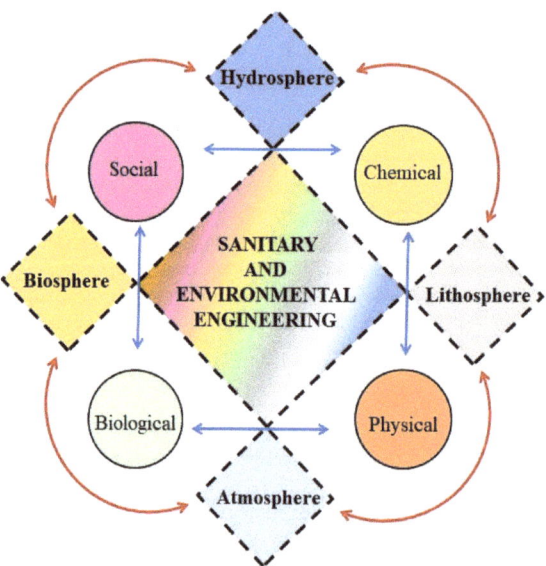

Figure 1. Conceptual figure of sanitary and environmental engineering subsystems and hazards.

Current sanitary and environmental engineering practices represent the basis for the One Health for All approach. Researchers, officials, and health professionals should collaborate to respond to global health threats, as environmental subsystems are interconnected, and threats spread through many of them. It is humanity's responsibility to take care of the environment and, by extension, health. Our presence on the planet is short-lived compared to other organisms, and we should be careful not to put a long-term strain on ecosystems. Sanitary and environmental engineering can help to comprehend this duty and provide answers to the challenges faced by modern society.

Funding: This research received no external funding.

Conflicts of Interest: The author declares no conflict of interest.

References

1. Prüss-Üstün, A.; Wolf, J.; Corvalán, C.; Bos, R.; Neira, M. *Preventing Disease through Healthy Environments: A Global Assessment of the Burden of Disease from Environmental Risks*; World Health Organization: Geneva, Switzerland, 2016.
2. Available online: https://www.worldwildlife.org/pages/living-planet-report-2022 (accessed on 5 March 2023).
3. Available online: https://www.un.org/sustainabledevelopment/sustainable-development-goals/ (accessed on 5 March 2023).
4. Yang, W.; Shen, P.; Ye, Z.; Zhu, Z.; Xu, C.; Liu, Y.; Mei, L. Adversarial Training Collaborating Multi-Path Context Feature Aggregation Network for Maize Disease Density Prediction. *Processes* **2023**, *11*, 1132. [CrossRef]
5. Jevšnik, M.; Pirc, L.; Ovca, A.; Šantić, M.; Raspor, P.; Torkar, K.G. A Multimethod Study on Kitchen Hygiene, Consumer Knowledge and Food Handling Practices at Home. *Processes* **2022**, *10*, 2104. [CrossRef]
6. Slabe, D.; Šparovec, E.D.; Jevšnik, M. Hygiene and Food Safety Habits among Slovenian Mountaineers. *Processes* **2022**, *10*, 1856. [CrossRef]
7. Galičič, A.; Rožanec, J.; Kukec, A.; Carli, T.; Medved, S.; Eržen, I. Identification of Indoor Air Quality Factors in Slovenian Schools: National Cross-Sectional Study. *Processes* **2023**, *11*, 841. [CrossRef]
8. Galičič, A.; Kranjec, N.; Rožanec, J.; Obid, I.; Grilc, E.; Gabrovec, B.; Fafangel, M. Spread of SARS-CoV-2 Infections in Educational Settings by Level of Education, Taking into Account the Predominant Virus Variant. *Processes* **2022**, *10*, 1947. [CrossRef]
9. Xia, B.; Zheng, L. Ecological Environmental Effects and Their Driving Factors of Land Use/Cover Change: The Case Study of Baiyangdian Basin, China. *Processes* **2022**, *10*, 2648. [CrossRef]
10. Zhang, Y.; Yan, Q. Application of Beetle Colony Optimization Based on Improvement of Rebellious Growth Characteristics in $PM_{2.5}$ Concentration Prediction. *Processes* **2022**, *10*, 2312. [CrossRef]
11. Wang, Q.; Li, S.; Yang, Y. Simulation Analysis of Implementation Effects of Construction Waste Reduction Policies. *Processes* **2022**, *10*, 2279. [CrossRef]
12. Zekanović, M.S.; Begić, G.; Mežnarić, S.; Jelovica Badovinac, I.; Krištof, R.; Tomić Linšak, D.; Gobin, I. Effect of UV Light and Sodium Hypochlorite on Formation and Destruction of Pseudomonas fluorescens Biofilm In Vitro. *Processes* **2022**, *10*, 1901. [CrossRef]
13. Piletić, K.; Kovač, B.; Planinić, M.; Vasiljev, V.; Karačonji, I.B.; Žigon, J.; Gobin, I.; Oder, M. Combined Biocidal Effect of Gaseous Ozone and Citric Acid on Acinetobacter Baumannii Biofilm Formed on Ceramic Tiles and Polystyrene as a Novel Approach for Infection Prevention and Control. *Processes* **2022**, *10*, 1788. [CrossRef]
14. Fink, R. Terpenoids as Natural Agents against Food-Borne Bacteria—Evaluation of Biofilm Biomass versus Viability Reduction. *Processes* **2023**, *11*, 148. [CrossRef]

Disclaimer/Publisher's Note: The statements, opinions and data contained in all publications are solely those of the individual author(s) and contributor(s) and not of MDPI and/or the editor(s). MDPI and/or the editor(s) disclaim responsibility for any injury to people or property resulting from any ideas, methods, instructions or products referred to in the content.

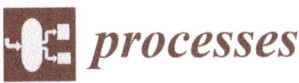

Article

Adversarial Training Collaborating Multi-Path Context Feature Aggregation Network for Maize Disease Density Prediction

Wei Yang [1,†], Peiquan Shen [2,†], Zhaoyi Ye [3,†], Zhongmin Zhu [1], Chuan Xu [3], Yi Liu [1] and Liye Mei [3,*]

1 School of Information Science and Engineering, Wuchang Shouyi University, Wuhan 430064, China
2 Electronic Information School, Wuhan University, Wuhan 430072, China
3 School of Computer Science, Hubei University of Technology, Wuhan 430068, China
* Correspondence: meiliye@hbut.edu.cn
† These authors contributed equally to this work.

Abstract: Maize is one of the world's major food crops, and its yields are closely related to the sustenance of people. However, its cultivation is hampered by various diseases. Meanwhile, maize diseases are characterized by spots of varying and irregular shapes, which makes identifying them with current methods challenging. Therefore, we propose an adversarial training collaborating multi-path context feature aggregation network for maize disease density prediction. Specifically, our multi-scale patch-embedding module uses multi-scale convolution to extract feature maps of different sizes from maize images and performs a patch-embedding operation. Then, we adopt the multi-path context-feature aggregation module, which is divided into four paths to further extract detailed features and long-range information. As part of the aggregation module, the multi-scale feature-interaction operation will skillfully integrate rough and detailed features at the same feature level, thereby improving prediction accuracy. By adding noise interference to the input maize image, our adversarial training method can produce adversarial samples. These samples will interfere with the normal training of the network—thus improving its robustness. We tested our proposed method on the Plant Village dataset, which contains three types of diseased and healthy maize leaves. Our method achieved an average accuracy of 99.50%, surpassing seven mainstream models and showing its effectiveness in maize disease density prediction. This research has theoretical and applied significance for the intelligent and accurate detection of corn leaf diseases.

Keywords: maize disease; adversarial training; context feature aggregation; patch embedding

1. Introduction

Crop yields are an instrumental factor in ensuring sustainable economic growth [1]. Maize has excellent adaptability, a wide planting area and distribution system, a variety of applications, and the potential to have its production increased [2,3]. As one of the most widely distributed crops in the world, it ranks second only to rice and wheat in terms of sowing area and production [4,5]. In spite of this, maize yield is impacted by many factors—including soil, heat, water, natural disasters, and disease—which result in a loss of 6–10% of corn production every year [6]. It is therefore crucial to detect and monitor diseases as early as possible during the growth of maize. Statistics indicate that there are more than 80 kinds of maize diseases in the world [7]. Among the most common maize diseases are large and small leaf spots, curved spore leaf spots, rust, brown spots, etc.—all of which adversely affect maize yield [8]. Presently, the identification of maize diseases is largely dependent on manual observations by growers [9]. This is time-consuming and laborious and can result in misjudgments due to a lack of professional knowledge [10]. At the same time, this makes it difficult to implement timely preventive and control programs. As a result, there is an urgent need for an intelligent and effective method that can be used for identifying maize diseases and increasing maize yields [11,12].

Up to now, many researchers have proposed various methods for crop disease identification. These methods are mainly divided into two categories: machine learning methods based on traditional features and automatic feature-learning methods based on deep learning [13–15]. For machine learning methods, an example is the work of Zhang et al. [16], in which a genetic support vector machine (SVM) was trained to classify six maize diseases with an average classification accuracy of 90.25%. Aravind et al. [17] used an SVM classifier to classify maize diseases and achieved an average accuracy rate of 83.7%. Zhang et al. [18] first segmented significant disease features from maize pictures, and then followed this by further classifying maize diseases using the k-nearest neighbor (KNN) with an accuracy of over 90%. Alehegn [19] applied an SVM to extract color, grain, and shape information from Ethiopian maize leaves, achieving an average accuracy of 95.63% in a dataset containing 800 maize leaves. Nonetheless, machine learning methods require training data and hand-designed features that are high quality, and thus the feature extraction ability for some data is poor and lacks robustness, which leads to unsatisfactory recognition accuracy. As for deep learning methods, they benefit from the powerful feature-extraction capabilities of convolution neural networks (CNNs). Waheed et al. [20] proposed an optimized dense CNN architecture (DenseNet) for the identification and classification of three types of diseased maize leaves in addition to healthy maize leaves. Gui et al. [21] proposed an improved CNN model for plant disease identification in the field by exploring the potential and generalization ability of CNN models, achieving a 72.03% accuracy. Qian et al. [22] explored the effect of a Transformer on maize disease identification, and then proposed an improved model on the basis of self-attention, which outperformed five mainstream CNN models. Dechant et al. [23] developed an automatic identification system for leaf blight detection in the field environment. Their method overcame the irregular leaf interference in the field environment and achieved 96.7% accuracy. For a four-class maize leaf recognition task, Xu et al. [24] implemented the Inception module in AlexNet, designed TCI-ALEXN, and avoided overfitting by using a global pooling layer. Ahila et al. [25] proposed a modified CNN-based LeNet method for diseased maize leaf identification and classification, and achieved 97.89% accuracy. Even though all of the above methods are capable of generating better detection results, the majority of them only use a CNN or a Transformer. This method does not consider detailed and long-range features, making it difficult to accurately predict and identify maize diseases [26]. This paper attempts to make maize disease density predictions by combining a depth convolution and a Transformer. Our main objective was to extract different features from various types of corn disease images with similar characteristics. At the same time, we needed to overcome the complex background noise to improve the prediction accuracy. To this end, we proposed an adversarial training collaborating multi-path context-feature aggregation network for maize disease density prediction. Specifically, we used multi-scale patch embedding to initially obtain multi-scale features in maize disease images, and multi-path context-feature aggregation to further obtain detailed and long-range feature information and aggregate it at the same feature level. Lastly, we used the adversarial training method to obtain adversarial samples by adding noise to the input maize images. This perturbed the training process—thus further improving the model's robustness and resistance to noise. The contributions of this paper are summarized as follows:

(1) We employ a multi-scale patch embedding module to extract multi-scale features from various types of maize images using multi-scale convolution with overlapping parts—thus adapting to different maize disease characteristics.
(2) Our proposed multi-path context feature aggregation module uses a depth convolution and Transformer encoder to further extract detailed features and long-range features, and allows these two to interact in the same dimension in order for the multi-scale features to effectively improve the network's ability to characterize features.
(3) We use the adversarial training method to generate adversarial samples by adding noise perturbations to the input maize images; this disrupts the normal training of the network—thus improving the robustness of the network.

2. Materials and Methods

2.1. Dataset

The experimental data used in this paper were primarily derived from the Plant Village international common dataset, which contains a large number of images depicting plant diseases. We used three kinds of diseased maize leaves as well as healthy maize leaves in this dataset as experimental data. The three maize disease species that were identified included leaf blight disease [27], gray leaf disease [28], and leaf rust disease [29]—with a total of 7701 images. Figure 1 illustrates some data images of the diseased and healthy maize leaves.

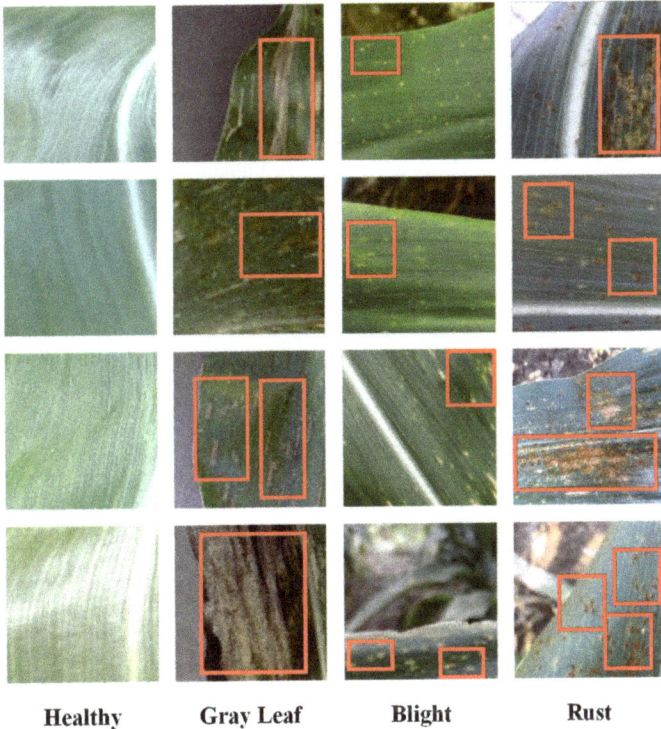

Figure 1. Depiction of diseased and healthy maize leaves from the Plant Village dataset. Note that the red rectangles correspond to maize disease characteristics.

Figure 1 illustrates the individual characteristics of the diseased maize leaves and healthy maize leaves. The leaf surfaces of healthy leaves are bright and smooth, showing no obvious disease symptoms; blighted leaves show gray or yellow–brown spots that do not expand, but spread parallel to the leaf veins; gray leaves have no obvious brown spots on the edges, but have more spots appearing parallel to the leaf veins; and rusted leaves show herpetic patches with colors from yellow to brown on both sides of the leaves, which are surrounded by yellow haloes.

The original resolution of the images in the dataset was 256 × 256 pixels, and in order to better fit our proposed network structure, we adjusted the images to be 224 × 224 pixels. In addition, the overall dataset was divided into a training set and a testing set. Specifically, the training set rate for leaf blight, gray leaf, healthy leaf, and leaf rust images was 78%, 75%, 75%, and 80%, respectively. Table 1 summarizes the number of images in the training set and testing set after the dataset division.

Table 1. Distribution details of the maize disease dataset.

Type	Leaf Blight	Gray Leaf	Healthy Leaf	Leaf Rust
Training Set	1743	750	1935	1523
Testing Set	500	250	500	500
Total	2243	1000	2435	2023

2.2. Overview of Network

Figure 2 shows the overview of the proposed adversarial training collaborating multi-path context feature aggregation network. The implementation process of our method was mainly divided into four steps, and each step was further divided into two parts: multi-scale patch embedding and multi-path context-feature aggregation, with the aim of obtaining multi-scale maize disease characteristics. Specifically, the multi-scale patch-embedding module extracted feature maps of different sizes by multi-scale convolution and performed a patch embedding operation. During the embedding of the multi-scale patch, it was flattened into tokens of different scales. Features with the same sequence length were output after adjusting the filling step of the convolution. In addition, the multi-path context feature aggregation module transferred the tokens with the same sequence length independently and simultaneously to the deep convolution and Transformer encoder through multiple paths for the further extraction of detailed features, and then performed a multi-scale feature interaction—thus identifying coarse and detailed feature representations at the same feature level. At the same time, our adversarial training module added noise to the input image to obtain the adversarial sample to improve the network's resistance to noise and ultimately improve its robustness.

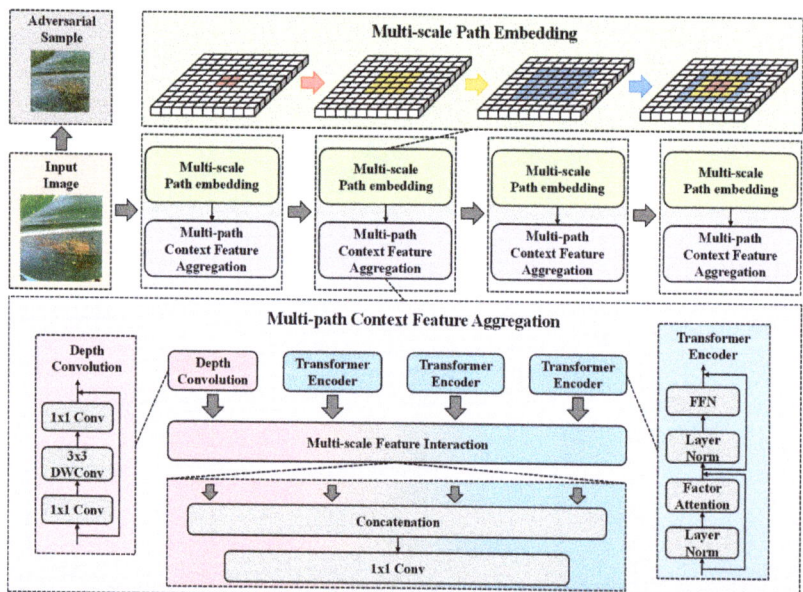

Figure 2. Overview of the proposed adversarial training, collaborating, multi-path context-feature aggregation network.

2.3. Multi-Scale Patch Embedding

Since the selected diseased maize leaves had small disease spots on the blighted leaves and large rust spots on the rusted leaves, conventional convolution could not take into account both detailed and large-scale disease features. To this end, we adapted multi-scale convolution—which is different from conventional convolution—to obtain multi-level disease-feature information. As shown in Figure 3, our multi-scale convolution was divided into overlapping 3×3, 5×5, and 7×7 parts.

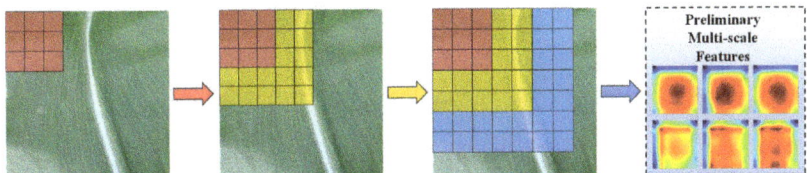

Figure 3. Schematic diagram of the multi-scale patch embedding.

The three convolution kernels were cascaded to obtain tokens with rich maize-disease information at multiple scales, and the height and width of the token feature map dimensions were calculated as follows:

$$H_i = \left[\frac{H_{i-1} - k + 2p}{s} + 1\right], W_i = \left[\frac{W_{i-1} - k + 2p}{s} + 1\right] \quad (1)$$

where k represents the size of the convolution kernel in a 2D convolution, s represents the stride, and p represents the padding. We can adjust the sequence length of the token by changing the stride and padding; this ensures that the output of different convolution kernel sizes attains the same size patch for embedding after convolution. In addition, the Hardswish activation function was executed once after each convolution.

2.4. Multi-Path Context-Feature Aggregation

Although multi-scale convolution can focus on locally connected information and retain a sense of local details, it tends to ignore correlations between patches. On the other hand, a Transformer is capable of obtaining long-range information. When detecting healthy leaves, it is imperative to ensure that local patches are in a healthy condition; this requires not only detailed information at the regional level, but also long-range information. Accordingly, our proposed multi-path context-feature aggregation module further processes multi-scale patches by performing depth convolution and Transformer encoder operations. Thus, local details and long-range information on maize leaves can be obtained simultaneously. Specifically, depth convolution is a composite component that consists of a 1×1 convolution, a 3×3 DW convolution, and a 1×1 convolution with the same channel size. Our Transformer encoder used FactorAtt, which was proposed for a CoAT in [30] and is calculated as follows:

$$\text{FactorAtt}(Q, K, V) = \frac{Q}{\sqrt{C}}(softmax(K)^T V) \quad (2)$$

where Q, K, and V are the linearly projected queries, keys, and values of the Transformer encoder, respectively. Since the pieces of extracted detailed and long-range feature information are currently independent of each other, we could not maximize their value. Therefore, we performed a multi-scale feature-interaction operation to allow for interactions between detailed and long-range features for enriched representations:

$$A_i = Concat([D_i, L_{i,0}, \ldots, L_{i,j}]) \quad (3)$$

where D_i represents the detailed feature at stage i, j represents the path of the Transformer encoder, and $L_{i,j}$ represents the long-range feature at stage i in path j. In our implementation, $j = 3$, which means that there are three Transformer encoder paths, and A_i refers to the final aggregated feature.

2.5. Loss Function

Since our maize disease prediction is actually a multi-classification task with four categories in total, we used cross-entropy loss—which is common in classification tasks—as the loss function. In our implementation, each class was compared against all others (as one). We used the softmax function to transform numerical results into probability values. Moreover, the predicted maize type was determined with the maximum probability values—thus achieving multi-classification. Cross-entropy loss was calculated as follows:

$$L(p_c) = -\sum_{c=1}^{K} y_c \log(p_c) \qquad (4)$$

where K is the total number of maize leaf species, c is the current predicted maize leaf species, y_c is the current actual maize leaf species, and p_c is the probability that our method will predict the current sample as maize leaf species c.

It is possible to smooth losses by using adversarial training under the given input conditions, which is also an effective technique for data enhancement. Training for deep learning is often sensitive to perturbing or noisy data. In the case of maize disease images, there are differences between samples due to the diversity of the data, which poses a challenge for the model training process. Thus, we adapted adversarial training loss for the purpose of regularization, which was calculated as follows:

$$L_{AT} = D[p(y|x), p(y|x + r_{adv}, \theta)] \qquad (5)$$

where r_{cn} represents the added counter noise to the input maize images; this was calculated as follows:

$$r_{cn} \equiv \underset{r}{\operatorname{argmax}}\{D[p(y|x), p(y|x + r, \theta)]; \|r\|_2 \leq \lambda\} \qquad (6)$$

In the above equations, x represents the input data and y represents the output results. D represents the non-negative measurement of the output after adding noise to the input maize data. $p(y|x)$ represents the conditional probability of the input x. $\|\cdot\|$ represents the L2 norm, limiting the noise value between 0 and 1. r represents the noise in the input maize image, and its distribution follows a mean value of 0 and a variance of 1. The specific noise value is 1×10^{-6}, and λ represents the tolerance value, which is set at 0.5.

KL divergence, sometimes referred to as information divergence, is basically a measure of the relative entropy between characteristics. It is an asymmetric measure that was employed to quantify the difference between the perturbed samples and the initially expected samples in the probability distribution. We calculated it as follows:

$$D_{KL}(P\|Q) \equiv \sum_{i=1}^{N} [P(x_i) \log P(x_i) - P(x_i) \log Q(x_i)] \qquad (7)$$

where N represents the number of input maize samples, $P(x_i)$ represents the actual prediction probability of sample i, and $Q(x_i)$ represents the prediction probability after noise has been added. It is noteworthy that this loss produces a perturbation for the output results of the network rather than the actual corn disease species. Then, the optimization process was performed by measuring the predicted probabilities before and after the addition of noise.

Therefore, we combined the cross-entropy loss and adversarial training loss as the loss function.

3. Experiments and Results

3.1. Experimental Settings

We performed all of our experiments on a tower server running the Ubuntu 20.04.2 LTS operating system on an Intel(R) Xeon(R) Gold 6226R CPU @ 2.90 GHz CPU (Santa Clara, CA, USA) and an Nvidia Tesla A100 with 80 GB of GPU (Santa Clara, CA, USA) memory. To speed up the training process, our experiments were implemented using the PyTorch deep learning framework. For training, all the experiments were run with a batch size of 32, and the total number of epochs was 200. Our input image size was resized to 224 × 224 pixels. We used the Adam optimizer with an initial learning rate = 0.00008 and a weight decay α = 0.00004 for the rest of the epochs. The specific settings for the hyperparameters during our adversarial training were a perturbation value of 1×10^{-6} and a tolerance value of 0.5.

3.2. Evaluation Metrics

We chose accuracy, precision, and recall metrics to evaluate the performance of each method in terms of accurate identification, missed detection, and false identification. These metrics were defined as follows:

$$Accuracy = \frac{TP + TN}{TP + TN + FP + FN} \tag{8}$$

$$Precision = \frac{TP}{TP + FP} \tag{9}$$

$$Recall = \frac{TP}{TP + FN} \tag{10}$$

where TP represents the number of true positives, TN represents the number of true negatives, FP represents the number of false positives, and FN represents the number of false negatives.

3.3. Quantitative Analysis

The receiver operating characteristic (ROC) and precision-recall (PR) curves are shown in Figure 4a,b, respectively, and both demonstrate the excellent prediction performance of our method. Since the values of the curves were close to 1, there was an overlap of the curves. Therefore, to facilitate observations with the experimental results, we further zoomed in on the images. The larger the area formed by the curve with the horizontal axis for either the ROC curve or PR curve, the better the performance. Clearly, our method generated near-perfect metric results, as the two curves were very close to the upper-left and upper-right corners. This shows that our method, which uses multi-scale patch embedding and multi-path context-feature aggregation, can further enhance the overall prediction performance for maize disease density prediction. It is evident that our method, which makes use of multi-scale patch embedding and multi-path context-feature aggregation, allows us to extract and characterize the features of diseased and healthy maize leaves more accurately.

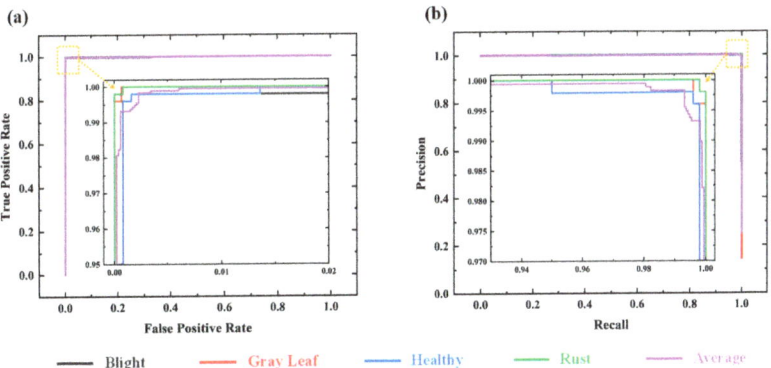

Figure 4. Results of the quantitative analysis. (**a**) ROC curve of maize disease prediction. (**b**) PR curve of maize disease prediction. Note that the yellow rectangle and arrow are for expanded display.

As shown in Figure 5a, we computed the confusion matrix to obtain explanatory insights into the maize disease density prediction results. The dark-colored squares on the diagonal indicate correct predictions, while the other light-colored squares indicate incorrect predictions. We can see that the diagonal prediction values were close to 1. It is evident from these results that our method was capable of obtaining the corresponding features for the three types of diseased maize leaves and the healthy maize leaves—thereby allowing us to make correct density predictions.

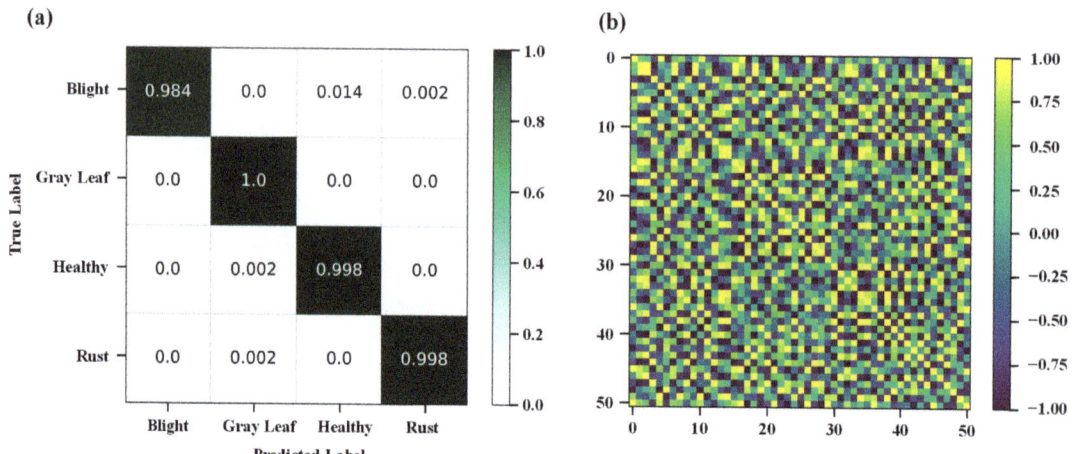

Figure 5. Results of the quantitative analysis. (**a**) Confusion matrix. (**b**) Correlation matrix of 51 randomly chosen testing maize samples.

Our network was divided into four stages, with each stage progressively refining the acquired features. At the final stage of the net process, we chose 51 random samples from the validation set; first, we clustered them, followed by calculating the Euclidean distances between each pair, computing similarity scores (ranging from 0 to 1), and finally, plotting the correlation matrix in Figure 5b. The highest value is highlighted on the diagonal of the correlation matrix, which indicates that the distance between the two feature maps was relatively close to zero. In addition to the diagonal data, the similarity scores for the remaining data were also high, which indicates that the feature representations learned by our method through multi-scale patch embedding and multi-path context-feature aggregation were very similar to the actual feature representations in the Euclidean distance space—demonstrating that our method can obtain robust representations of feature information.

As shown in Table 2, we compared the results of the various methods (VGG11 [31], EfficientNet [32], Inception-v3 [33], MobileNet [34], ResNet50 [35], ViT [36], and Improved ViT [22]) by using three metrics on the Plant Village dataset. Among them, VGG11, EfficientNet, Inception-v3, MobileNet, and ResNet50 had an average accuracy of 97.9%, 91.6%, 97.2%, 90.2% and 96.6%, respectively. Benefiting from the self-attentive mechanism in the Transformer, ViT, Improved ViT, and our method achieved an average accuracy of 93.9%, 98.7%, and 99.5%, respectively—which is much higher than that of other CNN-based methods. For the precision and recall metrics, we tested the results of predictive metrics for each of the three types of diseased maize leaves as well as the healthy leaves according to the distribution of the dataset. As a result of the clever combination of depth convolution and a Transformer encoder, we achieved precision and recall metrics of 98.6% and 99.8% on healthy leaves, respectively. In addition, our method detected gray leaves with a recall value of 100%; this is an encouraging result, indicating that our multi-scale patch embedding module can effectively extract gray leaves' disease characteristics.

Table 2. Comparison of three metrics to the results of other methods.

Metrics	VGG11	EfficientNet	Inception-v3	MobileNet	ResNet50	ViT	Improved ViT	Our Proposed Method
Accuracy	97.9%	91.6%	97.2%	90.2%	96.6%	93.9%	98.7%	99.5%
Precision								
Leaf Blight	99%	90%	97%	88%	99%	92%	99%	98.4%
Gray Leaf	100%	97%	99%	99%	100%	96%	100%	99.6%
Healthy Leaf	96%	88%	96%	88%	94%	91%	97%	98.6%
Leaf Rust	98%	94%	98%	92%	96%	98%	99%	99.8%
Recall								
Leaf Blight	96%	86%	94%	86%	91%	90%	97%	98.4%
Gray Leaf	97%	89%	98%	85%	97%	92%	99%	100%
Healthy Leaf	100%	92%	98%	93%	99%	95%	99%	99.8%
Leaf Rust	99%	98%	100%	96%	99%	97%	100%	99.8%

3.4. Interpretability Analysis

By utilizing the t-distributed stochastic neighbor embedding algorithm (t-SNE) [37], the regional variation in data density is represented by distance, and the size of the clustering set does not reflect the actual distance. Taking advantage of this nonlinear generative relationship, t-SNE is able to classify data results more accurately. As shown in Figure 6, the various colors indicated similarities between the three types of diseased maize leaves and the healthy leaves. Except for a small number of blight samples scattered far from the set, the other three types of samples were well grouped in their own neighborhoods. As a result, we can conclude that our proposed method is able to learn to identify similar representations from different maize samples.

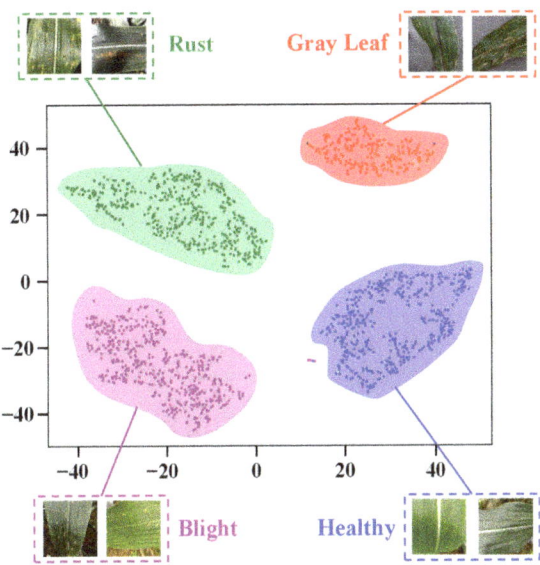

Figure 6. t-SNE visualization of the feature representations of the validation set.

4. Discussion

Maize disease recognition is of paramount importance in the agricultural field, and many researchers have studied a variety of algorithms for disease recognition; however, there are still defects. Traditional machine learning methods have a poor feature extraction ability, lack of robustness, and high requirements for training data quality—resulting in a low recognition accuracy. Deep learning methods are mostly based on neural networks; detecting and predicting maize diseases effectively and accurately is difficult because only local characteristics are taken into account and global information is not incorporated.

Despite the fact that we used images of three different varieties of diseased maize leaves in addition to healthy maize leaves, their appearance features were relatively similar—in particular, their predominant color was green. In terms of lesion characteristics, there were no significant differences between the three types of diseased leaves (mostly small spots), which presented an additional challenge for the detection method.

In our experiments, we tested eight methods: five CNN-based and three Transformer-based methods. CNN-based approaches rely primarily on convolutional methods for implementation and have the advantage of extracting local features. Our experimental results indicated that VGG-11 achieved an average accuracy of 97.6%. In addition, Thakur et al. [38] created a lightweight VGGNet to detect three crop diseases with an accuracy of 99.16%. Li et al. [39] combined inflated convolution and attention mechanisms to detect corn diseases in a field environment.

The CNN-based methods produced good results; however, the overall effect was not as effective as the Transformer-based methods due to the complex backgrounds of the corn images in natural environments and the close relationships between the spots—whereas convolution ignored long-range information, which is extremely important [40]. From our experimental results, we can see that the patch-embedding operation segmented the maize image into multiple patches and enhanced the correlation between the regions—thereby improving the feature representation of the disease. The Improved ViT and our method both achieved 100% recall metrics for two maize diseases—leaf rust and leaf blight—further demonstrating the Transformer's effectiveness for maize disease detection.

Based on the above discussion, our adversarial training collaborating multi-path context feature aggregation network is able to obtain tokens of different scales through multi-scale patch embedding, which can be independently input into Transformer encoders through multiple paths. In the process of multi-path context feature aggregation, multi-scale feature interactions can connect local features extracted by convolution with global features obtained by the Transformer, which can maximize the advantages of the local connectivity of convolution and the global relevance of the Transformer. Finally, the robustness and feature extraction ability of the model are further improved by the adversarial training method. On the Plant Village dataset—consisting of three diseases (blighted leaves, gray leaves, and rusted leaves) and healthy maize leaves—we achieved an average accuracy of 99.50%. Our method has a strong practical application value; it can help planters detect disease in a timely and accurate manner. It can also prevent and control pests and diseases, improve maize yield, and increase economic benefits.

5. Conclusions

In this paper, we proposed an adversarial training collaborating multi-path context feature aggregation network for maize disease density prediction. Multi-scale patch embedding is capable of extracting multiple tokens with corresponding features from various maize disease images, while multi-path context feature aggregation independently interacts with the extracted tokens at different scales through multiple paths—thus achieving effective multi-scale feature aggregation. Finally, we used the adversarial training method to reduce the problem of network overfitting and further improve the robustness and generalization of the model. We conducted quantitative analysis and interpretability analysis on the Plant Village dataset. As a result, we achieved high-quality results—with a recognition accuracy of 98.4%, 99.60%, 98.62%, and 99.80% for leaf blight, gray leaf, healthy leaf, and leaf rust images, respectively. In the future, we will further optimize the network structure to improve its recognition accuracy, and also apply it for the recognition of more kinds of plant diseases.

Author Contributions: Conceptualization, W.Y., P.S. and Z.Y.; methodology, W.Y.; software, Z.Z.; validation, C.X.; formal analysis, L.M.; investigation, L.M.; data curation, P.S.; writing—original draft preparation, Z.Y.; writing—review and editing, P.S.; visualization, Z.Z.; supervision, W.Y. and Y.L.; project administration, W.Y.; funding acquisition, W.Y., Z.Z. and C.X. All authors have read and agreed to the published version of the manuscript.

Funding: This research was funded by the National Natural Science Foundation of China (Nos. 41601443 and 42071353); Scientific Research Foundation for Doctoral Program of Hubei University of Technology (BSQD2020056); Science and Technology Research Project of Education Department of Hubei Province (B2021351); Natural Science Foundation of Hubei Province (2022CFB501); and University Student Innovation and Entrepreneurship Training Program Project (202210500028).

Data Availability Statement: Not applicable.

Conflicts of Interest: The authors declare no conflict of interest.

References

1. Upadhyay, M.K.; Shukla, A.; Yadav, P.; Srivastava, S. A review of arsenic in crops, vegetables, animals and food products. *Food Chem.* **2019**, *276*, 608–618. [CrossRef] [PubMed]
2. Hou, P.; Liu, Y.; Liu, W.; Liu, G.; Xie, R.; Wang, K.; Ming, B.; Wang, Y.; Zhao, R.; Zhang, W. How to increase maize production without extra nitrogen input. *Resour. Conserv. Recycl.* **2020**, *160*, 104913. [CrossRef]
3. Adisa, O.M.; Botai, J.O.; Adeola, A.M.; Hassen, A.; Botai, C.M.; Darkey, D.; Tesfamariam, E. Application of artificial neural network for predicting maize production in South Africa. *Sustainability* **2019**, *11*, 1145. [CrossRef]
4. Kaur, N.; Vashist, K.K.; Brar, A. Energy and productivity analysis of maize based crop sequences compared to rice-wheat system under different moisture regimes. *Energy* **2021**, *216*, 119286. [CrossRef]
5. Letsoin, S.M.A.; Purwestri, R.C.; Perdana, M.C.; Hnizdil, P.; Herak, D. Monitoring of Paddy and Maize Fields Using Sentinel-1 SAR Data and NGB Images: A Case Study in Papua, Indonesia. *Processes* **2023**, *11*, 647. [CrossRef]
6. Zhou, L.; Gu, X.; Cheng, S.; Yang, G.; Shu, M.; Sun, Q. Analysis of plant height changes of lodged maize using UAV-LiDAR data. *Agriculture* **2020**, *10*, 146. [CrossRef]
7. Zhang, Y.; Wa, S.; Liu, Y.; Zhou, X.; Sun, P.; Ma, Q. High-accuracy detection of maize leaf diseases CNN based on multi-pathway activation function module. *Remote Sens.* **2021**, *13*, 4218. [CrossRef]
8. Arora, J.; Agrawal, U. Classification of Maize leaf diseases from healthy leaves using Deep Forest. *J. Artif. Intell. Syst.* **2020**, *2*, 14–26. [CrossRef]
9. Ali, I.; HUO, X.-x.; Khan, I.; Ali, H.; Khan, B.; Khan, S.U. Technical efficiency of hybrid maize growers: A stochastic frontier model approach. *J. Integr. Agric.* **2019**, *18*, 2408–2421. [CrossRef]
10. Alemu, G.T.; Nigussie, Z.; Haregeweyn, N.; Berhanie, Z.; Wondimagegnehu, B.A.; Ayalew, Z.; Molla, D.; Okoyo, E.N.; Baributsa, D. Cost-benefit analysis of on-farm grain storage hermetic bags among small-scale maize growers in northwestern Ethiopia. *Crop Prot.* **2021**, *143*, 105478. [CrossRef]
11. Lv, M.; Zhou, G.; He, M.; Chen, A.; Zhang, W.; Hu, Y. Maize leaf disease identification based on feature enhancement and DMS-robust alexnet. *IEEE Access* **2020**, *8*, 57952–57966. [CrossRef]
12. Waldamichael, F.G.; Debelee, T.G.; Schwenker, F.; Ayano, Y.M.; Kebede, S.R. Machine learning in cereal crops disease detection: A review. *Algorithms* **2022**, *15*, 75. [CrossRef]
13. Chen, J.; Wang, W.; Zhang, D.; Zeb, A.; Nanehkaran, Y.A. Attention embedded lightweight network for maize disease recognition. *Plant Pathol.* **2021**, *70*, 630–642. [CrossRef]
14. Orchi, H.; Sadik, M.; Khaldoun, M. On using artificial intelligence and the internet of things for crop disease detection: A contemporary survey. *Agriculture* **2022**, *12*, 9. [CrossRef]
15. Fenu, G.; Malloci, F.M. Forecasting plant and crop disease: An explorative study on current algorithms. *Big Data Cogn. Comput.* **2021**, *5*, 2. [CrossRef]
16. Zhang, Z.; He, X.; Sun, X.; Guo, L.; Wang, J.; Wang, F. Image recognition of maize leaf disease based on GA-SVM. *Chem. Eng. Trans.* **2015**, *46*, 199–204.
17. Aravind, K.; Raja, P.; Mukesh, K.; Aniirudh, R.; Ashiwin, R.; Szczepanski, C. Disease classification in maize crop using bag of features and multiclass support vector machine. In Proceedings of the 2nd International Conference on Inventive Systems and Control, Coimbatore, India, 19–20 January 2018; pp. 1191–1196.
18. Zhang, S.; Shang, Y.; Wang, L. Plant disease recognition based on plant leaf image. *J. Anim. Plant Sci.* **2015**, *25*, 42–45.
19. Alehegn, E. Ethiopian maize diseases recognition and classification using support vector machine. *Int. J. Comput. Vis. Robot.* **2019**, *9*, 90–109. [CrossRef]
20. Waheed, A.; Goyal, M.; Gupta, D.; Khanna, A.; Hassanien, A.E.; Pandey, H.M. An optimized dense convolutional neural network model for disease recognition and classification in corn leaf. *Comput. Electron. Agric.* **2020**, *175*, 105456. [CrossRef]
21. Gui, P.; Dang, W.; Zhu, F.; Zhao, Q. Towards automatic field plant disease recognition. *Comput. Electron. Agric.* **2021**, *191*, 106523. [CrossRef]
22. Qian, X.; Zhang, C.; Chen, L.; Li, K. Deep learning-based identification of maize leaf diseases is improved by an attention mechanism: Self-Attention. *Front. Plant Sci.* **2022**, *13*, 864486. [CrossRef] [PubMed]

23. DeChant, C.; Wiesner-Hanks, T.; Chen, S.; Stewart, E.L.; Yosinski, J.; Gore, M.A.; Nelson, R.J.; Lipson, H. Automated identification of northern leaf blight-infected maize plants from field imagery using deep learning. *Phytopathology* **2017**, *107*, 1426–1432. [CrossRef] [PubMed]
24. Xu, Y.; Zhao, B.; Zhai, Y.; Chen, Q.; Zhou, Y. Maize diseases identification method based on multi-scale convolutional global pooling neural network. *IEEE Access* **2021**, *9*, 27959–27970. [CrossRef]
25. Ahila Priyadharshini, R.; Arivazhagan, S.; Arun, M.; Mirnalini, A. Maize leaf disease classification using deep convolutional neural networks. *Neural Comput. Appl.* **2019**, *31*, 8887–8895. [CrossRef]
26. Lee, Y.; Kim, J.; Willette, J.; Hwang, S.J. Mpvit: Multi-path vision transformer for dense prediction. In Proceedings of the IEEE/CVF Conference on Computer Vision and Pattern Recognition, New Orleans, Louisiana, USA, 19–24 June 2022; pp. 7287–7296.
27. Aregbesola, E.; Ortega-Beltran, A.; Falade, T.; Jonathan, G.; Hearne, S.; Bandyopadhyay, R. A detached leaf assay to rapidly screen for resistance of maize to Bipolaris maydis, the causal agent of southern corn leaf blight. *Eur. J. Plant Pathol.* **2020**, *156*, 133–145. [CrossRef]
28. Saito, B.C.; Silva, L.Q.; Andrade, J.A.d.C.; Goodman, M.M. Adaptability and stability of corn inbred lines regarding resistance to gray leaf spot and northern leaf blight. *Crop Breed. Appl. Biotechnol.* **2018**, *18*, 148–154. [CrossRef]
29. Wang, S.; Chen, Z.; Tian, L.; Ding, Y.; Zhang, J.; Zhou, J.; Liu, P.; Chen, Y.; Wu, L. Comparative proteomics combined with analyses of transgenic plants reveal Zm REM 1.3 mediates maize resistance to southern corn rust. *Plant Biotechnol. J.* **2019**, *17*, 2153–2168. [CrossRef]
30. Dai, Z.; Liu, H.; Le, Q.V.; Tan, M. Coatnet: Marrying convolution and attention for all data sizes. *Adv. Neural Inf. Process. Syst.* **2021**, *34*, 3965–3977.
31. Simonyan, K.; Zisserman, A. Very deep convolutional networks for large-scale image recognition. *arXiv* **2014**, arXiv:1409.1556.
32. Tan, M.; Le, Q. Efficientnet: Rethinking model scaling for convolutional neural networks. In Proceedings of the International Conference on Machine Learning, Long Beach, CA, USA, 10–15 June 2019; pp. 6105–6114.
33. Szegedy, C.; Vanhoucke, V.; Ioffe, S.; Shlens, J.; Wojna, Z. Rethinking the inception architecture for computer vision. In Proceedings of the IEEE Conference on Computer Vision and Pattern Recognition, Las Vegas, NV, USA, 27–30 June 2016; pp. 2818–2826.
34. Sandler, M.; Howard, A.; Zhu, M.; Zhmoginov, A.; Chen, L.-C. Mobilenetv2: Inverted residuals and linear bottlenecks. In Proceedings of the IEEE Conference on Computer Vision and Pattern Recognition, Salt Lake City, UT, USA, 18–23 June 2018; pp. 4510–4520.
35. He, K.; Zhang, X.; Ren, S.; Sun, J. Deep residual learning for image recognition. In Proceedings of the IEEE Conference on Computer Vision and Pattern Recognition, Las Vegas, NV, USA, 27–30 June 2016; pp. 770–778.
36. Dosovitskiy, A.; Beyer, L.; Kolesnikov, A.; Weissenborn, D.; Zhai, X.; Unterthiner, T.; Dehghani, M.; Minderer, M.; Heigold, G.; Gelly, S. An image is worth 16x16 words: Transformers for image recognition at scale. *arXiv* **2020**, arXiv:2010.11929.
37. Linderman, G.C.; Steinerberger, S. Clustering with t-SNE, provably. *SIAM J. Math. Data Sci.* **2019**, *1*, 313–332. [CrossRef] [PubMed]
38. Thakur, P.S.; Sheorey, T.; Ojha, A. VGG-ICNN: A Lightweight CNN model for crop disease identification. *Multimed. Tools Appl.* **2023**, *82*, 497–520. [CrossRef]
39. Li, E.; Wang, L.; Xie, Q.; Gao, R.; Su, Z.; Li, Y. A novel deep learning method for maize disease identification based on small sample-size and complex background datasets. *Ecol. Inform.* **2023**, *75*, 102011. [CrossRef]
40. Li, X.; Chen, X.; Yang, J.; Li, S. Transformer helps identify kiwifruit diseases in complex natural environments. *Comput. Electron. Agric.* **2022**, *200*, 107258. [CrossRef]

Disclaimer/Publisher's Note: The statements, opinions and data contained in all publications are solely those of the individual author(s) and contributor(s) and not of MDPI and/or the editor(s). MDPI and/or the editor(s) disclaim responsibility for any injury to people or property resulting from any ideas, methods, instructions or products referred to in the content.

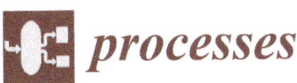

Article

A Multimethod Study on Kitchen Hygiene, Consumer Knowledge and Food Handling Practices at Home

Mojca Jevšnik [1,*], Lucija Pirc [1], Andrej Ovca [1], Marina Šantić [2], Peter Raspor [3,†] and Karmen Godič Torkar [1]

1 Sanitary Engineering Department, Faculty of Health Sciences, University of Ljubljana, SI-1000 Ljubljana, Slovenia
2 Faculty of Medicine, University of Rijeka, Braće Branchetta 20/1, 51000 Rijeka, Croatia
3 University of Ljubljana, SI-1000 Ljubljana, Slovenia
* Correspondence: mojca.jevsnik@zf.uni-lj.si; Tel.: +386-1-300-11-49
† Retired Emeritus Professor.

Abstract: The aim of the study was to identify consumers' food safety knowledge, practices, and hygiene status in the observed home kitchens. The results provide the starting point for evaluating progress or regression in this area compared to the past statewide study. Food safety knowledge was analyzed among 380 consumers with an online questionnaire. Additionally, 16 consumers were observed during their preparation of specified foods. The hygiene conditions in the kitchens were microbiologically examined using contact agar plates, while the cleaning adequacy was determined by measuring the ATP bioluminescence. A lack of knowledge on certain topics regarding food safety was established; the consumers aged from 36 to 55 in general and women demonstrated the highest level of knowledge. In some cases, the observed consumers did not take proper action when preparing the food. Increased total bacteria, coliform bacteria, and *Escherichia coli* counts were detected in 12.7% of the consumers' kitchens observed here. Eighty-three (74.1%) out of 112 surfaces examined with either hygiene test sheets or ATP swabs met the standards and were adequately or acceptably cleaned. The kitchen surfaces exceeded the recommended limits for 25% of consumers. Statistical differences in RLU and TCC levels on surfaces between older and younger consumers were not observed, although all (25%) inadequately cleaned kitchens belonged to older consumers. The greatest emphasis has to be put on the cleaning of home kitchens and personal hygiene. Even though consumers have some knowledge on food safety, they often fail to put that knowledge into daily practice.

Keywords: consumers; food safety; knowledge; practice; observation

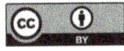

1. Introduction

Many consumers are unaware of the fact that their home environment poses a risk of foodborne disease outbreaks [1–3]. According to the EFSA and ECDC [4] report, the category "domestic setting" was the most commonly reported setting (N = 97; 39.1% of strong-evidence outbreaks) where foodborne outbreaks occurred. The research findings show that consumers most often associate foodborne disease (FBD) with the catering industry [5,6]. The recent Eurobarometer report [7] revealed that food hygiene is fifth place out of 15 topics that most concern European consumers (32%) when it comes to food and is at 10th place among Slovenian consumers (18%). Most food is prepared by consumers at home [2], so knowledge about food preparation in their home kitchens is all the more important, as it reduces the likelihood of FBD [8,9]. Proper consumer behavior in food preparation is—in addition to the knowledge of food hygiene—a key element in ensuring consumer safety [6,10–13]. The lack of knowledge and mishandling of food during preparation is more common in consumer groups of young adults (18 to 29 years of age), men, and people older than 60 years [5,14]. Irregularities in food handling at home are related to improper hand washing, the improper separation of equipment and utensils, inadequate cold food storage, cross-contamination, and the inadequate heat treatment of food [3,5,15–17]. Against such a background, there is a constant and still urgent need for improved domestic food hygiene knowledge and practice [2,17–19]. However, consumer education activities are expensive to organize, maintain, and evaluate. Thus, it is particularly important to correctly identify, target, and reach higher risk consumer groups [20–22].

The main purpose of our research was to assess and determine the level of food safety knowledge and food handling practices by consumers in the domestic milieu, including their behavior during the preparation of selected foods and the hygiene conditions in their home kitchens. The outcomes of this study also serve for a comparison with the data collected among Slovenian consumers in a nationwide study in 2008 [5] in order to evaluate the progress or regression of the results.

2. Materials and Methods

2.1. Consumer Food Safety Knowledge

To assess consumer food safety knowledge, we used a validated questionnaire, based on a questionnaire from the Food and Drug Administration (FDA) [23]. Some additional questions were added in order to compare the data with the previous Slovenian survey on consumer knowledge of food safety, carried out in 2008 [5]. The questionnaire was translated into the Slovenian language and tested among five experts in the food safety field and 20 consumers of different age groups and genders, resulting in minor modifications with the wording of questions.

The questionnaire was entered into an online survey application and a web link to the questionnaire was sent to consumers via e-mail and social networks. The questionnaire responses were analyzed using SPSS version 20.0 software (New York, NY, USA). To examine the relationships among and between the variables, a chi-square test for independence (χ^2 test) for categorical variables (nominal and dichotomous types) and an independent sample t-test or ANOVA for ordinal variables (5-point Likert-type measurement scale) treated as a continuous variable were used. Gender, age and educational level were used as independent variables. The significance level of $p < 0.05$ was used.

2.2. Observing Consumers' Food Handling Practices at Home

The sample for this qualitative research consisted of 16 people, selected based on the snowball principle [24]. Out of these, 8 consumers were more than 65 years of age and 8 were younger than 35 years with small children. We decided on such a sample because the elderly and children belong to a population group vulnerable to FBD. The responsible household member was informed about the general aim of the research. When a responsible household member agreed to participate, the date and hour were determined via the phone. During the home visit, the consumers' task was to prepare the raw food delivered to them into a roast chicken leg, rice with carrots and peas, and cabbage salad. Individual steps of their food handling were recorded in the observation checklist, which was prepared on the basis of a review of other similar studies [2,6]. We observed the frequency and method of hand washing; cleaning of equipment, utensils, and kitchen surfaces; prevention of cross-contamination; method of food preparation; and heat treatment of food. A Testo 106 food thermometer (measuring range −50 to +275 °C, ±0.5 °C accuracy at the range −30 to +99.9 °C) was used to measure the temperature of the air in the refrigerators. The air temperature was measured in the middle shelf in the refrigerator after the thermometer had been in the refrigerator for 15 min.

Moreover, participants were informed about the possibility to refuse their participation or to change their mind at any time during the home visit without any consequences. All the data were collected with consent.

2.3. Imprint and Swab Sampling to Establish the Microbiological Quality and Hygiene of Kitchen Surfaces

The microbiological conditions of work surfaces (Table 1) and utensils were established with RIDA®COUNT Total test hygiene sheets to determine the total aerobic mesophilic microorganism counts (total colony count—TCC), and RIDA®COUNT E. coli/Coliform test hygiene sheets to determine the number of coliform bacteria, including E. coli (R-Biopharm AG, Darmstadt, Germany). One sample per consumer was taken on a clean cutting board and service plate (Table 1). The sampling procedure was applied in accordance with ISO 18593 [25] and the manufacturer's instructions. The obtained results were compared to the guidelines for the microbiological safety of food intended for the final consumer [26] that define the criteria used to evaluate the cleanliness of surface samples.

Table 1. A table of the sample sites of test sheets for establishing the total number of aerobic mesophilic microorganisms and the number of coliform bacteria, including E. coli, and the sample sites of swabs taken to measure the ATP bioluminescence.

Method	Sample Sites
Test sheets RIDA®COUNT	Cutting board Service plate
Swabs taken to measure the ATP bioluminescence	Knife for cutting meat Work counter Refrigerator wall (shelf for delicacies) Dishwasher wall (rubber pad next to the filter) Salad servers

The cleanliness of the selected surfaces (Table 1) was evaluated by swabbing in order to measure the ATP bioluminescence (Hygiena, CA, USA). The swabs were taken according to the manufacturer's instructions from a 100 cm^2 surface area and from the whole surfaces of the cutlery and the knife used for cutting meat. The results were interpreted in relative light units (RLU). The limit values recommended by the swab and luminometer producer were used [27].

3. Results

3.1. Results of the Questionnaire

The online survey started in November 2018 and was completed in April 2019. Only the relevant units that were fully ($n = 260$) or partially completed ($n = 80$) were used for the analysis. The key results of the survey are presented separately according to content areas.

3.1.1. Demographic Data

Table 2 shows the demographic data for the surveyed consumers ($n = 340$), i.e., age group, level of education, and gender.

Table 2. Demographic data for the surveyed consumers ($n = 340$).

Variable		n	%
Gender	Men	63	19
	Women	277	81
Age group	1st age group (18 to 35 years)	171	50
	2nd age group (36 to 55 years)	107	31
	3rd age group (over 56 years)	62	19
Education level	Primary, secondary, and post-secondary *	185	55
	University education, master's degree, doctorate	155	45

Legend: * Post-secondary education includes a two-year post-secondary program of study.

3.1.2. Risk Perceptions

In our study, more than half (65%) of the consumers believed that FBD were rare in domestic households, and 62% of them claimed that people were more often infected or poisoned by food consumed in restaurants. The majority agreed that food contaminated with microorganisms posed a serious (50.5%) or very serious (38.6%) risk to consumers. However, some specific responses in this category were mainly influenced by age (Table 3).

Table 3. Overall results of the questionnaire analysis and statistical significance ($p < 0.05$) by gender, age, and education level.

Categories and Variables Studied	Overall Agreement Correctness/Rate	p-Values Gender	p-Values Age	p-Values Education	Subgroup with Statistically Significant Higher Rate *
Risk perception					
Certain groups of people are more susceptible to infections and/or food poisoning.	71%	0.352	**0.015**	**0.003**	Highly educated older consumers
Risk for infection and/or food poisoning is higher among the elderly.	71%	0.053	**0.033**	0.362	Younger consumers
Risk for infection and/or food poisoning is higher among people with poor hygiene habits.	57%	0.687	**0.041**	0.474	Middle-aged consumers
Eating hygienically prepared food cannot lead to infection or poisoning.	48%	0.923	**0.006**	0.291	Older consumers
Awareness of microorganisms existing on food and surfaces					
Prevention of infections from foods containing bacteria of the *Salmonella* genus by thorough heat treatment.	69%	0.892	**0.001**	0.112	Younger consumers
Agreeing with the fact that raw chicken contains pathogenic microorganisms.	63%	**0.030**	0.138	0.204	Women
Agreeing with the fact that that raw seafood contains pathogenic microorganisms.	52%	0.140	**0.008**	0.827	Middle-aged consumers
Washing hands					
Appropriate hand drying method (a paper towel or a kitchen towel only for wiping the hands).	63%	0.719	**0.036**	0.100	Middle-aged consumers
Appropriate hand washing technique (warm water and soap) before preparing food.	60%	0.632	**0.024**	0.885	Middle-aged consumers
Appropriate hand washing time (more than 20 s) before preparing food?	10%	**0.008**	0.415	0.678	Women
Handling utensils after contact with raw meat					
Washing the cutting board with detergent and warm water.	83%	**0.000**	0.095	0.167	Women
Using another knife or washing the knife with detergent and warm water.	78%	**0.019**	0.080	**0.033**	Highly educated consumers
Using another cutting board.	55%	0.064	0.27	0.060	Middle-aged consumers
Cold chain maintenance					
Control thermometer in the refrigerator.	30%	**0.014**	0.416	0.574	Women
Use of insulating bag after purchase of perishable food.	23%	0.137	**0.023**	0.176	Older consumers
Food thawing					
Appropriate thawing technique of frozen meat (in the refrigerator).	52%	0.509	0.105	**0.015**	Highly educated consumers
Food handling after heat treatment					
Appropriate reheating leftovers (until boiling and boil for a few minutes).	62%	0.906	**0.039**	0.115	Middle-aged consumers
Appropriate cooling method for heat-treated dishes (in less than two hours after heat treatment).	50%	0.622	**0.011**	0.071	Middle-aged consumers

Note: * Detailed information on the results of the subcategories can be found in Sections 3.1.2–3.1.8. Younger consumers (1st age group): 18–35 years; middle-aged consumers (2nd age group): 36–55 years; older consumers (3rd age group): over 56 years; higher level of education: university education, MSc., PhD.

Consumers in the 3rd age group were much more likely to agree (72.2%) that certain populations are more susceptible to food poisoning compared to the 2nd (62.8%) and 1st (47.9%) age groups. In contrast, elderly consumers (3rd age group) least agreed (56.4%) that elderly are at higher risk of foodborne infections compared to the 2nd and 1st age groups, with 73.4% and 75.0% agreement, respectively (Table 3). Elderly consumers (3rd age group) least agreed (43.6%) that people with poor hygienic habits are at higher risk of foodborne infections, while the 1st and 2nd age groups agreed at 56.0% and 64.9%, respectively.

3.1.3. Awareness of Microorganisms on Food and Surfaces

The awareness of microorganisms was highest among younger consumers in the first age group and lowest among older consumers in the third age group. When asked about specific microorganisms, the bacteria *Yersinia enterocolitica* (21%), *Bacillus cereus* (25%), and *Clostridium perfringens* (29%) were the least known, while *Salmonella* (96%), *E. coli* O157 (56%), and *Staphylococcus aureus* were among the best known. The respondents overall considered chicken to be riskier compared to seafood (Table 3). Women associated raw chicken meat with pathogenic microorganisms more than men, with 66.7% and 48.1% selecting the "very likely" option, respectively. On the other hand, the knowledge of how to prevent infections from food containing *Salmonella* was age-dependent (Table 3). Younger consumers were most likely (75.9% and 72.8% in the 1st and 2nd age groups, respectively) to see thorough cooking as the best course of action, while older consumers (3rd age group) saw this as an option only in 46.3%, while 44.4% no longer considered this type of food to be safe at all.

3.1.4. Washing Hands

The questionnaire revealed that 60% of consumers reported washing their hands always with warm water and soap before preparing food, while the rest reported washing their hands almost always (31%) or sometimes (9%). The technique of hand washing (with warm water and soap) was found to be age-dependent (Table 3), as in the 1st and 2nd age groups 67.7% and 65.5%, respectively, reported always washing their hands in this manner, while only 51.9% ($p = 0.024$) reported this in the 3rd age group. The handwashing time turned out to be the most critical element of hand hygiene. Among the 290 consumers, 26% reported washing their hands for 10 s or less, 46% for 11 to 20 s, and 10% for 20 s or more, while the others gave no consideration to the washing time. Significantly more males (43%) than females (23%) washed their hands for only 10 s or less. The statistical analysis (Table 3) revealed that women reported washing their hands for longer than men ($p = 0.008$). After washing their hands, 37% of the consumers reported using a kitchen towel that was only for drying hands, followed by those who used paper towels (26%) and those who used a kitchen towel that was also used for drying dishes (22%). The proper technique of hand drying was reported (Table 3) significantly more frequently by older (78.3% and 77.1% in the 2nd and 3rd age groups, respectively) consumers than by the 1st age group, who reported a proper technique of hand drying in 63.2% of respondents.

3.1.5. Handling Utensils after Contact with Raw Meat

Overall, 17% of the consumers (Table 3) reported risky practices with potential for cross-contamination, while washing the cutting board after use (cutting raw meat) with water only was more frequent in males (35.3%) than females (13.5%) ($p < 0.001$). Similarly, after using the knife (cutting raw meat), males were more likely (35.3%) than females (19.1%) to wash it with water only. After cutting red meat or poultry, 61.2% of consumers in the 2nd age group and 56.8% in the 1st age group used a second cutting board for vegetables, while only 39.7% of consumers in the 3rd age group reported this practice ($p = 0.027$).

On the other hand, after cutting raw meat, a large share (44%) of the consumers reported to washing the cutting board with detergent and warm water (38% of all female and 27% of all male consumers).

3.1.6. Cold Chain Maintenance

Of all the categories studied, the lowest food safety performance was found in maintaining the cold chain (Table 3). Thirty percent of respondents reported having a thermometer in their refrigerator at home, with females reporting this more often (33%) then males (18.5%) (Table 3). More than half of the respondents (51%) did not know the temperature in their refrigerator. Of those who said they had a thermometer, slightly more than half (54%) knew the temperature. As many as 40% of consumers reported never checking the temperature or only checking it when food felt too hot or too cold (32%), while the rest checked the temperature daily, once a month, or weekly (28%). The consumers were asked to indicate the temperature in their home refrigerator. The mean value of the temperatures reported was 5.4 °C. Most consumers (31%) indicated that the temperature was 5 °C. After a purchase, the use of an insulated bag to maintain the cold chain was found to be age-specific (Table 3), and was most commonly used by the third age group, who reported always using it (33.3%), followed by the second (21.7%) and first (19.3%) age groups.

3.1.7. Food Thawing

Frozen meat was reported to be properly defrosted by 52% of the consumers (34% in the refrigerator, 11% under cold running water, and 7% in the microwave), while 42% and 6% of the consumers defrosted meat on the kitchen counter and never defrosted frozen meat, respectively. The defrosting of frozen meat was related to the level of education (Table 3), with those with low education most likely (47.3%) to defrost frozen meat on the kitchen counter, while 36.8% of those with higher education reported this practice ($p = 0.015$).

3.1.8. Food Handling after Heat Treatment

Half of the 250 consumers reported allowing the prepared dish to cool at room temperature for less than two hours, 28% of them for more than two hours, and 21% did not pay attention. The majority (88%) handled the roasted meat correctly after heat treatment, as they did not place it in the container where the raw meat had been stored. Reheating (heating food quickly to 75 °C or hotter by stirring to distribute the heat over the entire surface) was reported by 62% to be done until the food is boiling, followed by 26.1% who reheated only until the food is warm enough and suitable for immediate consumption. The rest indicated that reheating was not necessary as leftovers were thrown away or given to animals.

The methods of cooling heat-treated dishes (cooling to a temperature of about 20 °C within a maximum of two hours, then refrigerating up to 5 °C or freezing −18 °C immediately afterwards) and reheating leftovers were age-dependent (Table 3). The proper cooling method was applied in 25.8%, 18.8%, and 10.3% of age groups 2, 3, and 1, respectively. Similarly, the method of reheating was applied in 71.4%, 65.5%, and 53.2% in age groups 2, 3, and 1, respectively.

3.2. The Results of Observing Consumers and Their Food Handling Practices

Observations of the preparation of the selected foods were carried out with prior arrangements at the consumers' homes. We observed 16 consumers, 8 of whom were over 65 years old and 8 under 35 years old with children aged 5 years or younger. We observed 8 women, 4 being under 35 years of age, and 8 men, 4 being over 65 years of age, preparing selected foods.

3.2.1. Hand Washing

Through the observations of consumers' food handling, it was found out that 8 of 16 washed their hands properly with soap and warm water, out of which 2 were over 65 years and 6 were younger than 35 years. Four consumers did not wash their hands and another 4 did not wash them correctly. The latter were over 65 years old (2 men and 2 women); they did not use soap or used cold water when washing their hands.

The differences between genders were not obvious. After contact with raw poultry meat, 8 consumers washed their hands correctly, with half of them being younger than 35 years and half of them being older than 65 years. Women demonstrated much better conduct after handling raw poultry meat, since 5 women washed their hands correctly (out of which 4 were over 65 years and 1 was younger than 35 years), while 3 men did so (2 younger and 1 older).

After washing, 3 consumers correctly wiped their hands, namely 1 older and 1 younger consumer, who both used paper towels, as well as 1 younger consumer who used a kitchen towel for this purpose. The others did not wipe their hands or wiped them incorrectly with a kitchen towel that was used for wiping hands, surfaces, and dishes.

The duration of washing hands for the surveyed consumers before starting to prepare food and after handling raw poultry meat and raw vegetables was too short, since none of the surveyed consumers washed their hands for more than 12 s.

3.2.2. Cleaning the Cutting Board after Its Use

Nine out of 16 consumers, of which 6 were younger and 3 were older consumers, correctly cleaned the board used for cutting raw poultry meat. The consumers cleaned the board with warm water and detergent and rinsed it with warm water ($n = 6$) or they put the board in the dishwasher ($n = 3$). Two male consumers over 65 years only washed the board with cold water and without detergent, and five consumers did not clean the cutting board (4 of them did not use the board, while 1 younger consumer subsequently used the same board without washing it to cut vegetables). No significant differences between genders were detected.

3.2.3. Measurements of Air Temperature in Refrigerators

At the time of measurement, only 2 of 16 refrigerators were operating below the recommended temperature (5 °C) for consumer refrigerators [28]. Nine out of 16 refrigerators operated above 7.0 °C, while the rest operated within the tolerance range (5 ± 2 °C). The highest measured temperature in a refrigerator was 12.9 °C, while the lowest 4.1 °C. The average temperature in the refrigerators of consumers younger than 35 years was 7.1 °C (max 9.2 °C; min 4.1 °C), while for consumers over 65 years it was somewhat higher, namely 7.6 °C (max 12.9 °C; min 4.5 °C).

3.2.4. The Risks of Cross-Contamination during Food Preparation

Fourteen consumers did not use separate boards and knives to prepare meat and vegetables. Only 2 male consumers separated items correctly. Ten consumers correctly separated raw poultry meat from other food types, 5 of whom were over 65 years. The others did not separate them consistently. We also paid attention to the separation of raw foods from ready-made foods, which was respected by the majority (14) of consumers. Two younger male consumers separated them inconsistently. The majority of the observed consumers (14 out of 16 observed) did not wash poultry meat before preparation, which is in line with the recommendations (28). Before using it, the meat was washed by 3 women, namely 2 younger than 35 years (out of 8) and 1 older than 65 years (out of 8).

Seven consumers washed carrots before cutting them. Nine consumers did not wash carrots, out of these 5 were younger and 4 were older consumers. Only one younger consumer peeled the carrots before cutting and washed the cabbage before preparation, while the other 15 consumers did not wash them but instead only removed the outer leaves.

3.3. The Microbiological Quality Results and the Cleanliness of Surfaces

3.3.1. Hygiene Test Sheets

The presence of presumptive coliform bacteria, including *E. coli*, on the cutting boards was detected in one surveyed consumer. According to the manufacturer's instructions (R-Biopharm, Germany), the lowest detection limit for the total colony count and coliform bacteria (*E. coli*) is 1 CFU/20 cm^2, while the maximum number of colonies per sheet is

250 CFU/20 cm². Since only two characteristic colonies grew on the medium and were not further identified in this sample, this result cannot be used to interpret the adequacy of the surfaces examined here. In the other 15 consumers, *E. coli* and other coliform bacteria were not detected, which means that the samples from the mentioned surfaces complied with the parameters from the guidelines for the microbiological safety of food intended for the final consumer [26], stipulating that no *E. coli* bacteria are found in a swab.

Based on the TCC values, we classified each surface into one of three groups: adequately cleaned, acceptable, and inadequately cleaned. The acceptable level for the TCC on kitchen utensils is 100 CFU/20 cm² or 2.0 log CFU/20 cm² according to the guidelines [26]; thus, we assessed surface contamination above these levels as inadequate. Surfaces with TCC levels below log 1.0 CFU/20 cm² were defined as adequately cleaned. Surfaces were classified as acceptably cleaned when the TCC values were between log 1.1 and log 2.0 CFU/20 cm². The TCCs were above log 2.0 CFU/20 cm² on two cutting boards (12.5%), while the plates of all consumers were adequately (n = 12, 75%) or acceptably (4, 25%) cleaned.

According to the TCC limits of the two tested utensils as a whole, we divided the individual consumers into four classes as follows: 1st class: cutting board and plate were adequately cleaned; 2nd class: one of the tested surfaces was adequate and the other was acceptable; 3rd class: both surfaces were acceptable; 4th class: one or both tested surfaces were inadequately cleaned (Table 4).

3.3.2. ATP Swabs

The measurements of ATP bioluminescence were used to evaluate the cleanliness of the selected surfaces (knife for cutting meat, work counter, refrigerator walls, dishwasher wall, and salad servers). The manufacturer's recommended limits were used to interpret the results obtained as adequately cleaned (pass, 0 to 10 RLU), acceptably cleaned (caution, 11 to 30 RLU), and inadequately cleaned (fail, 31 RLU and above)/100 cm² of surface [29]. No less than 26 (40.6%) of the surfaces tested were inadequately cleaned according to these criteria. The average RLU values were the highest on knives used for cutting meat (163.68 ± 266.28). These utensils were inadequately cleaned by half (n = 8) of the 16 consumers surveyed, while only 31% (n = 5) were rated as adequately clean. The highest RLU value/total area of the knife was exceeded by more than 100 times (Table 4, Figure 1).

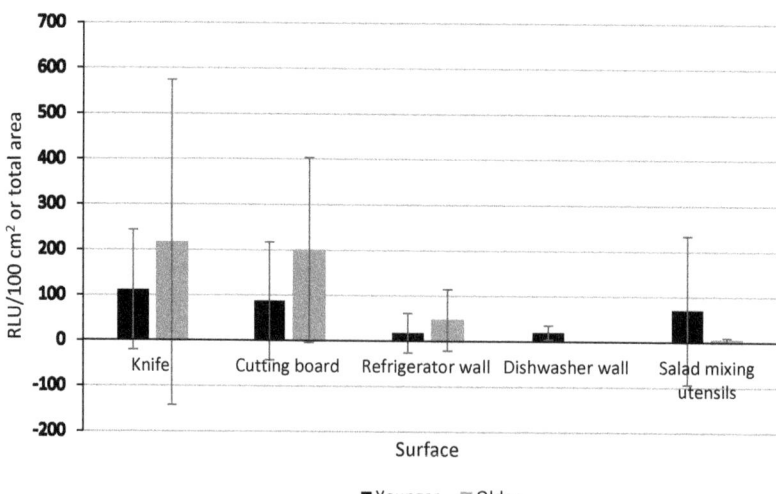

Figure 1. Average RLU values of the kitchen surfaces referring to older and younger consumers, measured via ATP bioluminescence (n = 16). Note: The measurements of dishwasher walls referring to older consumers were not included because most of them did not have this appliance.

Table 4. Cleanliness of surfaces and utensils used by the observed consumers based on the ATP bioluminescence and total colony count results.

Consumer Group	ATP Bioluminescence				*	TCC (log CFU/20 cm^2)		**
	Knife (RLU/Total Area)	Working Counter (RLU/100 cm^2)	Refrigerator Wall (RLU/100 cm^2)	Salad Mixing Utensils (RLU/Total Area)		Cutting Board	Plate	
Y1	8	64	1	3	3	1.90	0.60	2
Y2	116	401	8	58	4	1.25	0.30	2
Y3	317	25	0	1	3	1.51	0	2
Y4	306	101	1	9	4	0.90	0	1
Y5	0	43	0	3	3	1.30	0.30	2
Y6	115	5	2	7	3	1.51	1.23	3
Y7	11	38	125	472	4	1.25	0	2
Y8	18	22	6	7	2	0	0	1
O1	51	104	6	3	4	2.31	0.84	4
O2	12	81	9	15	3	0	0	1
O3	7	251	37	9	4	0.30	1.04	1
O4	4	96	2	1	3	0.60	1.45	2
O5	0	11	80	0	3	0.48	0	1
O6	484	359	5	1	4	1.71	1.88	3
O7	1003	620	201	6	4	1.30	1.53	3
O8	167	76	32	3	4	2.60 ^{en}	0.85	4
Average	163.68	143.56	23.19	37.38		1.18	0.63	
SD	266.28	174.84	56.86	116.17		0.77	0.65	

Note: Y: group of younger consumers; O: group of older consumers; RLU: relative light units—the bold black values mean that the cleanliness of the sampled surface is inadequate; TCC: total colony count. * Degree of surface cleanliness was estimated according to the producer' instructions (Hygiena, 2021) as a pass (adequate, 0 to 10 RLU), caution (acceptable, 11 to 30 RLU), and fail (inadequate, 31 and more) per 100 cm^2, and four classes were formed: 1st class: three or four surfaces belong according the RLU values to pass; 2nd class: two surfaces belong to pass according the RLU values and two surfaces belong to caution; 3rd class: three surfaces belong to pass or caution according to the RLU values and only one belongs to fail; 4th class: two or more surfaces belong to fail according to the RLU values. ** Degree of surface contamination was estimated according to Guidelines (2019) with the compliant limit values of the TCC on kitchen utensils under 2.0 log CFU/20cm^2 and four classes were formed: 1st class: the TCC on the cutting desk and plate was below log 1.0 CFU/20cm2; 2nd class: TCC of one surface was below log 1.0 CFU/20cm^2 and the TCC of the other was between 1.1 log CFU and 2.0 log CFU/20cm^2; 3rd class: TCC of both surfaces was between 1.1 log CFU and 2.0 log CFU/20cm^2; 4th class: TCC of one or both tested surfaces was above 2.0 log CFU/20cm^2; en: estimated number.

According to the ATP bioluminescence measurements, the work counter was rated as inadequately clean for the majority (75%, $n = 12$) of the consumers surveyed, while only one (young) consumer (6.3%) had an adequately clean working counter (Table 4).

The refrigerator walls were found to be inadequately clean for 5 (31.3%) consumers, although the average RLU values were the lowest compared to the other surfaces tested (32.19 ± 56.86 RLU/100 cm^2) (Table 4, Figure 1).

The samples taken from the walls of the dishwasher (rubber pad on the filter) were less numerous because 44% of the consumers surveyed (7 elderly) did not have a dishwasher at home, so they were not included in further calculations. About 55.6% ($n = 6$) of 9 samples showed acceptable cleanliness for the dishwasher walls, while 22.2% ($n = 2$) each were adequate and inadequate, respectively.

The ATP bioluminescence results for salad utensils (forks, spoons, stirring spoons) were encouraging, as 81.2% ($n = 13$) of the samples could be rated as adequately cleaned, while one sample was acceptably cleaned and 12.6% ($n = 2$) were inadequately cleaned. The RLU levels were highest on the surfaces in kitchens mainly belonging to the older consumers, except for the salad mixing utensils (Figure 1).

Following the same principle of classifying consumers based on TCC limits, we did the same based on RLU limits, as follows: 1st class: three or four surfaces were adequate according to the RLU values, none were inadequate; 2nd class: two surfaces were adequate according to the RLU values and two surfaces were acceptable, none were inadequate; 3rd class: three surfaces were adequate or acceptable according to the RLU values, only one was inadequate; 4th class: two or more surfaces were inadequate.

After classifying the hygienic adequacy of the surfaces based on the RLU and TCC values, we calculated the sum of the classes for each individual consumer and defined the overall hygienic conditions in their kitchen. In 4 (25%) kitchens, the surfaces were inadequately cleaned, and all of them belonged to the older consumers. The hygiene levels of the observed kitchen surfaces and utensils were acceptable and adequate in 9 (56.3%) and 3 (18.8%) of the observed consumers, respectively. Statistical differences in RLU and TCC values on the surfaces when using the t-test for independent samples between older and younger consumers were not observed (p = 0.33).

4. Discussion

It was assumed that consumers with a higher level of education would have more food safety knowledge, but was not be fully confirmed, as it was found that there were only certain areas where consumers with a higher level of education showed better performances than those with a lower level of education. However, this is not a surprising result, since food safety is part of regular education only in primary schools and in professional education in the field of food science. The Food Safety Survey by the FDA [23] found that food was handled the least safely by the youngest American consumers, by the oldest, and by those with the highest level of education. In studies that gathered data through questionnaires and by observing consumers during food preparation, it was established that many consumers correctly answered questions about food safety and good hygiene practices, but they often acted contrary to what they stated in the questionnaires [1,18,19,22]; the chances of FBD are, thus, much higher than shown in the epidemiological data [2,10,21].

One of the reasons for violations of good housekeeping practices according to Redmond and Griffith [30] is optimistic bias related to the perceptions of risk in the context of food safety from the foods people prepare. The unhygienic food handling conditions at home in the current study contradict the lowest ranked risk perceptions according to Redmond and Griffith [30]. In our study, more than half of the consumers believed that FBD were rare in domestic households and claimed that people were more often infected or poisoned by food consumed in restaurants. Although the last Eurobarometer report [7] revealed that food hygiene ranks 5th considering the topics on food that most concern European consumers, food hygiene is rated as last (18%) among Slovenian consumers. Our study also pointed out that the elderly consumers least agreed about the elderly being at higher risk of foodborne infections compared to younger ones and about people with poor hygienic habits being at higher risk of foodborne infections.

Proper hand washing before and during food preparation according to the survey was done more consistently by female consumers than by male ones. When comparing the results with a previous similar study among Slovenian consumers [5], we can see that 86% of consumers always washed their hands before preparing food. Our present research illuminated the fact that the situation is not improving; on the contrary, we found that only 60% of consumers always washed their hands before preparing food. The study by Jevšnik et al. [5] found that more than half of consumers washed their hands for less than 10 s. In our recent study about one-quarter reported a hand washing duration of less than 10 s. Furthermore, 67% of consumers washed their hands with soap and warm water after handling raw red meat, chicken, or fish, which was more than in the study by Jevšnik et al. [5], where the relevant share was 57%.

The questionnaire results showed that slightly less than half of the consumers defrosted food at room temperature, while the rest carried out the procedure correctly in the refrigerator, under running cold water, or in a microwave oven. Lower results were reported by Sterniša et al. [31] and Jevšnik et al. [5], where almost three-quarters (73%) or half (50%) of the consumers thawed frozen meat at room temperature. Studies from abroad found that meat was thawed at room temperature by 44% of Nigerian consumers [32], 47%

of African and Asian consumers [3], and 73% of consulted Belgian consumers [9], as well as more than a half of Turkish consumers [16].

The best knowledge of microorganisms that can cause FBD was shown by younger consumers, which can be attributed to the fact that they have better access to information than older consumers. In general, the knowledge of pathogenic microorganisms was poor. More than half of the surveyed consumers knew only two types of bacteria, namely *Salmonella* and *E. coli*, which was more than noted by Gong et al. [33], as more than half of Chinese consumers had never heard of these bacteria. Borda et al. [34] established that Romanian consumers did not recognize some of the pathogens, especially those that may affect their health in the present day and are categorized as emerging pathogens.

While observing consumers, we found many irregularities that can cause the microbiological contamination of surfaces. A higher risk of microbiological contamination of food was evident in consumers older than 65 years. Raw poultry meat must be kept in the refrigerator, as this prevents the growth of pathogenic microorganisms and cross-contamination during storage. It must be kept at temperatures of up to 5 °C on the lowest shelf in the refrigerator to prevent possible dripping on other foods [1]. We found that most of surveyed consumers (94%) paid no attention to the place in the refrigerator where they stored packed or unpacked foods. Only 1 younger man was attentive in this respect. Incorrect practices with storing foods in refrigerators were found by Janjić et al. [35], who noted that almost half of consumers stored foods incorrectly (raw food above prepared food, inconsistent separation of raw and prepared foods). In the home refrigerators of the surveyed consumers, we measured the cold air temperatures and established that the average temperature amounted to 7.4 °C, which was 1.5 °C higher then recently reported by Ovca et al. [36] after 24 h refrigerator measurements in Slovenian households. A Serbian study of consumers by Janjić et al. [35] demonstrated poorer results, with an average temperature of 9.3 °C, which was above those recommended (5 ± 2 °C) (NIJZ, 2011).

In our recent study, it was found that 30% of the consumers claimed they had a thermometer in their home refrigerator to check the temperature. However, it could also be possible that consumers mistakenly thought their refrigerator's built-in display was a control thermometer. The recent study by Ovca et al. [36] among Slovenian households proved that none of the analyzed refrigerators were equipped with a control thermometer and only few (16%) had a built-in display. Better results were shown in a survey of American consumers, where 42% of consumers had a thermometer in the refrigerator, with an average temperature of 3.6 °C [23].

The question of how the surveyed consumers checked the heat-treated poultry meat was answered by majority that they cut the meat or evaluated its color, and only some of them measured the core temperature [31]. Studies of American [19] and Belgian consumers [1] gave similar results. Visual control is not always a reliable indicator that the meat has received appropriate thermal treatment. Only the core temperature of the meat can attest to this with certainty [16]. In the current study, none of the surveyed consumers used a thermometer during the heat treatment of meat; rather, they evaluated the color of the poultry meat and the baking time, and some cut through the poultry leg.

Most of them (69%) kept leftovers on the kitchen counter, others in the refrigerator (12%), or others gave leftovers to animals to be eaten (19%). Two foreign studies also showed similar results, since 24% of Italian [37] and 17% Chinese [33] consumers let foods cool down at room temperature and then stored them in the refrigerator.

Consumers younger than 35 years and older than 56 years were less informed about the methods of ensuring food safety than consumers aged between 36 and 55 years, meaning they could, thus, more often cause FBD. Due to having weaker immune systems and more diseases, the elderly are more prone to infections or food poisoning [14]. The knowledge of the elderly was acceptable in some areas; however, they often failed to transfer it into practice, since the consumers older than 65 years fared worse when preparing food than the consumers younger than 35 years. We further established that weaker knowledge and practices regarding ensuring food safety were demonstrated by male consumers, which was also stated in studies performed abroad [16,17,20,22].

Most surfaces (93.8%) sampled with hygiene test sheets used to assess the microbiological quality of surfaces met the guidelines [26] for both standards (total aerobic mesophilic microorganism and coliform bacteria counts, including *E. coli*), indicating that the consumers were adequately cleaning their cutting boards and serving plates. The results of the swabs used for measuring ATP bioluminescence showed poorer hygiene conditions.

Bukhari et al. [38] reported that meat slicers and cutting boards were the most contaminated surfaces in restaurant kitchens (60% and 50%, respectively), whereas washed serving dishes were the least contaminated (18%). The same situation was observed in our study, where more than half of the ATP swabs taken from the surfaces of the knives used to cut meat were inadequately cleaned. Therefore, the surfaces that came into contact with raw food, especially foods of animal origin such as meat, were more contaminated, as the concentrations of faulty microbiota in meat can quickly reach 6.5–7.0 log CFU/g, depending on the handling and storage conditions [39].

Additionally, twelve (75%) working surfaces failed to meet the producer standards [29]. The reasons could be inadequate cleaning, the use of contaminated sponges for cleaning, and the fact that these surfaces were not exposed to higher temperatures or were not rinsed with clean water. Indeed, about 72% of sponges from household kitchens contained more than 7.0 log CFU for the TCC [40]. The lowest average number of RLUs was found on the surfaces of the delicacies drawer in the refrigerator, which can be explained by the inhibition of microorganism growth due to low refrigeration temperatures. Only about 56% of surfaces inside the dishwashers were acceptably clean. The manufacturers recommend regular cleaning of the grates, rubber linings, and filters with a degreaser and additional rinsing with hot water. According to our previous observations in some households, the dishes in the dishwasher were washed only with warm water (only 40 °C to 50 °C), which is not sufficient to kill microorganisms. Therefore, the improper cleaning and maintenance of the dishwasher could pose a risk for the microbiological contamination of kitchen utensils during washing. The poorer results from the ATP swabs in comparison to the results of test sheets could be linked to the fact that the ATP swabs detected all cells (microbial, plant, and animal cells) and also residues of organic origin (e.g., food leftovers), while the test sheets detected only microbial cells [27].

We can conclude that eighty-three (74.1%) of the 112 surfaces examined with either hygiene test sheets or ATP swabs met the standards and were adequately or acceptably cleaned (Table 4). The kitchen surfaces of 4 (25%) consumers exceeded the recommended limits. Statistical differences in RLU and TCC levels on surfaces between older and younger consumers were not observed, although all (25%) inadequately cleaned kitchens belonged to older consumers.

To sum up all of the results obtained with all of the methods used, we found differences between what the consumers mentioned in the survey questionnaire and the way they handled food during its preparation. More than half (60%) of the consumers claimed that they always washed their hands before food handling, i.e., more elderly than younger consumers. Through observing the consumers, we established that half of the consumers washed their hands correctly, but only 25% of the elderly did so. In the survey questionnaire, more than half claimed that they correctly wiped their hands with kitchen or paper towels after washing, while our observations revealed that more than half of the consumers wiped their hands with a kitchen towel that was also used for wiping dishes or the counter. Differences were seen also with handwashing after contact with raw poultry meat, since 67% of the consumers claimed that they always washed their hands with soap and warm water, while through observations we identified a smaller share of correct handwashing after contact with raw poultry meat (50%). We found out that more than half of the surveyed consumers (56%) correctly washed the cutting board after cutting raw poultry meat. The majority of the surveyed consumers (87%) did not separate utensils, such as knives and boards, while the survey results showed a different picture, since 55% of the consumers claimed that they separated their cutting boards. Differences were observed in washing vegetables before consumption, since 97% of the consumers claimed that they always washed tomatoes before consumption. The results obtained through observation were poor, since less than half of the surveyed consumers washed the carrots before cutting and only 1 consumer washed the cabbage.

5. Conclusions

Deficiencies were found in the consumers' knowledge regarding food defrosting procedures, temperatures in refrigerators, food handling practices, hand hygiene, knowledge about pathogenic microorganisms in food, and the use of thermometers for checking the internal temperature of food during heat treatment. Similar findings were also reported by some other analyzed studies. Moreover, we identified a lack of knowledge in the same content areas as in the previous Slovenian survey [5], which indicates an inadequate emphasis on food safety content.

The biggest drawbacks were identified in the field of cold chain maintenance, where a lack of knowledge identified with the questionnaire was also evident during the observation study. Risky practices (with potential cross-contamination) reported in the questionnaire in reference to the use of cutting boards and knifes were evident during the microbiological study, where the highest loads were identified primarily on theses surfaces. The highest level of knowledge and skills was shown by consumers aged from 36 to 55; in particular, female consumers performed much better than men, regardless of education. The consumers, especially the older ones, were largely convinced that FBD occurred primarily in restaurants and not at home, which is not in concordance with the actual EFSA statistics.

An increased total bacterial count was detected in 12.5% of the observed consumers' kitchens. The results of the ATP measurements showed that about 40% of the surfaces were cleaned inadequately. An increased emphasis has to be put on the cleaning of home kitchens and on personal hygiene, especially on washing hands more often and more thoroughly. Even though consumers have some knowledge of food safety, they often fail to put that knowledge into daily practice.

It is, therefore, necessary to raise food safety awareness in all consumers with an emphasis on vulnerable groups and to provide formal food safety education about ensuring food safety measures during purchasing and when handling food at home. This very complex field of activities clearly shows that the performance of consumers, as human beings, is constantly under the challenge of traditional beliefs about their skills, which they believe are improving with regular daily practice; this study, however, indicates that human beliefs represent one side of the coin of consumer performance, while the reality is much different and is changing with age and technological advancements in the kitchen.

Author Contributions: Conceptualization, M.J., P.R. and M.Š.; methodology, M.J., K.G.T. and A.O.; software, A.O.; formal analysis, L.P.; investigation, L.P.; data curation, A.O. and K.G.T.; writing—original draft preparation, M.J., K.G.T. and A.O.; writing—review and editing, M.Š. and P.R.; visualization, A.O. and K.G.T. All authors have read and agreed to the published version of the manuscript.

Funding: This research was funded by the Slovenian Research Agency (research core funding No. P3-0388).

Data Availability Statement: The data presented in this study are available on request from the corresponding author.

Acknowledgments: The authors would like to acknowledge all participating consumers and the participating households for making this research possible.

Conflicts of Interest: The authors declare no conflict of interest.

References

1. Sampers, I.; Berkvens, D.; Jacxsens, L.; Ciocci, M.; Duomulin, A.; Uyttendaele, M. Survey of Belgian consumption patterns and consumer behaviour of poultry meat to provide insight in risk factors for campylobacteriosis. *Food Control* **2012**, *26*, 293–299. [CrossRef]
2. Byrd-Bredbenner, C.; Berning, J.; Martin-Biggers, J.; Quick, V. Food safety in home kitchens: A synthesis of the literature. *Int. J. Environ. Res. Public Health* **2013**, *10*, 4060–4085. [CrossRef] [PubMed]
3. Odeyemi, A.O.; Sani, N.A.; Obadina, A.O.; Saba, C.K.S.; Bamidele, F.A.; Abughoush, M.; Asghar, A.; Dongmo, F.F.D.; Macer, D.; Aberoumand, A. Food safety knowledge, attitudes and practices among consumers in developing countries: An international survey. *Food Res. Int.* **2019**, *116*, 1386–1390. [CrossRef] [PubMed]
4. EFSA; ECDC. The European Union One Health 2020 Zoonoses Report. *EFSA J.* **2021**, *19*, 6971.
5. Jevšnik, M.; Hlebec, V.; Raspor, P. Consumers' awareness of food safety from shopping to eating. *Food Control* **2008**, *19*, 737–745. [CrossRef]
6. Jevšnik, M.; Ovca, A.; Bauer, M.; Fink, R.; Oder, M.; Sevšek, F. Food safety knowledge and practices among elderly in Slovenia. *Food Control* **2013**, *31*, 284–290. [CrossRef]
7. EFSA. Special Eurobarometer–Wave EB91.3–Kantar, Food safety in the EU. 2019. Available online: https://www.efsa.europa.eu/sites/default/files/corporate_publications/files/Eurobarometer2019_Food-safety-in-the-EU_Full-report.pdf (accessed on 15 February 2021).
8. Meysenburg, R.; Albrecht, J.A.; Litchfield, R.; Ritter-Gooder, P.K. Food safety knowledge, practices and beliefs of primary food preparers in families with young children. A mixed method study. *Appetite* **2014**, *73*, 121–131. [CrossRef]
9. Stratev, D.; Odeyemi, O.A.; Pavlov, A.; Kyuchukova, R.; Fatehi, F.; Bamidele, F.A. Food safety knowledge and hygiene practices among veterinary medicine students at Trakia University, Bulgaria. *J. Infect. Public Health* **2017**, *10*, 778–782. [CrossRef]
10. Kendall, H.; Kuznesof, S.; Seal, C.; Dobson, S.; Brennan, M. Domestic food safety and the older consumer: A segmentation analysis. *Food Qual. Prefer.* **2013**, *28*, 396–406. [CrossRef]
11. Ovca, A.; Jevšnik, M.; Raspor, P. Food safety awareness knowledge and practices among students in Slovenia. *Food Control* **2014**, *42*, 144–151. [CrossRef]
12. Gkana, E.N.; Nychas, G.-J.E. Consumer food safety perceptions and self-reported practices in Greece. *Int. J. Consum. Stud.* **2018**, *42*, 27–34. [CrossRef]
13. Bolek, S. Consumer knowledge, attitudes, and judgments about food safety: A consumer analysis. *Trends Food Sci. Technol.* **2020**, *102*, 242–248. [CrossRef]
14. Leal, A.; Ruth, T.K.; Rumble, J.N.; Simonne, A.H. Exploring Florida residents' food safety knowledge and behaviors: A generational comparison. *Food Control* **2017**, *73*, 1195–1202. [CrossRef]
15. Ovca, A.; Jevšnik, M. Maintaining a cold chain from purchase to the home and at home: Consumer opinions. *Food Control* **2009**, *20*, 167–172. [CrossRef]
16. Ergönül, B. Consumer awareness and perception to food safety: A consumer analysis. *Food Control* **2013**, *32*, 461–471. [CrossRef]
17. Burke, T.; Young, I.; Papadopoulos, A. Assessing food safety knowledge and preferred information sources among 19–29-year-olds. *Food Control* **2016**, *69*, 83–89. [CrossRef]
18. Clayton, D.; Griffith, C. Observation of food safety practices in catering using notational analysis. *Brit. Food J.* **2004**, *106*, 211–227. [CrossRef]
19. Mazengia, E.; Fisk, C.; Liao, G.; Huang, H.; Meschke, J. Direct observational study of the risk of cross-contamination during raw poultry handling: Practices in private homes. *Food Prot. Trends* **2015**, *35*, 8–23.
20. Lazou, T.; Georgiadis, M.; Pentieva, K.; McKevitt, A.; Iossifidou, E. Food safety knowledge and food-handling practices of Greek university students: A questionnaire-based survey. *Food Control* **2012**, *28*, 400–411. [CrossRef]
21. Lange, M.; Goranzon, H.; Marklinder, I. Self-reported food safety knowledge and behaviour among home and consumer studies student. *Food Control* **2016**, *67*, 265–272. [CrossRef]
22. Tomaszewska, M.; Trafialek, J.; Suebpongsang, P.; Kolanowski, W. Food hygiene knowledge and practice of consumers in Poland and in Thailand—A survey. *Food Control* **2017**, *85*, 76–84. [CrossRef]
23. Food and Drug Administration (FDA). Food Safety Survey. 2010. Available online: https://www.fda.gov/media/89145/download (accessed on 13 January 2021).
24. Hartnoll, R.; Griffiths, P.; Taylor, C.; Vincent, H.; Blanken, P.; Nolimal, D.; Weber, I.; Toussirt, M.; Ingold, R. *Handbook on Snowball Sampling*; Pompidou Group, Council of Europe: Strasbourg, France, 1997.
25. *ISO 18593*; Microbiology of the Food Chain—Horizontal Methods for Surface Sampling. International Standard Organization: Brussels, Belgium, 2018; pp. 1–11.
26. National Laboratory of Health, Environment and Food and Veterinary Faculty, University of Ljubljana. Guidelines for the Microbiological Safety of Food Intended for the Final Consumer. 2019. Available online: https://www.vf.uni-lj.si/sites/www.vf.uni-lj.si/files/smernice_mb_2019_ver4.pdf (accessed on 3 June 2022).
27. Hygiena. Surface ATP Test. Available online: https://www.hygiena.com/food-and-beverage-products/ultrasnap-food-and-beverage.html (accessed on 3 November 2021).

28. NIJZ (National Institute of Public Health). Hygienic Recommendations for Food Safety for Consumers. Available online: https://www.nijz.si/sites/www.nijz.si/files/publikacije-datoteke/higienska_priporocila_za_varnost_zivil_za_potrosnike_2011.pdf (accessed on 5 September 2021).
29. Hygiena. Lower and Upper RLU Limits for ATP Monitoring Programs. Available online: https://d163axztg8am2h.cloudfront.net/static/doc/c1/b1/d472875da397448c7747d185c9e2.pdf (accessed on 6 October 2021).
30. Redmond, E.C.; Griffith, C.J. Consumer perceptions of food safety risk, control and responsibility. *Appetite* **2004**, *43*, 309–313. [CrossRef] [PubMed]
31. Sterniša, M.; Smole Možina, S.; Levstek, S.; Kukec, A.; Raspor, P.; Jevšnik, M. Food safety knowledge, self-reported practices and attitude of poultry meat handling among Slovenian consumers. *Brit. Food J.* **2018**, *120*, 1344–1357. [CrossRef]
32. Adebowale, O.O.; Kassim, I.O. Food safety and health: A survey of rural and urban household consumer practices, knowledge to food safety and food related illnesses in Ogun state. *Epidemiol. Biostat. Public Health* **2017**, *14*, 1–7.
33. Gong, S.; Wang, W.; Yang, Y.; Bai, L. Knowledge of food safety and handling in households: A survey of food handlers in Mainland China. *Food Control* **2016**, *64*, 45–53. [CrossRef]
34. Borda, D.; Mihalache, O.A.; Dumitraşcu, L.; Gafiţianu, D.; Nicolau, A.I. Romanian consumers' food safety knowledge, awareness on certified labelled food and trust in information sources. *Food Control* **2021**, *120*, 107544. [CrossRef]
35. Janjić, J.; Katić, V.; Ivanović, J.; Bošković, M.; Starčević, M.; Glamočlija, N.; Baltić, M.Ž. Temperatures, cleanliness and food storage practices in domestic refrigerators in Serbia, Belgrade. *Int. J. Consum. Stud.* **2015**, *40*, 276–282. [CrossRef]
36. Ovca, A.; Škufca, T.; Jevšnik, M. Temperatures and storage conditions in domestic refrigerators—Slovenian scenario. *Food Control* **2021**, *123*, 107715. [CrossRef] [PubMed]
37. Langiano, E.; Ferrara, M.; Lanni, L.; Viscardi, V.; Abbatecola, A.M.; De Vito, E. Food safety at home: Knowledge and practices of consumers. *J. Public Health* **2012**, *20*, 47–57. [CrossRef]
38. Bukhari, M.A.; Banasser, T.M.; El-Bali, M.; Bulkhi, R.A.; Qamash, R.A.; Trenganno, A.; Khayyat, M.; Kurdi, M.A.; Al Majrashi, A.; Bahewareth, F. Assessment of microbiological quality of food preparation process in some restaurants of Makkah city. *Saudi J. Biol. Sci.* **2021**, *28*, 5993–5997. [CrossRef] [PubMed]
39. Shao, L.; Chen, S.; Wang, H.; Zhang, J.; Xu, X.; Wang, H. Advances in understanding the predominance, phenotypes, and mechanisms of bacteria related to meat spoilage. *Trends Food Sci. Technol.* **2021**, *118*, 822–832. [CrossRef]
40. Chen, F.C.; Godwin, S.L.; Kilonzo-Nthenge, A. Relationship between cleaning practices and microbiological contamination in domestic kitchens. *Food Prot. Trends* **2011**, *31*, 672–679.

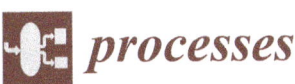

Article

Hygiene and Food Safety Habits among Slovenian Mountaineers

Damjan Slabe, Eva Dolenc Šparovec and Mojca Jevšnik *

Sanitary Engineering Department, Faculty of Health Sciences, University of Ljubljana, Zdravstvena pot 5, 1000 Ljubljana, Slovenia
* Correspondence: mojca.jevsnik@zf.uni-lj.si

Abstract: The study provides a deeper insight into Slovenian mountaineers' and excursionists' habits regarding food safety knowledge, food handling practices, and hygiene on expeditions. The objective of the study is to identify gaps in food safety knowledge and food handling practice at home and during mountaineers' activities. Data were collected using an anonymous online questionnaire (n = 330) and eight semi-structured interviews. The research participants take most of their food with them when they set off, mountaineers more often than excursionists ($p < 0.05$, p = 0,000). Few interviewees indicated that it is important to them that food is safe while consuming it. Almost 90% of mountaineers and excursionists believe they can identify food safety by smell and taste. Significantly more mountaineers prioritise food enjoyment over hygiene compared to excursionists ($p < 0.05$, p = 0.001). Mountaineers also feel that they are more resistant to foodborne diseases and are much less concerned about foodborne disease than excursionists ($p < 0.05$, p = 0.011). The respondents highlighted the need for the Alpine Association of Slovenia to organise food safety education for its members. The greatest emphasis has to be put on food safety education material that has to be put in general training programme for mountaineers. Informing mountaineers and excursionists about food safety requirements needs to be improved with target strategy.

Keywords: food safety; hygiene; mountaineers; excursionist

1. Introduction

The burdens of foodborne diseases (FBD) on public health, welfare, and the economy have often been underestimated due to underreporting because they cause short-term diseases or asymptomatic infections. Outbreaks of FBD occurring in private homes are less likely to be reported than those in commercial and public premises, and it is believed that infections attributed to private homes are three times more frequent than those attributed to canteens [1]. However, studies in recent years have highlighted gaps in food safety knowledge and critical safety violations regarding food handling at home [2–4].

According to Al-Sakkaf [5], the main factors influencing consumers' food handling are personal. They can be divided into psychological, demographical, and socio-economical. The psychological factors include the so-called optimism control and habit bias. The optimism bias is defined as follows: an individual exposed to risk is aware that a certain factor may pose a risk but believes that the probability of this happening to them is lower than the probability of it happening to someone else [5].

The perceived impact of FBD on individuals can depend on perceptions of risk, experiences, trade-offs, and heuristics [6]. According to Zanetta et al. [7], the risk perceptions were not associated with the risk assessment of the restaurants. Performance, time, and health were the consequences with higher risk perceptions. Consumers underestimate the risk of FBD in their home kitchen [8] and when they eat away from home [7]. They believe it is less likely that they perform inadequate food handling practices than others do. Most investigations of food FBD outbreaks state that the consumers have more positive memories

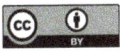

of food consumed away from their homes and blame food prepared by their friends or a restaurant as the main cause of FBD. The consumers identify the food industry and food processing plants as the most high-risk places for food contamination. Consequently, they are less motivated to change their own poor food handling practices [9,10]. The consumer is the last link in the food supply chain, which the European Food Safety Authority believes is inadequately addressed, as the largest proportion of foodborne outbreaks is related to consumers' domestic environment [11]. Lack of knowledge and misconduct in food preparation is more prevalent among consumer groups such as young adults (18 to 29 years), men, and individuals over 60 years of age [8,12,13].

Automatic behaviour patterns regularly occurring without special thought are called 'habits', and individuals do not pay special attention to them [5]. They get used to the behaviour; consequently, the cognitive effort needed for certain behaviours is reduced. For many individuals, food preparation can be described as usual behaviour as it is a frequently repeated act. If the behaviour is repeated regularly, individuals react to it without deep thought. As a result, their practice follows its goal without further ado. The practise becomes a habit, and as the behaviour had been performed often in the past, it becomes increasingly automated [5,9]. Age and gender demographic factors significantly impact people's behaviour when preparing food at home and on trips. Some studies have shown that older consumers follow safe food preparation processes more consistently than younger consumers do and that young consumers have less knowledge about food safety [10]. Gender is important for the perception of risk. Women place greater importance on health risk prevention than men. Because women are mothers and educators, they give more importance to health. Women also have more knowledge about safe food preparation than men do [5,14,15].

Among different groups of athletes, actual nutrition [16] and food safety knowledge [9,17] does not always comply with the official recommendations because of a lack of general nutrition and food safety knowledge, mistaken beliefs, lack of interest or motivation, practical problems, or perhaps intuition [18]. Food safety knowledge and beliefs can influence food safety behaviour [9,19], even if the relationship is not necessarily obvious. Improved food safety and nutritional knowledge and practices during sport activities play an important role in changing already established habits among mountaineers and climbers' [19]. Better insight into food safety and nutrition knowledge and behaviour is of importance for adapting guidelines in view of improving compliance [2,16,17].

Mountaineers perform their sports activity in demanding conditions that increase the risk of FBD and are an interesting target group for researching food safety knowledge and practice [17]. They are organised within the Alpine Association of Slovenia, which is the largest sports organization in Slovenia. A member of the alpine association can take part in a variety of mountaineering activities: hiking, sport climbing, mountaineering, ski touring, mountain biking [20]. Due to the lack of satisfactory data in Slovenia and worldwide, a pilot study among mountaineers in Slovenia was carried out to investigate food safety knowledge and practices and their experience with FBD during mountaineering activities.

The objective of the study was to identify gaps in food safety knowledge and critical safety violations regarding food handling at home and during mountaineering activities.

2. Materials and Methods

2.1. Research Protocol

We used a combination of qualitative and quantitative data collection methodologies. Data were collected using an anonymous online questionnaire and semi-structured interviews. Informed consent was obtained for semi-structured interviews. In addition, the privacy rights of participants were observed.

2.2. Data Collection and Statistical Analysis of the Questionnaire

A link to the online questionnaire (see Appendix B) was sent to Slovenian mountaineers of various profiles. Alpinists, mountaineers, sport climbers, and mountain guides were combined into a group named 'mountaineers'. A second group (control group) was 'excursionists' which are people who are not mountaineers but spend time in nature and do not take part in mountaineering activities (e.g., campers, mushroom pickers, nature visitors). The link was sent via e-mail to alpine, climbing, hiking, and mountaineering clubs and was posted on various websites and social media sites whose potential users are people who go on nature trips. The purpose of the questionnaire was explained. The questionnaire was designed based on the authors' pre-existing empirical research [2,17] dealing with various aspects of food safety. The pre-tested questionnaire included 21 closed-ended questions divided into sections: demographic data, dietary information, knowledge and concern about food safety, the attitude towards it, and experience with FBD. The survey was administered online from 25 March to 25 May 2020, via the web platform 1 ka™. In total, 898 participants responded to the invitation (clicked on the questionnaires' link), whereby 345 completed the questionnaire, and 15 were excluded (because they selected the answers 'other' and were not part of a target group, e.g., cyclists). Finally, 330 participants were included in data analyses. According to their answers about activity, we divided the sample into two groups: 64.2% were mountaineers, and 35.8% were excursionists.

The IBM SPSS Statistics for Windows, version 26 (IBM Corp., Armonk, N.Y., USA) was used for statistical analysis. The demographic data were shown using descriptive statistics. We performed preliminary analyses for normality. Given that the distribution was not normal, we used Mann–Whitney U test to investigate statistically significant differences between the groups. Nevertheless, we presented results with averages and standard deviations for a more straightforward interpretation and comprehensibility of results. A p-value of less than 0.05 was considered significant for all analyses. The statistically significant differences between the different groups of categories were determined with the χ^2 square test. Finally, the level of statistical significance was adjusted ($p < 0.05$).

2.3. Data Collection and Analysis of the Semi-Structured Interviews

This qualitative study used semi-structured interviews to explore gaps in food safety knowledge and critical safety violations regarding food handling at home and during mountaineers' activities. We followed the 32-item consolidated criteria checklist for reporting qualitative research [21]. Through purposeful sampling, participants were recruited from the population of Slovenian mountaineers. The following sampling criteria were applied: participants from different age groups and the various mountaineering activities in which they engage. We introduced the researchers to them and explained the purpose of the research. The purposeful sample size was determined by theoretical saturation, which is the point in the data collection process at which new data no longer offer additional insights for the research question [22]. The final number of interviews conducted was 8 (Table A1 in Appendix A).

In line with the research goals, we decided to conduct interviews to explore mountaineers' attitude towards food safety and their experiences with FBD during their activities. A semi-structured questionnaire (see Appendix C) was prepared and developed through a literature review. It was additionally redesigned after pilot interviews. The interviews were conducted by a doctoral student of Public Health at the Faculty of Medicine of the University of Ljubljana and an assistant professor at the Sanitary Engineering Department, Faculty of Health Sciences. The interviews were held face to face between September and November 2020. They took place at the interviewees' homes. They were recorded digitally (audio), transcribed verbatim, and anonymised. Some field notes were made during and after interviews and included in the final analysis. Transcripts were not returned to participants. No repeat interviews were made.

The authors of the study conducted a qualitative content analysis. The interview transcripts were read, qualitatively coded, reviewed, and labelled, using inductive content analysis. Each interview was analysed by the authors independently. After that, the authors reached a consensus on categories and themes. Themes and categories were defined in an inductive process after establishing codes to condense observations from the data. To provide anonymity, interviewees' names were changed, but they did not provide feedback on the findings. Because of the amount of data obtained through interviews, this part of the results introduces only excerpts from interview transcripts, with the sharpest and most interesting quotes reflecting each interviewee's positions/opinions/experience.

2.4. Demographic Data

A total of 330 respondents participated in the study (64.2% mountaineers and 35.8% excursionists). Approximately 40% of the respondents were under the age of 30, and the same percentile was between 30 and 50 years of age. A good half (57%) of the respondents were university graduates. Meat eaters represented 88.8% of all respondents. The largest share (41.7%) of the surveyed mountaineers had been physically active for over 15 years. Slightly over three-fourths of the mountaineers were often physically active.

We conducted 8 interviews. Each of them lasted about 30 min on average (Table A1 in Appendix A).

3. Results and Discussion

In the following, we present the results obtained from the analysis of survey questionnaires (hereafter respondents) and the qualitative analysis of interviews (hereafter interviewees).

3.1. Eating Habits

The surveyed mountaineers and excursionists most often eat food that they bring with them from home. Typically, mountaineers eat food that they bring from home more often than excursionists do ($p < 0.05$, $p = 0.000$), or they combine that food with eating meals in mountain huts ($p < 0.05$, $p = 0.016$). Mountaineers and excursionists most often bring the beverages they consume from home, however, mountaineers do it more often ($p < 0.05$; $p = 0.030$) than excursionists, who tend to ($p < 0.05$; $p = 0.001$) purchase (additional) beverages from a restaurant, shop (Table 1).

Table 1. Eating habits and water supply on nature trips.

	Mountaineers $\bar{x}$, (σ)	Excursionists $\bar{x}$, (σ)	*p*-Value
Eating habits			
Only with the food I took from home. *	3.05 (0.7)	2.8 (0.7)	0.000
By combining my food and eating in a mountain hut. *	2.6 (0.8)	2.3 (0.8)	0.016
In a mountain hut.	2.3 (0.6)	2.2 (0.6)	0.208
In bars where they serve food (inn, farm tourism, etc.). *	1.9 (0.6)	2.1 (0.5)	0.006
By self-cooking on a portable stove.	1.5 (0.6)	1.4 (0.7)	0.010
Water supply			
I bring all the necessary drinks with me from home. *	3.4 (0.6)	3.3 (0.7)	0.030
If I run into a water source, I pour myself a drink.	2.8 (0.9)	2.7 (1)	0.010
I buy a drink (up to) in a restaurant, shop. *	1.8 (0.6)	2.1 (0.7)	0.001
If I pour water from a source in nature, I filter it or add disinfectant tablets.	1.1 (0.4)	1.1 (0.3)	0.494

Legend: Average grades for both groups of the respondents are expressed as means (and standard deviations); a score means: 1 = never; 2 = sometimes; 3 = often; 4 = always; *—statistically significantly ($p < 0.05$) different when compared groups; $\bar{x}$—average; σ—standard deviation.

From the interviews, we defined three key themes related to the mountaineers' and excursionists' eating habits during their activities in nature T: T1 eating habits, T2 experience with FBD, T3 ensuring health compliance of foodstuffs (Table 2).

Table 2. Theme and categories of qualitative analysis.

THEMAS	Eating Habits	Experience with Foodborne Diseases	Ensuring Health Compliance of Foodstuffs
CATEGORIES	(1) dietary concept, (2) foodstuffs, (3) what is important in a diet	(1) location, (2) cause, (3) consequence (4) what helped	(1) types of foods, (2) no risk/risk for health, (3) food processing, (4) better resilience of mountaineers, (5) hygiene of hands, (6) hygiene of food, and (7) role of alpine society

Under Theme T1, 'eating habits', we identified three categories with associated sub-categories: (1) dietary concept, (2) foodstuffs, and (3) what is important in a diet. In the interviews, the mountaineers highlighted that during their activities, they adapt their diet to the season, length of their tour (half-day, day, several-day long expedition), risk in the country they are travelling to (domestic tours, Europe, other countries), location of accommodations (mountain lodge, camping, bivouac), as well as the available personnel (a hired cook, cooking for themselves). They eat according to how they feel in the moment (1.1.13.5.M3 'intuitively'), modestly (1.1.3.1.M1 'spartan'), and whether they are meat-eaters or vegetarian.

The results of the quantitative analysis show that a total of 74% of the surveyed mountaineers and 78% of excursionists often or regularly take fresh fruit and vegetables; 70.8% of mountaineers and 66.1% of excursionists take dried fruit and nuts. They often or always take beverages or tea prepared at home (69.4% of mountaineers and 55.9% of excursionists). About half of mountaineers and excursionists take cured meats (salami, prosciutto etc.); 47.1% of mountaineers take chocolate bars, energy bars and similar products, with 37.9% of excursionists doing the same. A little less than a third consume different tinned food on their trips (30.7% of mountaineers and 29.7% of excursionists); 28.3% of mountaineers and 24.5% of excursionists consume dairy products (cheese, spreads). Often, mountaineers (21.2%) and excursionists (28%) bring homemade pastries on the trip. Mountaineers never or rarely (99.8%) take fresh milk with them, and it is much the same for excursionists (98.3% do not bring fresh milk). Less than 5% of mountaineers and excursionists take soft-boiled eggs or store-bought pastries with them.

During interviewees' activities in the mountains, we established that they consume very diverse foodstuffs: grains, fresh vegetables, fresh or dried fruit, nuts, dairy products, cured meat, spreads, deserts, eggs, and even mushrooms. Liquids are very important to them: water, water with lemon, tea, homemade tea, or tea with honey. They take water from the springs, streams, or snowmelt to obtain fluids. Schnapps was also mentioned (1.2.11.11 M5 'My flask accompanies me everywhere, with homemade schnapps inside'.). Interviewee (1.2.11.11 M1) stressed that liquids are more important to them than food: 'If I run out of liquids, I will overheat, but I can do without food, providing I have enough to drink'. Interviewee PB (1.3.8.2.M6) highlighted the great role of food during activities: 'It is almost better to forget socks than food'. Several interviewees mentioned that it is important to them that the meal fills them (1.3.2.1.M6: 'It takes up little space, but is still nourishing'), that it is light and with the smallest possible volume, yet has sufficient energy value so that they consume enough carbohydrates, which give them enough strength and energy, and also that the food makes them feel full and that they are sufficiently hydrated at the same time. They also said it is important they enjoy the food (tasty food, that they like it, that it is good: 1.3.4.2.M7 'I like the food to be tasty'), and that the food is homemade (1.3.7.1.M5: 'I swear by homemade food'). Very few individuals highlighted that it is important to them that food is safe (shelf life, reliable food, non-perishable, safe so they do not get sick, and food they have tested), easy to digest, or that they consume a warm meal. For some, it was important they consume food without meat. Others pointed out the psychological (reward, motivation, pleasure) or social (ritual, learning about the culture, sharing, socialising) aspects of eating. The latter was emphasised by 1.3.5.1.M3: 'For me, it is the pleasure on the top of the hill when you eat that sandwich and share some sweets with others'.

3.2. Safety of Food

Almost 90% of respondents (mountaineers and excursionists) believe they can judge food safety by taste and smell. Compared to excursionists, a six-times larger share of mountaineers prioritise food enjoyment over hygiene, which is also statistically significantly ($\chi^2 = 14.348$; $p < 0.05$) higher. Mountaineers also consider themselves more resistant to FBD ($\chi^2 = 8.978$; $p < 0.05$) and worry about possible FBD in a significantly lower proportion ($\chi^2 = 6.008$) than excursionists do (Table 3).

Table 3. Beliefs about food safety.

Statements	Mountaineers		Excursionists		p-Value
	% of Agreement	I Do Not Know	% of Agreement	I Do Not Know	
I can tell by the smell and taste that the food is safe to eat.	88.7	4.7	89.8	2.5	0.596
The most important thing is that the food suits me, and only then is hygiene important. *	26.4	5.2	9.3	4.2	0.001
Mountaineers are more resistant to possible foodborne poisonings. *	13.7	21.2	5.1	32.2	0.011
I am often worried that I would be poisoned with spoiled food during activity in nature. *	9.4	3.3	15.3	7.6	0.048
The food in the mountain huts is safe. *	83.0	15.1	66.1	28.8	0.002
I have good experience in ensuring food safety with food providers when I go to nature, the mountains.	82.5	14.6	73.7	21.2	0.155
Employees in mountain huts do not pay enough attention to clean hands.	10.8	62.3	10.2	66.1	0.778

Legend: The percentage of agreement with the statement according to the number of all respondents in each group are shown; *—statistically significantly ($p < 0.05$) different when compared groups.

The respondent group of mountaineers ranked their knowledge about the safety of food on a scale of 1 to 5 (1-insufficient knowledge, 5-excellent knowledge) with an average grade of 3.58 and excursionists with 3.71; there were no significant differences between the groups in the average self-assessment of their knowledge ($p > 0.05$; $p = 0.136$). The mountaineers acquired the most knowledge through their education (average 2; 1 means no knowledge, 2 medium and 3 a lot of knowledge), the least in mountaineering school (average 1.6) or in newspapers (average 1.6). The majority of the respondent group of excursionists also acquired most of this knowledge through education or online (both average 2.2; where 1 means no knowledge, 2 medium, and 3 a lot of knowledge). Most of the food is prepared by consumers at home [23], so knowledge about food preparation in their home kitchens is definitely more important, as it reduces the likelihood of FBD [24].

With qualitative analysis, we identified seven categories and associated subcategories: (1) types of foods, (2) no risk/risk for health, (3) food processing, (4) better resilience of mountaineers, (5) hygiene of hands, (6) hygiene of food, and (7) role of alpine society. Some interviewees highlighted the importance of consuming properly conserved food or sufficiently thermally processed food. Although mountaineers take a wide variety of food with them in the mountains (see theme 1, category 2), they said that it is important for them that food is non-perishable (3.1.2.2.M8: 'non-perishable'; 3.1.2.3 'perhaps food that does not spoil easily'). In contrast, M7 (3.1.3.4.M7) states: 'Even if food is past the best-before date, it is not that bad'. Some are aware of health risks due to FBD during mountaineering activities. They believe that contaminated water and food can present health risks. They explained that FBD has an undesired effect on a mountaineer's body, which is especially problematic since they are active in demanding conditions (heat/cold), and they cannot cope with the effort required when sick.

Foodborne diseases make the body more vulnerable, leading to hypothermia and dehydration, as well as the inability to think rationally, which can result in improper actions. This can pose an additional danger of slipping or falling.

3.2.3.1.M3 had the following thoughts on the subject: 'When I get sick, I am done for. I can no longer think well or rationally. I can no longer withstand such strain and deal with nature, such as it is in the mountains. I cannot imagine being up there on 5K and get seriously ill?! How will I get down? There is a greater likelihood I will slip or fall'. In addition, the opinion of 3.2.3.2M3 was that a person can die of an FBD.

There are, however, those among the interviewees who feel that food does not pose a health risk due to FBD. For example, 3.2.4.1.M7 said: 'Well, it is not great, no, but I would not say it is a serious threat'. Others prioritise other things before food safety (3.2.4.1.M5): 'I do not complicate things with food; there are other more important things when mountain climbing. There are a lot more dangerous things in the mountains than food—there are rocks and slips and cliffs, avalanches, rock walls'.

The surveyed mountaineers doubt that they are more resilient to FBD than people in general. They link this 'hardiness' of their bodies is due to the fact that they are often exposed to risks and poor conditions. 3.4.2.1.M7: 'Because mountaineers spend a lot of time in a wild environment, they consume more bacteria and bad things. In the mountains, it very often happens that we drink water from whatever stream is there. I feel that the more things pass through your stomach, the more you strengthen your immunity, flexibility to be creative'.

However, interviewee 3.4.1.12.M3 warned about the trap of such a 'brave' posture: 'A couple of times it happened that I thought, it is okay, nothing will happen, or some food was questionable, and I ate it, but I was later sorry, when my stomach hurt, when I felt ill or when I vomited. Every time I said to myself, how stupid you are when you know you should not have!'

3.3. Ensuring Food Safety When Processing Food at Home

When buying food in a shop and preparing food at home, the respondent group of mountaineers takes measures for ensuring food safety less often than excursionists ($p < 0.05$; Table 4). In addition to the knowledge of food hygiene, proper consumer behaviour in food preparation is a key element in ensuring consumer safety [8,25,26]. The lack of knowledge and mishandling of food during preparation is more common in consumer groups of young adults (18 to 29 years), men, and people older than 60 years [2,12]. Irregularities in food handling at home are related to improper handwashing, improper separation of equipment and utensils, inadequate cold food storage, cross-contamination, and insufficient heat treatment of food [2,13,27–29].

Table 4. Measures for purchasing food and preparing food at home.

	Mountaineers $\bar{x}, (\sigma)$	Excursionists $\bar{x}, (\sigma)$	p-Value
WHEN SHOPPING IN A STORE			
Shelf life of the food. *	2.8 (1.9)	3.1 (1)	0.017
(Non) damage to the packaging. *	2.9 (1.1)	3.2 (1)	0.036
Temperature in the refrigerators in the store when buying dairy or meat products and desserts. *	1.2 (0.6)	1.4 (0.8)	0.030

Table 4. Cont.

	Mountaineers x̄, (σ)	Excursionists x̄, (σ)	p-Value
WHEN PREPARING FOOD AT HOME			
Washing hands before preparing food.	3.4 (0.9)	3.6 (0.7)	0.082
Checking the shelf life of food before preparation.	2.9 (1)	3 (1)	0.065
Checking the cleanliness of the packaging in which you store food (thermos, container, …). *	3.7 (0.6)	3.8 (0.4)	0.027
Additional cooling of perishable food with freezers. *	1.8 (1)	2.6 (1.1)	0.000

Legend: Average grades for both groups of the respondents are expressed as means (and standard deviations); a score means: 1 = neve; 2 = sometimes; 3 = often; 4 = always; *—statistically significantly ($p < 0.05$) different when compared groups; x̄—average; σ—standard deviation.

3.4. Ensuring Food Safety during Activities in Nature

The surveyed mountaineers observe food safety measures more infrequently than excursionists while eating during activities in nature ($p < 0.05$) (Table 5).

Table 5. Measures regarding hand hygiene in nature.

	Mountaineers x̄, (σ)	Excursionists x̄, (σ)	p-Value
I rub my hands against my pants or T-shirt. *	2.3 (1)	1.9 (0.9)	0.001
I wash my hands with running drinking water. *	2.1 (0.8)	2.7 (0.9)	0.000
I wipe my hands with wet (factory-prepared) wipes. *	1.9 (0.8)	2.4 (0.9)	0.000
I wipe my hands with a paper towel. *	1.5 (0.7)	1.9 (0.8)	0.000
I wash my hands with running drinking water and soap. *	1.4 (0.6)	1.8 (1)	0.000
I clean my hands with disinfectant (spray, etc.). *	1.4 (0.7)	1.7 (0.9)	0.001

Legend: Average grades for both groups of the respondents are expressed as means (and standard deviations); a score means: 1 = never; 2 = sometimes; 3 = often; 4 = always; *—statistically significantly ($p < 0.05$) different when compared groups; x̄—average; σ—standard deviation.

Proper handwashing before and during food preparation is important to prevent cross-contamination. In our survey, only 11% of all respondents always or often wash their hands with soap and water before consuming a meal in nature. If we compare the results with a previous study among general Slovenian consumers [2], we see that 86% of consumers always wash their hands before preparing food. In the study by Jevšnik et al. [2], it was found that more than half of respondents washed their hands for less than 10 s, and 57% of respondents washed their hands with soap and warm water after handling raw red meat, chicken, or fish.

The interviewees presented different opinions about the importance of hand hygiene while consuming food during activities in nature. Some believe hand hygiene is of significant importance and recognise it as a preventive measure to reduce the risk of infection. They wash their hands using water from streams, plastic bottles, with soap and warm water in mountain lodges, or they 'wash' their hands with snow (3.5.4.3.M2: 'I also wipe them in snow'.). They also stressed that during mountaineering activities, the opportunities for hand hygiene are often limited, or it is even impossible to wash their hands, for example, when there is no water available for several days, or it is half an hour's hike away, or the only water available was needed for hydration. 3.5.1.1.M2 had the following thoughts on the topic: '… She came straight from the toilet without washing her hands. You cannot do things like that! If you have the opportunity, of course, you wash your hands, and even if there is not an opportunity, there is always some way. Often, when I see water running somewhere, I say to myself, oh, right, great, I can wash my hands. Sometimes, I even wash them with water from my bottle if I know I have enough." 3.5.4.3.M2 described hand washing: 'Sometimes you wash them in snow, or some dew, sometimes you wipe them on your trousers. Soap is rare—you usually do not have it'. It was also highlighted that the hand hygiene issue had become more popular during the SARS-CoV-2 pandemic. Some people use disinfecting/hygiene wipes (3.5.3.1.M1: 'If I have to relieve myself, I use the alcohol wipes I carry with me'.). Some are against using them (3.5.3.3.M2 'I am not a fan', 3.5.3.4.M3 'I never have them with me'). Some do not find hand hygiene important while touching 'natural things', as illustrated by the following statement by 3.5.2.1.M1: 'If my hands are dirty from soil, rocks, anything, it means I have touched natural things while climbing, and before I start eating, I do not wash my hands. It is nature—it cannot be poisonous'.

The interviewed mountaineers take care of food hygiene by wiping the food against their trousers or in snow and stress that it suffices. (3.6.3.3.M3 'It is a different feeling'). They avoid direct contact with their hands by using packaging (3.6.2.3.M4: 'If my sandwich is wrapped in plastic wrap, I wrap it so that I hold it by the wrapper'.), or they hold the food with a paper tissue (3.6.2.1.M2 'I hold a sandwich with a tissue'). When cleaning their utensils, much like when cleaning hands, they use any resource available (3.6.3.2M8 'rubbed the spoon in snow and wiped it off a bit'. and 'We cleaned the food off mechanically'). BH (3.6.3.3.M5) gave an interesting description of washing the dishes: 'You only wash the dishes in nearby streams. Cows may be grazing nearby. First, you wipe off the food remains with a paper towel. No dishwashing liquid—no way—it must not go into the environment. You wash more carelessly'.

3.5. Experience with Foodborne Diseases

Regarding FBD during a trip in nature or in the mountains, a small group of respondent (9.9% mountaineers, 4.2% excursionists) have experienced it; there was no significant difference in shares between the groups. ($p > 0.05$; $p = 0.104$). As the most likely reason for FBD, the interviewees identified poor options for personal hygiene (56% of the interviewees), food in alpine lodges (52%), or perishable food prepared at home (34%); 30% see drinking water from natural sources as a plausible reason because the water was not filtered (disinfected).

Within the analysed theme 'Experience with foodborne diseases', we identified four categories with associated subcategories: (1) location, (2) cause, (3) consequence, and (4) what helped. Some of the interviewees experienced FBD during their mountaineering activities. These happened in domestic or foreign mountains; they also reported getting FBD from eating a meal in an alpine lodge. The cause of FBD were beverages (water, cold drinks, ginger ale), food, especially desserts (strawberry cake with cream), meat (leftover meat, sausage, bean soup and cured meat), or food coming in contact with animals (2.2.3.2. M8 'soup, and the container had been nibbled on'; 2.2.3.3. M6 'contaminated water, an animal carcass was in it'). They faced the following health issues: indigestion (vomiting, diarrhea, lack of appetite), dehydration, overall weakness (weight loss, they were confined to bed, exhausted or unable to walk), pain (in the abdomen, stomach, kidneys), and cramps; the consequences also manifested in their psyche (they were frightened). M1 vividly described his food poisoning: 'I got sick in Bolivia when we were climbing Ilimani in Cordillera Real. Before the ascent, we went to a hotel to have a good meal. It was a three-star restaurant, and we had a big meal. It was good, too. Then, I saw some strawberry cakes with cream. I had passed them about three times, and I could not stop myself, and I ordered one. Then, my friend had one, too. They were good, I must say. We ate them, but then before dawn, I do not know who had to go to the toilet first, and then it started [. . .] After three days, we were very weak [. . .]'.

M4: 'I got really sick in Peru. I drank the water up there. It was high up, almost below the glaciers. I knew I must not drink it downstream because there are cows and cow patties, but I did not know cows can get so high up such steep slopes; also I saw a porter, a local, drink that water. They are immune; they can do many things we tourists may not. Well, I got sick overnight. I vomited something awful. We thought it was the altitude, but I knew it was the water. I had trouble for a while; I am thin as it is, and then I came home looking like a skeleton. Weak. On the way back, they put me on a horse, because I could not walk. I was a bit delusional, and my pal got infected by some sweets, but that was in India, and he had the opposite. He got so constipated that he had a belly like a pregnant woman. Imagine not going to the toilet for a week or more'.

In some cases, people needed to be hospitalised. Some of them had positive insights from the otherwise bad experience, as they learned something about more appropriate food handling during their future activities in nature. (2.3.6.1.M2: 'It will not happen to me again'.; 2.3.6.2.M3: 'You really have to be very careful […] put chlorine tablets in it.") When dealing with health issues due to FBD, they were given medicine, select food (2.4.2.1.M1 'coca tea'), hospitalisation, and rest.

Respondents attached great importance to the alpine association in terms of educating about the health status of foods, especially in the area of member education and training (in schools for 'alpinists and mountaineers, in exams, training courses, online, and before visiting more 'exotic' states) because in their opinion this is an important and wide-ranging topic. They also warn about the problem of less-experienced mountaineers going on longer expeditions, especially abroad or to less developed countries (3.7.5.1. 'You have to be more careful'), and they do not even know how to use chlorine tablets, for example. They believe that the SARS-CoV-2 pandemic is a good opportunity to warn them, especially where there are larger groups of people (in lodges, on busses). They also see a role for the alpine association in raising awareness among mountain visitors about the dangers of FBD and contamination risks, preventive measures, and ensuring hygiene standards in mountain lodges (e.g., placing hand disinfectants, monitoring if measures are observed). In the respondents' opinion, this is necessary because of the mass of visitors (3.7.5.2.M4: 'Just think about one and a half million people eating breakfast together and then driving for an hour to some starting point, where they "leave their mark". That is a million and a half of those "marks", and then there are the animals who contaminate them'.). They also highlighted the individuals' responsibility to learn about preventive actions and to have the means to take the basic hygiene measures while eating when travelling. They also note that there always needs to compromise between sufficient gear and weight. They concluded that personal hygiene is important and that disinfectant wipes can help provide it and that you can get seriously ill if you do not follow the preventive measures. Respondent M3 warned about individuals' responsibility: 'You need to be careful, this is your free time, your vacation, your holiday, and it would be really bad if you got sick'. Common sense needs to be applied, because it is impossible to guarantee 100% food safety in the mountains, especially on longer tours that last several days. Against such a background, there is a constant and urgent need to improve domestic food hygiene knowledge and practice [30–32]. However, consumer education activities are expensive to organise, maintain, and evaluate. Thus, it is particularly important to identify, target, and reach higher risk consumer groups correctly [30–34].

4. Conclusions

With our analysis we established that:

1. The respondents take most of the food on tour with them. The energy density of food and sufficient hydration are important for them.
2. Almost 90% of mountaineers and excursionists believe that they can recognise food safety by smell and taste. Statistically significantly more mountaineers prioritise food enjoyment to safety compared to excursionists. Mountaineers also believe they are more resilient to FBD and are significantly less worried about FBD than excursionists. Nevertheless, some interviewed mountaineers also stressed the importance of properly preserved or sufficiently cooked food being aware of health risks due to FBD while mountaineering. To others, food safety poses no additional concern, and they usually disregard best-before date of the foods.

3. When buying food in stores and preparing food at home, the mountaineers in comparison to the excursionists, less often observe food safety measures and less often consider food safety while consuming food during their outdoor activities. Their attitude and perception reflect their belief that they cannot contract FBD during mountaineering. Such a behaviour presents a high risk and could lead to serious health issues during expeditions.
4. A small share of the participating mountaineers and excursionists reported a history of FBD during their tour in nature or in the mountains due to poor possibilities of maintaining adequate personal hygiene, keeping food in mountain lodges, and consuming home-prepared perishable food and water from natural sources.
5. The majority of food safety knowledge was obtained during regular schooling by mountaineers and by excursionists. The respondents stressed the necessity that the alpine association organise training courses and educate about food safety. They also believe that the SARS-CoV-2 pandemic is a good opportunity to raise awareness about the dangers of FBD infection risk among people visiting mountains.

Author Contributions: D.S.—conduct and analysis of interviews, investigation, presentation of interview results; E.D.Š.—methodology, software, formal analysis, presentation of results, conduct and analysis of interviews, editing form; M.J.—literature review, theoretical background, discussion, conceptual design, writing—review and editing, project administration, supervision. All authors have read and agreed to the published version of the manuscript.

Funding: The authors acknowledge the financial support from the Slovenian Research Agency (research core funding No. P3-0388).

Data Availability Statement: The data presented in this study are available on request from the corresponding author. The data are not publicly available due to data file sizes.

Acknowledgments: The authors would like to acknowledge to all participated mountaineers and excursionists for making this research possible.

Conflicts of Interest: The authors declare no conflict of interest.

Appendix A

Table A1. Demographic characteristics of respondents and interviewees.

Characteristics	RESPONDENTS Data Sample			
	Mountaineers ($n = 212$)		Excursionists ($n = 118$)	
	n	%	n	%
SEX				
Male	95	44.8	35	29.7
Female	117	55.2	83	70.3
AGE GROUPS				
<31	93	43.9	38	32.2
31–50	85	40.1	50	42.4
>50	34	16.0	30	25.4
EDUCATION				
Primary school	4	1.9	5	1.5
High school	49	23.1	92	27.9
college, university, university program	124	58.5	188	57.0
specialisation, master's degree, doctorate of science	35	16.5	45	13.6

Table A1. Cont.

Characteristics	RESPONDENTS			
	Mountaineers (n = 212)		Data Sample Excursionists (n = 118)	
	n	%	n	%
DIET				
Omnivorous	185	87.2	108	91.5
Vegetarian	15	7.1	8	6.8
Vegan	12	5.6	2	1.7
YEARS ENGAGING WITH MOUNTAINEERING				
1 to 5	40	19		
5 to 10	54	25.6		
10 to 15	29	13.7		
>15	88	41.7		
FREQUENCY OF ENGAGING WITH MOUNTAINEERING				
very often, at least twice a month	163	77.3		
often, once a month	34	16.1		
occasionally, less than once a month	14	6.6		

INTERVIEWEES				
Characteristics (n = 8)				
Label of the interviewee	Sex	Age (years)	Time of engaging with (years)	Kind of diet
M1	M	70	36	omnivorous
M2	Ž	61	16	vegetarian
M3	Ž	31	31	omnivorous
M4	M	48	21	vegetarian
M5	M	26	15	omnivorous
M6	Ž	35	10	omnivorous
M7	M	28	8	omnivorous
M8	M	56	35	omnivorous

Appendix B

Survey questionnaire

Q1—How often do you eat in the ways listed below during your most popular outdoor activity (walking, hiking, sport climbing, mountaineering) (mark as appropriate)?

Q2—How often do you take the following food with you on a trip to nature, a climbing area or the mountains . . . (mark as appropriate)?

Q3—How often do you check when you buy food for a trip, to a climbing area, hills . . . (mark as appropriate)?

Q4—How important do you think it is that we pay special attention to the appropriate (quality) PACKAGING (mark accordingly) when storing/packaging an individual food that we take with us into nature?

Q5—How do you usually get liquid (mark accordingly) during a trip to nature, in a climbing area or in the mountains?

Q6—When preparing food at home (e.g., sandwich) for a trip to nature, climbing or mountains, do you take care of . . . (mark as appropriate)?

Q7—How often and with what do you clean your hands before eating a meal during a trip in nature, in a climbing area, hills or in the mountains (mark as appropriate)?

Q8—Do you agree, are the following statements correct . . . ?

Q9—What do you understand by the term "FOOD SAFETY" (write the answer)?

Q10—Have you ever had a foodborne disease during a nature trip or in the mountains (mark as appropriate)?

Q11—Briefly describe your experience with this foodborne disease (where, with what …).
Q12—How likely is it that the cause was the factor listed below (mark as appropriate)?
Q13—Please rate your knowledge of food safety in general, with "1" meaning "insufficient" and "5" meaning "excellent knowledge" (mark as appropriate).
Q14—Where did you gain the most knowledge in the field of food safety when preparing food in nature, in a climbing area or in the mountains (mark as appropriate)?
DEMOGRAFIC QUESTIONS:
Q15—Gender (mark as appropriate)
Q16—Age (mark as appropriate)
Q17—Highest education attainment (mark as appropriate)
Q18—What activity do you mainly do? (mark as appropriate)
Q19—How many years have you been doing these activities? (mark as appropriate)
Q20—How often do you engage in this activity? (mark as appropriate)
Q21—What kind of diet you have? (mark as appropriate)

Appendix C

Interview questions
INTRODUCTION

1. Please tell me how you eat during mountain activities? Describe to me your meal. (With sub-questions: What does this look like while climbing, in winter, abroad?).
2. What if you go for several days. What does food preparation and eating itself look like?

FOODBORNE DISEASE

1. Have you ever had a foodborne disease on a tour in domestic mountains?
2. IF YES1: Tell me more about it. (with relevant sub-questions: What was the main reason, signs and symptoms, consequences, possible health threats)
3. What about abroad? (with relevant sub-questions: Where was it? What was the main reason signs and symptoms, consequences, possible health threats?)

IF YES 2: Tell me more about this. (with relevant sub-questions: What was the main reason, signs and symptoms, consequences, possible health threats?)

IF NOT 1, 2: What do you attribute to the fact that you avoided never getting sick from food on tour?

4. Do you know any other cases that occurred during the tour, on an expedition, when someone else got sick from food? Do you know anything more about this?
5. Have you acted differently from this case (s) since then? Are you paying more attention to yourself?

FOOD SAFETY ASSURANCE

6. What is important to you in terms of food and nutrition during mountain activities?
7. Do you think that people who engage in activities like you are more resistant to possible foodborne diseases? Why?
8. How dangerous do you think spoiled food can be for you?
9. How do you take care of washing your hands before eating in the mountains?

CONCLUSION

10. Do you have any ideas or suggestions on how to improve hygiene conditions during mountain activity? (with relevant sub-questions: What could you do yourself, What could organisations do about it?)

DEMOGRAPHIC QUESTIONS:
Gender:
Age:
Mountaineering status:
Time of activity:

References

1. Scott, E. Food safety and foodborne disease in 21st century homes. *Can. J. Infect Dis. Med. Microbiol.* **2003**, *14*, 277–280. [CrossRef]
2. Jevšnik, M.; Hlebec, V.; Raspor, P. Consumers' awareness of food safety from shopping to eating. *Food Control* **2008**, *19*, 737–745. [CrossRef]
3. Wills, W.J.; Meah, A.; Dickinson, A.M.; Short, F. I don't think I ever had food poisoning'. A practice-based approach to understanding foodborne disease that originates in the home. *Appetite* **2015**, *85*, 118–125. [CrossRef]
4. Taché, J.; Carpentier, B. Hygiene in the home kitchen: Changes in behaviour and impact of key microbiological hazard control measures. *Food Control* **2014**, *35*, 392–400. [CrossRef]
5. Al-Sakkaf, A. Domestic food preparation practices: A review of the reasons for poor home hygiene practices. *Health Promot. Int.* **2013**, *30*, 427–437. [CrossRef]
6. Sharot, T. The optimism bias. *Curr. Biol.* **2011**, *21*, R941–R945. [CrossRef]
7. Zanetta, L.D.; Hakim, M.P.; Stedefeldt, E.; de Rosso, V.V.; Cunha, L.M.; Redmond, E.C.; da Cunha, D.T. Consumer risk perceptions concerning different consequences of foodborne disease acquired from food consumed away from home: A case study in Brazil. *Food Control* **2022**, *133*, 108602. [CrossRef]
8. Ovca, A.; Jevšnik, M.; Raspor, P. Food safety awareness knowledge and practices among students in Slovenia. *Food Control* **2014**, *42*, 144–151. [CrossRef]
9. Young, I.; Waddell, L. Barriers and Facilitators to Safe Food Handling among Consumers: A Systematic Review and Thematic Synthesis of Qualitative Research Studies. *PLoS ONE* **2016**, *11*, e0167695. [CrossRef]
10. Ruby, G.E.; Ungku Zainal Abidin, U.F.; Lihan, S.; Jambari, N.N.; Radu, S. A cross sectional study on food safety knowledge among adult consumers. *Food Control* **2019**, *99*, 98–105. [CrossRef]
11. EFSA (European Food Safety Authority) and ECDC (European Centre for Disease Prevention and Control). The European Union One Health 2019 Zoonoses Report. *EFSA J.* **2021**, *19*, 6406. [CrossRef]
12. Leal, A.; Ruth, T.K.; Rumble, J.N.; Simonne, A.H. Exploring Florida residents' food safety knowledge and behaviors: A generational comparison. *Food Control* **2017**, *3*, 1195–1202. [CrossRef]
13. Ergönül, B. Consumer awareness and perception to food safety: A consumer analysis. *Food Control* **2013**, *32*, 461–471. [CrossRef]
14. Sterniša, M.; Smole Možina, S.; Levstek, S.; Kukec, A.; Raspor, P.; Jevšnik, M. Food safety knowledge, self-reported practices and attitude of poultry meat handling among Slovenian consumers. *Br. Food J.* **2018**, *120*, 1344–1357. [CrossRef]
15. Tabrizi, J.; Nikniaz, L.; Sadeghi-Bazargani, H.; Farahbakhsh, M.; Nikniaz, Z. Determinants of the food safety knowledge and practice among Iranian consumers. *Br. Food J.* **2017**, *119*, 357–365. [CrossRef]
16. Spendlove, J.K.; Heaney, S.E.; Gifford, J.A.; Prvan, T.; Denyer, G.S.; O'Connor, H.T. Evaluation of general nutrition knowledge in elite Australian athletes. *Br. J. Nutr.* **2012**, *107*, 1871–1880. [CrossRef]
17. Slabe, D.; Dolenc, E.; Jevšnik, M. Hygienic aspect of nutrition among trekkers, alpinists and sport climbers. *Šport* **2013**, *61*, 74–80.
18. Praz, C.; Granges, M.; Burtin, C.; Kayser, B. Nutritional behaviour and beliefs of ski-mountaineers: A semi-quantitative and qualitative study. *J. Int. Soc. Sports Nutr.* **2015**, *12*, 46. [CrossRef]
19. Worsley, A. Nutrition knowledge and food consumption: Can nutrition knowledge change food behaviour? *Asia Pac. J. Clin. Nutr.* **2002**, *11*, S579–S585. [CrossRef]
20. Alpine Association of Slovenia. Introduction. Available online: https://en.pzs.si/vsebina.php?pid=1 (accessed on 4 July 2022).
21. Tong, A.; Sainsbury, P.; Craig, J. Consolidated criteria for reporting qualitative research (COREQ): A 32-item checklist for interviews and focus groups. *Int. J. Qual. Health Care* **2007**, *19*, 349–357. [CrossRef]
22. Glaser, B.; Strauss, L.A. *The Discovery of Grounded Theory: Strategies for Qualitative Research*, 4th ed.; AldineTransaction: New Brunswick, NJ, USA; London, UK, 1999; pp. 61–62.
23. Byrd-Brebenner, C.; Berning, J.; Martin-Bigggers, J.; Quick, V. Food safety in home kitchens: A synthesis of the literature. *Int. J. Environ. Res.* **2013**, *10*, 4060–4085. [CrossRef]
24. Meysenburg, R.; Albrecht, J.A.; Litchfield, R.; Ritter-Gooder, P.K. Food safety knowledge, practices and beliefs of primary food preparers in families with young children. A mixed methods study. *Appetite* **2014**, *73*, 121–131. [CrossRef]
25. Jevšnik, M.; Ovca, A.; Bauer, M.; Fink, R.; Oder, M.; Sevšek, F. Food safety knowledge and practices among elderly in Slovenia. *Food Control* **2013**, *31*, 284–290. [CrossRef]
26. Kendall, H.; Kuznesof, S.; Seal, C.; Dobson, S.; Brennan, M. Domestic food safety and the older consumer: A segmentation analysis. *Food Qual. Prefer.* **2013**, *28*, 396–406. [CrossRef]
27. Bearth, A.; Cousin, M.; Siegrist, M. Poultry consumers' behaviour, risk perception and knowledge related to campylobacteriosos and domestic food safety. *Food Control* **2014**, *44*, 166–176. [CrossRef]
28. Gong, S.; Wang, X.; Yang, Y.; Bai, L. Knowledge of food safety and handling in households: A survey of food handlers in Mainland China. *Food Control* **2016**, *64*, 45–53. [CrossRef]
29. Burke, T.; Young, I.; Papadopoulos, A. Assessing food safety knowledge and preferred information sources among 19–29-year-olds. *Food Control* **2016**, *69*, 83–89. [CrossRef]
30. Clayton, D.; Griffith, C. Observation of food safety practices in catering using notational analysis. *Br. Food J.* **2004**, *106*, 211–227. [CrossRef]

31. Mazengia, E.; Fisk, C.; Liao, G.; Huang, H.; Meschke, J. Direct observational study of the risk of cross-contamination during raw poultry handling: Practices in private homes. *Food Prot. Trends* **2015**, *35*, 8–23.
32. Lazou, T.; Georgiadis, M.; Pentieva, K.; McKevitt, A.; Iossifidou, E. Food safety knowledge and food-handling practices of Greek university students: A questionnaire-based survey. *Food Control* **2012**, *28*, 400–411. [CrossRef]
33. Lange, M.; Goranzon, H.; Marklinder, I. Self-reported food safety knowledge and behaviour among home and consumer studies student. *Food Control* **2016**, *67*, 265–272. [CrossRef]
34. Tomaszewska, M.; Trafialek, J.; Suebpongsang, P.; Kolanowski, W. Food hygiene knowledge and practice of consumers in Poland and in Thailand—A survey. *Food Control* **2017**, *85*, 76–84. [CrossRef]

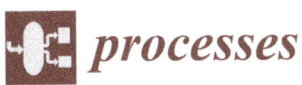

Article

Identification of Indoor Air Quality Factors in Slovenian Schools: National Cross-Sectional Study

An Galičič [1,2,*], Jan Rožanec [1], Andreja Kukec [1,2], Tanja Carli [1,2], Sašo Medved [2,3] and Ivan Eržen [1,2]

1. National Institute of Public Health, Trubarjeva ulica 2, SI-1000 Ljubljana, Slovenia
2. Faculty of Medicine, University of Ljubljana, Vrazov trg 2, SI-1000 Ljubljana, Slovenia
3. Faculty of Mechanical Engineering, University of Ljubljana, Aškerčeva cesta 6, SI-1000 Ljubljana, Slovenia
* Correspondence: an.galicic@nijz.si

Abstract: Poor indoor air quality (IAQ) in schools is associated with impacts on pupils' health and learning performance. We aimed to identify the factors that affect IAQ in primary schools. The following objectives were set: (a) to develop a questionnaire to assess the prevalence of factors in primary schools, (b) to conduct content validity of the questionnaire, and (c) to assess the prevalence of factors that affect the IAQ in Slovenian primary schools. Based on the systematic literature review, we developed a new questionnaire to identify factors that affect the IAQ in primary schools and conducted its validation. The questionnaires were sent to all 454 Slovenian primary schools; the response rate was 78.19%. The results show that the most important outdoor factors were the school's micro location and the distance from potential sources of pollution, particularly traffic. Among the indoor factors, we did not detect a pronounced dominating factor. Our study shows that the spatial location of schools is key to addressing the problem of IAQ in schools.

Keywords: primary school; indoor air quality factors; outdoor air quality factors; questionnaire; cross-sectional study

---

Citation: Galičič, A.; Rožanec, J.; Kukec, A.; Carli, T.; Medved, S.; Eržen, I. Identification of Indoor Air Quality Factors in Slovenian Schools: National Cross-Sectional Study. *Processes* **2023**, *11*, 841. https://doi.org/10.3390/pr11030841

Academic Editor: Chi He

Received: 31 January 2023
Revised: 28 February 2023
Accepted: 9 March 2023
Published: 11 March 2023

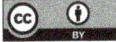

Copyright: © 2023 by the authors. Licensee MDPI, Basel, Switzerland. This article is an open access article distributed under the terms and conditions of the Creative Commons Attribution (CC BY) license (https://creativecommons.org/licenses/by/4.0/).

1. Introduction

Research shows [1] that people spend around 90% of their time in indoor environments (housing, public buildings, educational settings, etc.). Data show that school-aged children and adolescents spend almost 12% of their lives in the school environment, significantly more time than in any other indoor environment except the indoor living environment at home [2]. Indoor air is known to have equal or greater impacts on health than outdoor air [3]. Indoor air quality (IAQ) in schools is recognized as one of the most important risk factors affecting pupils' health and learning performance [2]. Children and adolescents are more susceptible to the effects of air pollution than adults, because they typically have a higher respiratory rate due to a faster metabolism, which means higher exposure to pollutants in relation to body weight compared to adults [4]. Their lungs and immune systems are still not fully developed, which makes children more prone to frequent respiratory infections. Therefore, children and adolescents, aged 13 years or younger, are classified as a vulnerable population group [5].

Several international studies have been conducted in Europe on the quality of the school environment and its impact on children's health. Simoni et al. [6] reported that in observed schools (Italy, France, Norway, Sweden, and Denmark), the mean concentrations of CO_2 exceeded 1000 ppm in 66% of the included classrooms and the mean concentrations of PM_{10} were elevated over 50 µg·m^{-3} in 78% of the classrooms. Respiratory symptoms were more frequently self-reported and parent-reported for children from poorly ventilated classrooms. Szabados et al. [7] have measured concentrations of $PM_{2.5}$ above the World Health Organization recommended levels in 85% of schools (Czech Republic, Hungary, Italy, Poland, and Slovenia). About 80% of schools had concentrations of CO_2 above

1000 ppm. For 31% of school buildings, it was found that exposure to indoor air pollutants could present a significant health risk. In addition, the median lifetime cancer risk value exceeded the acceptable value for radon and formaldehyde.

From a public health perspective, there is a need to improve the IAQ in schools. As IAQ in schools is not always monitored, it is important to consider the identified factors on IAQ at all stages of the design, construction, and management of school buildings [7]. To improve the indoor environment quality of buildings, it is important to obtain data directly from the users. At the international level, the post-occupancy evaluation methodology is one of the methods used to identify the factors that affect the indoor environment [8]. The benefits of such an assessment include obtaining feedback from users about problems in buildings and in identifying solutions; the feed-forward of the positive and negative lessons learned into the next building cycle; and the creation of databases and designing protocols [9]. In this way, a post-occupancy evaluation can be used to support technical measures to improve the performance of indoor environments. The most common way of obtaining information using the post-occupancy evaluation is through the use of questionnaires [8].

Our research aimed to identify the factors that affect the IAQ in primary schools, so we set the following objectives: (a) to develop a questionnaire to assess the prevalence of factors in primary schools, (b) to conduct content validity of the questionnaire, and (c) to assess the prevalence of factors that affect the IAQ in Slovenian primary schools. The contribution to the related literature that this article intends to offer is a new approach to identifying factors that affect the IAQ in primary schools and the example of its application in Slovenian primary schools. In addition, in the discussion, the article explains how identified factors may affect IAQ in schools, thereby contributing to a better understanding of the indoor environment. Last but not least, the article suggests possible measures that could be taken to improve the quality of the school's indoor environment to protect children's health in the future.

2. Materials and Methods

2.1. Identification of the Factors That Affect the Indoor Air Quality and Development of a Questionnaire to Identify These Factors

The development process was performed in two phases. In the first phase, we identified the factors that affect the IAQ, followed by the development of the questionnaire.

First phase: the identification of the factors that affect the IAQ was based on a systematic literature review in the ScienceDirect database. The purpose of the literature review was to identify the factors that affect the IAQ in the school environment. The search term used was "IAQ" OR "IAP" OR "indoor air" AND "school" OR "classroom" OR "kindergarten" OR "primary education" AND "risk factors" OR "environmental factors" for the period from 2010 to 2019. The literature was selected based on inclusion and exclusion criteria, which were designed according to the purpose of the literature review. The screening of the results of the selected search term was completed in five steps and according to the Preferred Reporting Items for Systematic review and Meta-Analysis (PRISMA) [10]. The inclusion and exclusion criteria for each step are shown in the online Supplementary Materials, Table S1. Of the 514,905 studies in first step of the systematic review, we included 72 that were relevant. More detailed results are shown in the online Supplementary Materials, Figure S1. The most frequently identified sources of indoor air pollution were the proximity to busy roads ($n = 57$) and the classroom activity of the users ($n = 46$). In addition to traffic, the researchers also identified the following outdoor factors that affect the IAQ: commercial and industrial establishments ($n = 29$); meteorological conditions ($n = 25$); emissions from heating buildings ($n = 20$); compounds from the natural environment ($n = 17$); atmospheric reactions and secondary emissions ($n = 11$); unpaved school playgrounds ($n = 6$); and smoking ($n = 3$). For the indoor factors that affect the IAQ, besides the classroom activity, they also identified: ventilation ($n = 35$); cleaning processes ($n = 33$); age and number of children/occupation rate ($n = 30$); technical characteristics of the classroom/building

(n = 29); and materials and equipment (n = 28). See the online Supplementary Materials, Table S2.

Second phase: The questionnaire has been prepared based on the identified factors that affect the IAQ. The questionnaire included the following three sections: (1) school building and school location information, (2) 3rd grade classroom information and IAQ in the classroom, and (3) natural ventilation of the classroom (Table 1).

Table 1. Content of the developed questionnaire in Slovenian primary schools.

Section 1: School Building and School Location Information	Section 2: 3rd Grade Classroom Information and Indoor Air Quality in the Classroom	Section 3: Natural Ventilation of the Classroom
Location (statistical region, micro location); building (year of construction, year of last extension or renovation, purpose of construction); sources of outdoor air pollution (potential sources within 200 m, proximity to a major road); heating (type of heating, period of the heating season).	Classroom (year of construction, year of the last renovation, number of pupils during class time, type of flooring, the height of the ceiling, window surface, orientation); materials (flooring, window frames); equipment (type of board and writing equipment, humidifiers, air fresheners); cleaning (frequency, method, cleaning schedule, ventilation during cleaning); classroom damage (damp spots, mold growth); classroom activity (school breakfast); perceived air quality (according to season and heating season).	Ventilation frequency (heating season, non-heating season); ventilation efficiency (ventilation duration, window opening method); human factor (giving incentive for the ventilation by children, the reason for less ventilation by opening windows).

2.2. Content Validation of the Questionnaire

The questionnaire was validated in terms of its content validity [11] and face validity [12]. Content validation was performed among 6 experts (4 public health experts, 1 expert in the field of ventilation, and 1 in the field of school infrastructure) who were asked to give a score of either 0 (item not relevant) or 1 (item very relevant). Of the Content Validity Indices (CVIs), we calculated: the scale content validity index (S-CVI/Ave), scale universal agreement validity index (S-CVI/UA), and a face item validity index (I-FVI). This was followed by response process validation among 12 raters who were asked to give a score of 0 or 1 based on the clarity and comprehensibility of the questionnaire. For the indices, the following threshold was set: I-CVI $\geq$ 0.78 [11] and S-CVI/Ave $\geq$ 0.90 [13], and S-CVI/UA a value of $\geq$ 0.80 [14,15] and I-FVI above $\geq$ 0.83 [12].

The questionnaire was clear to all participants. On average, it took 20 min to answer all the questions. The final version of the questionnaire included 38 questions. The I-CVI and S-CVI/Ave reached a value of 1.00 and the S-CVI/UA reached a value of 0.97, while the I-FVI reached a value of 0.85.

Therefore, during the content validation of the questionnaire, we gave the whole questionnaire to 12 3rd grade teachers to complete. We checked with them their understanding of the whole questionnaire and the correctness of the answers. In accordance with their minor comments, we upgraded the questionnaire to make it fully understandable for the teachers.

2.3. Assessment of the Prevalence of Factors That Affect the Indoor Air Quality

The national cross-sectional study on IAQ and natural ventilation of classrooms in Slovenian primary schools (3rd grade) was carried out between 7 January 2020 and 6 February 2020. The population surveyed included all 454 Slovenian primary schools in the school year 2019/2020. The observation unit was the 3rd grade classroom of each primary school. We selected the 3rd grade because pupils in the 3rd grade in Slovenia are in the same classroom for the entire duration of classes.

The request for participation, a participation/informed consent form, and study questionnaires were sent to all primary schools by traditional mail. In the informed consent form, they agreed that they were aware of the purpose and meaning of the study and that they were willing to participate in it. They had the opportunity to ask questions or ask for help in completing the questionnaire via the researcher's email address. The questionnaire was addressed to the headmasters of the primary schools who selected the 3rd grade teachers who filled out the questionnaire with the assistance of the caretaker. The questionnaires were sent to the primary schools on 7 January 2020 and the collection was completed when the last questionnaire was received on 6 February 2020.

The response rate was 78.19%, which represents a response from 355 out of 454 primary schools in Slovenia.

The distribution of values of the technical characteristics of classrooms is shown by the statistical parameters minimum and maximum, quartile 1, median, quartile 3, average, and standard deviation. With a univariate statistical analysis, we assessed the association between the outdoor factors of IAQ and the micro location in Slovenian primary schools, the association between the indoor factors of IAQ and the year of construction, and the association between the outdoor factors (classroom discomfort, IAQ, and outdoor noise) and the micro location. A univariate statistical analysis was performed using the Pearson, Chi-Square, or Fisher's exact test. The statistical significance was defined at $p \leq 0.05$. Data analyses were made in SPSS (version 27).

The research was approved by the Medical Ethics Committee of the Republic of Slovenia (No. 0120-548/2019/4).

3. Results

3.1. School Building and School Location Information

The data from the first section on the characteristics of the school building and school location show that most schools are located in villages/rural areas, of which most were built between 1960 and 1979 and mainly expanded/renovated in the period from 2010 to 2019. More detailed information on school buildings and school location is shown in Table 2, and the technical characteristics of the 3rd grade classrooms are shown in Table 3.

Table 2. School building and school location information in Slovenian primary schools.

Variables	Description of Variables	Number	Prevalence [%]
Primary school micro location (n = 334)	City center	49	14.67
	Suburbs/small town	124	37.13
	Village/rural area	161	48.20
Year of school construction (n = 320)	Until 1959	98	30.63
	1960–1979	147	45.94
	1980–1999	50	15.63
	2000–2019	25	7.81
Year of extension and/or last renovation (n = 286)	Until 1959	1	0.35
	1960–1979	9	3.15
	1980–1999	40	14.00
	2000–2019	236	82.52
Was the school building built for the purpose of education? (n = 350)	Yes	347	99.14
	No	3	0.86
The floor where the 3rd grade classroom is located (n = 353)	Ground floor	151	42.78
	1st floor	157	44.48
	2nd floor	39	11.05
	3rd floor	5	1.42
	Mansard	1	0.28

Table 3. Technical characteristics of the 3rd grade classrooms in the Slovenian primary schools.

Technical Characteristic	Min	Q1	Average	Q3	Max	SD
Flooring surface [m^2]	20.00	50.55	59.70	62.50	96.00	10.71
Ceiling height [m]	2.10	3.00	3.30	3.60	5.50	0.52
Window surface * [m^2]	1.00	8.88	12.00	16.00	40.00	6.39

* Total ventilation area of all windows in the classroom; Min—minimum, Q1—first quartile, Q3—third quartile, Max—maximum, SD—standard deviation.

3.2. The Outdoor Factors of Indoor Air Quality

The results of the outdoor IAQ factors show that within 200 m from the school, the most frequent potential source is a busy road and a residential area with individual wood-burning stoves. Over half of the schools (56.43%) are located within 100 m of a busy road. The prevalence of outdoor IAQ factors and the association between them and the micro location is shown in Table 4.

3.3. The Indoor Factors of Indoor Air Quality

The results of the indoor IAQ factors show data on the materials used in the classrooms, cleaning characteristics, the occurrence of moisture-related factors, and the location of the school breakfast, either in the classroom or in the dining hall. The prevalence of indoor IAQ factors and the association between them and the year of construction is shown in Table 5.

Table 4. Prevalence of outdoor factors of indoor air quality and the association between the outdoor factors of indoor air quality and the micro location in Slovenian primary schools.

Variables	Description of Variables	City Center: Number (Prevalence [%] for This Micro Location)	Suburbs/Small Town: Number (Prevalence [%] for This Micro Location)	Village/Rural Area: Number (Prevalence [%] for This Micro Location)	Total: Number (Prevalence [%])	p
Are there potential sources of air pollution located within 200 m from the primary school? (n = 350) **	Busy road	39 (45.35)	86 (42.16)	97 (39.59)	222 (63.42)	0.030
	Industrial zone	6 (6.98)	10 (4.90)	2 (0.82)	18 (5.14)	0.003
	Individual industrial installations	8 (9.30)	18 (8.82)	12 (4.90)	38 (10.86)	0.088
	Residential areas with individual wood-burning stoves	24 (27.91)	71 (34.80)	106 (43.27)	201 (57.43)	0.076
	No potential sources of pollutants can be identified in the school's surroundings	8 (9.30)	14 (6.86)	21 (8.57)	43 (12.29)	0.670
	Other	1 (1.16)	5 (2.45)	7 (2.86)	13 (4.39)	*
Distance from the nearest thoroughfare (not the access road to the primary school) (n = 350)	0–100 m	28 (65.12)	60 (53.10)	81 (56.25)	169 (48.29)	<0.001
	101–200 m	7 (16.28)	16 (14.16)	23 (15.97)	46 (13.14)	<0.001
	201–500 m	6 (13.95)	25 (22.12)	26 (18.06)	60 (17.41)	<0.001
	501–1000 m	2 (4.65)	8 (7.08)	8 (5.56)	18 (5.14)	<0.001
	>1000 m	0 (0.00)	4 (3.54)	6 (4.17)	10 (2.86)	*
Energy source used to heat the school building (multiple answers) (n = 355) **	Natural gas	18 (36.73)	61 (49.19)	40 (24.84)	119 (33.52)	<0.001
	Fuel oil	7 (14.29)	22 (17.74)	40 (24.84)	69 (19.44)	0.167
	Solar cells	7 (14.29)	22 (17.74)	31 (19.25)	60 (16.90)	0.728
	Heat pump	0 (0.0)	1 (0.81)	0 (0.0)	1 (0.28)	0.669
	Firewood	2 (4.08)	16 (12.90)	49 (30.43)	67 (18.87)	<0.001
	Wood pellets, wood chips, wood briquettes	22 (44.90)	20 (16.13)	19 (11.80)	61 (17.18)	<0.001

Table 4. Cont.

Variables	Description of Variables	City Center: Number (Prevalence [%] for This Micro Location)	Suburbs/Small Town: Number (Prevalence [%] for This Micro Location)	Village/Rural Area: Number (Prevalence [%] for This Micro Location)	Total: Number (Prevalence [%])	p
Orientation of the classroom ($n = 353$) **	Towards a traffic road	7 (14.29)	18 (14.52)	25 (15.53)	50 (14.16)	0.962
	Towards a road with moderate traffic	19 (38.78)	31 (25.0)	40 (24.84)	90 (25.50)	0.130
	Towards the school car park	5 (10.20)	24 (19.35)	26 (16.15)	55 (15.58)	0.339
	Towards school playground	13 (26.53)	35 (28.23)	51 (31.68)	99 (28.05)	0.717
	Towards school grounds park	11 (22.45)	38 (30.65)	36 (22.36)	85 (24.08)	0.246
	Other	5 (10.20)	13 (10.48)	19 (11.80)	37 (10.48)	*

* Data not provided; ** There were multiple possible answers to this question.

Table 5. Prevalence of indoor factors of indoor air quality and the association between the indoor factors of indoor air quality and the year of construction in Slovenian primary schools.

Variables	Description of Variables	Number	Prevalence [%]	p
Flooring material ($n = 355$) **	Parquet	151	42.54	<0.001
	Laminate	6	1.69	0.674
	Synthetic materials (linoleum panels, vinyl panels, PVC, etc.)	197	55.49	<0.001
	Other	2	0.56	*
Type of board and writing equipment ($n = 346$) **	Green chalkboard and chalk	282	81.50	0.339
	Plastic whiteboard and markers	169	48.84	0.035
	Interactive whiteboard and associated digital pen	142	41.04	0.620
Frequency of classroom cleaning ($n = 353$)	Several times a day	28	7.93	*
	Once a day	324	91.78	*
	Every other day	1	0.28	*
Classroom cleaning method ($n = 346$)	Wet cleaning of floors and surfaces	274	79.19	*
	Dry cleaning of floors and surfaces	43	12.43	*
	Combination	29	8.38	*
Classroom cleaning term ($n = 349$)	In the morning before classes	1	0.29	*
	Afternoon after classes	345	98.85	*
	Combination	3	0.86	*
Opening windows during classroom cleaning ($n = 330$)	Yes	180	54.55	*
	Not in winter, yes in summer	128	38.79	*
	No	22	6.67	*
Presence of damp patches on walls, ceiling or floor ($n = 355$)	Yes	7	1.97	*
	No	348	98.03	*
Presence of visible mold growth in the classroom ($n = 355$)	Yes	2	0.56	*
	No	353	99.44	*
Location of the school breakfast ($n = 351$)	In classroom	208	59.26	0.508
	In dining hall	143	40.74	0.570

* Data not provided; ** There were multiple possible answers to this question.

3.4. Ventilation of Classrooms

The data from the third section on the natural ventilation of schools shows data on the prevalence and ventilation characteristics in the heating and non-heating seasons, with 30.00% of classrooms being ventilated for more than 45 min in the heating season, while 29.88% of classrooms are ventilated for more than 180 min in the non-heating season (Table 6).

Table 6. Prevalence and ventilation characteristics in the heating and non-heating seasons in Slovenian primary schools.

Variables	Description of Variables	Heating Season		Non-Heating Season	
		Number	Prevalence [%]	Number	Prevalence [%]
Ventilation frequency (*n* = 353) **	Classroom is ventilated before the class	200	56.66	198	56.09
	Classroom is ventilated during every break	180	50.99	144	40.79
	Classroom is ventilated during every other break	60	17.00	18	5.10
	Classroom is ventilated once in the morning	24	6.80	13	3.68
	Classroom is ventilated during class	192	54.39	177	50.14
	Classroom is ventilated after school breakfast	127	35.98	89	25.21
	Classroom is ventilated after the end of the class	129	36.54	110	31.16
	Classroom is not ventilated	1	0.28	2	0.57
	Classroom is ventilated continuously or most of the time during class	54	15.30	181	51.27
Average total ventilation time per day (*n* = 340) **	Less than 20 min	124	36.47	25	7.40
	25–45 min	114	33.53	43	12.72
	50–90 min	66	19.41	74	21.89
	95–135 min	19	5.59	60	17.75
	140–180 min	9	2.65	35	10.36
	More than 180 min	8	2.35	101	29.88
How do you mostly open the windows? (*n* = 349)	Opening wide	170	48.71	151	44.15
	Opening on ventus/horizontally	148	42.41	119	34.80
	Combination	31	8.88	72	21.05

** There were multiple possible answers to this question.

The initiative to ventilate the classroom is usually given by the teacher (309; 91.15%), the pupils (4; 1.18%), or both (26; 7.67%). The reasons why the teacher chooses to open the windows less frequently than normally would be thermal discomfort in the classroom (cold in heating season, heat in non-heating season) (252; 71.39%); outside noise (100; 29.50%), draughts (86; 25.37%), safety concerns (40; 11.80%), and bad outdoor air quality (33; 9.37%). Among the outdoor factors (classroom discomfort, IAQ, and outdoor noise), only outdoor noise has a statistically significant association with micro location ($p = 0.001$).

4. Discussion

In our cross-sectional study in Slovenian primary schools, we found the occurrence of some pollutant sources and factors that affect the IAQ to be statistically significant: the association between the frequency of the factors that affect the IAQ and the micro location of the primary school for a distance of 200 m from the major road and an industrial zone; the distance from the nearest major road for the distances of 0–100 m, 101–200 m, 201–500 m, and 501–1000 m; and the energy source used to heat the school building for wood pellets, wood chips, wood briquettes, firewood, and natural gas. An association between the frequency of the factors that affect the IAQ and the year of construction of the primary school was found for the classroom flooring materials for parquet and synthetic materials, and the type of board and writing equipment for the plastic whiteboard and markers.

4.1. School Building and School Location Information

Almost half of the participating Slovenian primary schools are located in villages/rural areas, which is associated with the dispersed and sparse settlements in Slovenia [16]. Almost half of the buildings in the participating primary schools were built between 1960 and 1979. More than 80% of the participating primary schools have renovated their buildings in the last 20 years. Yang et al. [17] found that newer and renovated buildings compared to older buildings have higher emissions of materials and equipment and are more airtight. However, the older buildings were more prone to outdoor pollution, due to the wear and tear of the materials used, worse installation techniques, and consequently more infiltration of outdoor air into the indoor spaces [18]. Most primary schools in Slovenia (99.14%) were built for education purposes. Most of the observed 3rd grade classrooms included in our study were located in the basements, ground floors, and first floors of the school buildings. Studies show that rooms on the lower floors tend to have higher concentrations of volatile organic compounds (VOC) [19] and radon [20] than rooms on the higher floors. Furthermore, Branco et al. [21] found elevated levels of nitrogen dioxide in ground floor classrooms facing toward the road.

4.2. The Outdoor Factors of Indoor Air Quality

Most of the participating schools identified a busy road and a residential area with individual wood-burning stoves as potential sources of air pollution within 200 m from the school. Additionally, in other studies, the most frequently indicated outdoor source of indoor air pollution was proximity to busy roads [22–26]. The results of our study show that the busy roads are statistically significantly associated with the micro locations of the participating primary schools, as are the industrial zones. This association is confirmed by other studies, where higher concentrations of traffic pollutants have been reported in urban kindergartens and schools, compared to kindergartens and schools located in the suburbs or rural areas [24,26–28]. However, the concentrations of traffic pollution in outdoor air are not distributed evenly throughout the urban area. In areas with lower traffic density, lower concentrations of pollutants in outdoor air were measured and therefore better IAQ in classrooms [29]; particle number concentrations also decreased with distance from the city center (the main source of traffic emissions) [22]. Schools located more than 5 km from the city had lower and more stable concentrations of traffic pollutants compared to urban schools [26]. Meanwhile, the highest concentrations of industry pollutants have been recorded in schools around the industrial zones and urban areas [30]. Due to the long-range transport of industry emissions, emissions can also be detected in rural areas or the industry is located in areas close to rural areas [27]. In our study, most of the participating schools report being located within 0–100 m of the nearest major road, followed by 201–500 m, 101–200 m, 501–1000 m, and over 1000 m. Rim et al. [23] also pointed out that many schools are located in close proximity to major roads and located less than 100 m away from them. The results of our study show that the distance to the major road is statistically significantly associated with the micro location of the school. Rim et al. [23] found that schools located closer to main roads had higher concentrations of $PM_{2.5}$, PM_{10}, and black carbon compared to schools located further away. The greater distance of schools from the road also had a significant impact on indoor concentrations of carbon monoxide and nitrogen dioxide [31]. The most commonly used energy source for the heating of school buildings in Slovenia is natural gas, followed by firewood, fuel oil, wood pellets, wood chips and wood briquettes, solar panels, and heat pumps. Natural gas and firewood are statistically significantly associated with school micro location. Therefore, in rural areas, Canha et al. [32] found a higher impact of emissions from heating surrounding buildings with wood biomass compared to urban environments. Replacing old wood-burning stoves with modern heating systems that are more ecologically friendly in schools does not show a measurable improvement in IAQ [33]. From this, we can conclude that the IAQ in primary school classrooms during the heating season depends mainly on the type of heating systems in the area and not so much on the type of energy used to heat the school building.

The largest proportion of Slovenian primary schools had the 3rd grade classroom oriented towards the school playground, followed by the school grounds park and the road with moderate traffic. As many as 14.73% of the 3rd grade classrooms were oriented toward the busy road. The position and orientation of the classroom relative to the outdoor source of the pollutant have a significant impact on changes in IAQ [34]. Reche et al. [19,21] found that traffic pollutant concentrations were higher in classrooms, which were oriented toward the street than in classrooms oriented toward schoolyards. Further, the orientation of the building relative to the playground contributed to the differences in PM concentrations. Amato et al. [35] detected higher concentrations of PM when the room was oriented towards an unpaved playground compared to a paved one. Despite this, PM concentrations were higher in classrooms that were oriented towards the street. Almeida et al. [36] detected higher concentrations of PM in classrooms where the classroom door opened directly onto the playground compared to those where the door opened into the building interior.

In total, 77.42% of Slovenian schools are located within 200 m of a major road. The major road is identified by 67.14% schools as a potential source of IAQ pollution. The traffic-related factors are associated with the micro location of the school. This makes the major road the most important outdoor factor, especially in schools in the city center. From this, we can conclude that, of all the outdoor factors, pupils and teachers in urban schools are the most exposed to pollutants generated by traffic. Especially exposed to traffic pollutants are occupants of classrooms that are oriented towards major roads. Pupils and teachers in suburbs/small towns are most likely to be exposed to pollutants from the industrial zones, to which, of course, they are also exposed in the cities. The exposure of pupils and teachers in villages/rural areas is significantly different, as they are most often exposed to pollutants from individual wood-burning stoves. The results of our study and their evaluation suggest that in order to reduce the impact of outdoor factors that affect IAQ, it is necessary to design measures that target the micro location of the school, including the distance from the major road and other potential sources in the school surroundings. When planning the location of new schools, it is necessary to take into account the sufficient distance from the potential sources of pollution and take great care when locating new activities in the areas and proximity of schools.

4.3. The Indoor Factors of Indoor Air Quality

The results of our study showed that in Slovenian primary schools, the most commonly used materials for flooring are synthetic materials and parquet. The building materials used, as well as the furniture and equipment in the classrooms, have a significant association with VOC concentrations [30,37,38]. Poulhet et al. [38] found that building materials have higher formaldehyde emissions in classrooms compared to furnishing materials. The building materials have not always been made of the most emissive materials, but due to their high-volume use and coverage of large areas in space, they consequently have a strong impact on concentrations of pollutant emissions. The main source of formaldehyde emissions at all school locations was the classroom ceiling, which contributed on average around 50% of the total indoor formaldehyde emissions. Flooring materials contributed 4–9% of the total formaldehyde emissions. The results of our study also show that the most commonly used board and writing equipment during lessons are green chalkboards and chalk, which have been linked by researchers to PM emissions [34,39]. This is followed by the use of plastic whiteboards and markers, which researchers have linked to total volatile organic compounds (TVOC) emissions [30,37].

The materials of the flooring, synthetic materials, and parquet, as well as the presence of plastic boards and markers, in our study are associated with the age of the school building. For the indoor factors such as building materials (e.g., flooring, walls, and windows) and interior furnishings (e.g., furniture, type of board, and writing instruments), it is difficult to find a significant association with the building age, as more than 80% of Slovenian primary school buildings have been renovated in the last 20 years. Similar findings were reported by Rivas et al. [18], who noted that although window type is related to the age of the building at installation, the age of the building itself cannot be related to the type of windows, due to frequent renovation activities.

The most commonly used method for cleaning classroom floors and surfaces in Slovenian primary schools is wet cleaning. Less than 21% of primary schools clean the floors of their classrooms with dry cleaning, i.e., by sweeping, vacuuming, and wiping the dust from surfaces with a dry cloth. The classrooms in almost all schools are cleaned once per day in the afternoon after the end of classes. In Slovenia, 54.55% of schools have their windows open during cleaning, while 38.79% of schools ventilate during cleaning only in the summer. This presents a risk as wet cleaning, which is the most common cleaning method in schools, due to the use of cleaning products, results in higher concentrations of TVOCs and are a potential source of polycyclic aromatic hydrocarbons (PAH) [27,40]. Mishra et al. [41] found that the use of cleaning products in schools contributes up to 41% of indoor TVOC concentrations. Wet cleaning can therefore especially affect the concentrations of limonene and p-tolualdehyde, but also the concentrations of some other hydrocarbons [19,30,37,42,43]. In addition, the use of cleaning products can lead to the formation of new particles, such as secondary organic aerosols, which affect PM concentrations [44]. The formation of secondary particles is caused by the reaction between the ozone and terpenes emitted by cleaning products [22]. As a consequence of cleaning with cleaning products, Viana et al. [45] also traced chlorine emissions in indoor dust. In comparison to wet cleaning, dry cleaning resuspends more PM particles into the air, but we should note that dry cleaning does not result in the additional emissions of cleaning products. Cleaning can lead to increases in PM_{2-10} concentrations [44].

The results of our study showed that 1.97% of classrooms have damp patches on the walls, ceilings, or floors and 0.56% of classrooms have visible mold growth. Mainka et al. [46] point out that the presence of mold on walls has a significant impact on the concentration of fungi in indoor air.

The results of our study showed that the majority of the participating schools in Slovenia have their school breakfast in classrooms and not in the dining hall. This is probably due to the lack of space in schools to accommodate the dining hall in the building or the dining hall capacity being too low for the number of pupils attending school breakfasts. When children have their school breakfast in the classroom, food odors are released into the room, and if children are in the classrooms during break time, this has an effect on higher concentrations of carbon dioxide in the classroom [37]. During breaks, there are usually also children playing in the classrooms with lots of moving and running, which also has the effect on the re-suspension of particulate matters (PM) in the air and a consequent increase in PM concentrations [44,47]. During occupied periods, PM_{10} concentrations can be three to five times higher compared to when pupils are not present in the classroom [44].

The results of our study and their evaluation showed that there are a number of indoor factors that affect IAQ in schools, with some of them being controlled by certifications (e.g., materials and equipment used in the classrooms have to comply with the requirements of the certificate). The results of our study and their evaluation show that there is a need to reduce the impact of indoor factors that affect IAQ in schools. It would be necessary to develop measures that are mainly organization-oriented, which can be controlled by the schools themselves (e.g., by organizing school breakfast and lunch in the dining hall, the sufficient ventilation of classrooms, and preventing damp patches).

4.4. Ventilation of Classrooms

The results of our study show that during the heating season, classrooms are ventilated for less time compared to the non-heating season. Only 30.00% of classrooms are ventilated for more than 45 min per day during the heating season, while in the non-heating season, more than half of the classrooms are ventilated continuously or most of the time during the school day. The results of our study also show that the way a classroom is ventilated depends on the ventilation time itself and the outside temperature in relation to the heating and non-heating seasons. For the heating season in Slovenian primary schools, it is typical that the classroom is ventilated for less time but also more intensively by opening the windows wide, a little less on the ventus/horizontally, but still used for the thermal comfort of the classroom users. Compared to the heating season, the prevalence of combined ventilation (ventilation by opening the windows wide and to the ventus/horizontally) increases significantly in the non-heating season, due to the longer ventilation time of the classroom. Other studies have also found an association between the frequency and method of classroom ventilation by season and indoor/outdoor temperature. Kalimeri et al. [37] have recorded two different ventilation patterns. During the heating season, windows were opened for short periods and at a low frequency. The windows were closed during school hours and only partially opened or even closed during breaks, while in the non-heating season the windows were open most of the time. Laiman et al. [48] found that the air exchange in classrooms was 20% higher during the non-heating season as opposed to what was measured during the heating season. Therefore, the frequency of window opening was primarily related to the indoor/outdoor temperature and, consequently, to the thermal comfort of individuals in the classroom. Elbayoumi et al. [49] observed a lower frequency of ventilation by opening windows when the outside temperature was between 28 °C and 32 °C and when outside temperatures were much higher than indoor temperatures. Ventilation of the classroom through opening windows and doors increased when the outside temperature was between 18 °C and 28 °C and when the indoor temperature was significantly higher than the outside temperature. However, when the outside temperature was below 15 °C and the difference between the indoor and outdoor temperature was high, ventilation was adjusted according to the air quality. The studies show that the researchers' findings on the frequency and method of ventilation are consistent with our findings. It is important to emphasize the importance of ventilation during the non-heating season, as a reduced air exchange in the classroom leads to the accumulation of indoor pollutants [31,32]. The results of our study show that teachers have a major role in classroom ventilation. In only 8.85% of the cases of natural ventilation of classrooms, pupils initiated the opening of the windows. The major role of teachers in classroom ventilation was also found by Korsavi et al. [2], who observed that in 16% of cases of natural ventilation, pupils in 3rd–6th grades would open windows on their own. In comparison to our study, a higher proportion of pupils participated in the ventilation of classrooms, but we should be aware that the results of our study are encouraging, as 3rd grade pupils in Slovenian schools have already suggested the ventilation initiative. The most common reasons given by Slovenian teachers for less ventilation in classrooms were thermal discomfort and outside noises. At the same time, it is important to understand that teachers have a higher comfort temperature compared to pupils and therefore ventilation occurs later [2]. This is particularly evident during the heating season, where lower outdoor temperatures and less frequent ventilation increase carbon dioxide concentrations in the classroom [2,31]. Madureira et al. [50] also reported noise problems as a reason for the lower frequency of opening windows in schools. In Slovenian primary schools, we found that external noise is statistically significantly associated with the micro location of the school.

High classroom occupancy, low classroom volume, and inadequate ventilation during classes can lead to excessive levels of carbon dioxide in classrooms [51]. Several researchers have reported average CO_2 concentrations exceeding the recommended carbon dioxide level of 1000 ppm [52] in educational settings in England [2], Portugal [3,50,53], Poland [46], and France [44]. It is important to bear in mind that natural ventilation by opening windows depends on the good ventilation habits of the occupants [2]. Ventilating rooms with mechanical ventilation can help to improve IAQ. Schools with central mechanical ventilation allow for continuous ventilation through mechanical ventilation units and ventilation independent of occupants' good habits [51]. Moreover, natural ventilation by opening windows is not always an appropriate ventilation strategy in kindergartens and schools located in polluted environments or close to significant outdoor sources of pollutants [23]. Majd et al. [31] found that the number of opened windows in classrooms was significantly associated with the concentration of traffic emissions in the classrooms. Each opened window contributed to an 8.2% increase in the average daily concentration of carbon monoxide in the room. Rim et al. [23] observed that the natural ventilation of kindergarten rooms reduced carbon dioxide concentrations but increased indoor air concentrations of black carbon and particulate matter. Some other authors have also found that ventilation increases the concentrations of pollutants in the indoor environment. Elbayoumi et al. [49] observed a positive association between ventilation and indoor carbon monoxide concentrations. Zhang et al. [54] linked $PM_{2.5}$ and nitrogen dioxide emissions to ventilation and air infiltration in classrooms. Rim et al. [23] observed an association between high indoor concentrations of ultrafine particles, particle number, and black carbon indoors and the ventilation of classrooms (in schools located near busy roads).

The results of our study show different approaches to the natural ventilation of classrooms, where teachers have a major role in classroom ventilation. To improve the effectiveness of natural ventilation in terms of IAQ in the classroom, it is necessary to design a natural ventilation strategy that takes into account the heating/non-heating season. This strategy should also take into account the characteristics of the school micro location with identified outdoor sources of IAQ pollution (e.g., rush traffic hours in the urban area), the most efficient ventilation methods, and the ventilation frequency. The implementation of such a strategy would limit the infiltration of outdoor pollutants into the classrooms through open windows and reduce the concentrations of indoor pollutants from classroom indoor air. Such a strategy would also have an impact on reducing the spread of common respiratory viruses (including SARS-CoV-2) indoors, where pupils and teachers are a potential source.

4.5. Limitations and Strengths of Our Study

The studies for the development of the questionnaire were obtained from the ScienceDirect bibliographic database. Perhaps better-quality data could have been obtained if more databases were included. Nevertheless, we assess that the data collected are of sufficient quality to develop the questionnaire, as researchers in this field have in the past already conducted literature reviews in several databases, identifying a large number of duplicates. To date, we have not found such a systematic approach to identifying the factors that affect the increase in indoor concentrations of pollutants. In addition, no cross-sectional study has been conducted to assess the prevalence of these factors in Slovenian primary schools. Our national study is characterized by a high response rate of 78.19% and a large study population, representing all 454 primary schools in Slovenia in the 2019/2020 school year. Validation of the questionnaire at the national level is also an important advantage. Therefore, a first analysis of the IAQ situation at the level of the factors that affect the IAQ was prepared. Our study results will contribute to the approach of improving IAQ in schools at the level of factors that affect the IAQ, since in schools often only the risk factors are analyzed (i.e., pollutants). Knowing the factors that affect the IAQ gives us important insights into the discussed issues and gives us focus on the most pressing questions about reducing the concentrations of pollutants in school classrooms. As a part of the study, we have developed a questionnaire that has been validated, giving it scientific weight. The questionnaire may also be used in other countries, with certain adaptations (e.g., season characteristics).

5. Conclusions

The main findings of our national cross-sectional study in Slovenia showed that among the outdoor factors, the most important were the micro location of the school and the distance from potential sources of pollution, particularly the main roads. Among the indoor factors, we did not detect a pronounced dominating factor. This is probably because the indoor environment is equipped with elements that meet the quality standards and safety ratings. Due to the numerous renovations over the last 20 years, the age of the building does not have a major impact on IAQ. This suggests that in Slovenia, the spatial location of schools is key to addressing the problem of the IAQ in schools. This means that school location planning needs to take into account the sufficient distance from potential sources of pollution and take great care when locating new activities in the areas and proximity of schools. To improve the effectiveness of ventilation in classrooms, where natural ventilation is used, it is necessary to design a natural ventilation strategy that takes into account the characteristics of the school micro location (identified outdoor sources of IAQ pollution), the most effective ventilation methods, the ventilation frequency, and the heating/non-heating season. Where a natural ventilation strategy would not be able to provide adequate air quality in the classroom, it is reasonable to include mechanical ventilation, which also requires proper design, use, and maintenance.

Supplementary Materials: The following supporting information can be downloaded at: https://www.mdpi.com/article/10.3390/pr11030841/s1, Table S1: Systematic literature review process; Figure S1: A flow chart of the selection of articles for the systematic literature review; Table S2: The results of the literature review of the factors that affect Indoor Air Quality.

Author Contributions: Conceptualization, A.G.; methodology, A.G., J.R. and A.K.; T.C.; statistical analysis, A.G.; writing—original draft preparation, A.G. and J.R.; writing—review and editing, A.K. and T.C.; visualization, A.G. and J.R.; supervision, I.E. and S.M. All authors have read and agreed to the published version of the manuscript.

Funding: This article is funded by the project "Measures to manage the spread of COVID-19 with a focus on vulnerable groups of population", which is co-financed by the Republic of Slovenia and the European Union under the European Social Fund in the framework of the EU response to the COVID-19 pandemic (Grant No. C2711-20-054101). The content of this article represents the views of the authors only and is their sole responsibility; it cannot be considered to reflect the views of the European Commission or any other body of the European Union. The European Commission does not accept any responsibility for the use that may be made of the information it contains. The study was conducted also as part of a Slovenian Research Agency (ARRS) project, entitled "Development of the prognostic model of exposure to indoor air pollutants in schools and preparation of evidence-based measures for planning of efficient natural ventilation of the classrooms (No. V3-1904)" and grant No. P3-0429.

Institutional Review Board Statement: The research was approved by the Medical Ethics Committee of the Republic of Slovenia (No. 0120-548/2019/4).

Informed Consent Statement: Not applicable.

Data Availability Statement: Data supporting the findings of this study are available from the corresponding author upon reasonable request.

Acknowledgments: We would like to thank all headmasters of the participating primary schools for their high response to the request to participate in the study. We would like to thank the 3rd grade teachers and the caretakers of the participating primary schools for their time and for accurately filling in the questionnaires. We would also like to thank all the colleagues and other members of the project "Development of the prognostic model of exposure to indoor air pollutants in schools and preparation of evidence based measures for planning of efficient natural ventilation of the classrooms (No. V3-1904)" who contributed to the development of our study.

Conflicts of Interest: The authors declare no conflict of interest.

References

1. Bennett, J.; Davy, P.; Trompetter, B.; Wang, Y.; Pierse, N.; Boulic, M.; Phipps, R.; Howden-Chapman, P. Sources of Indoor Air Pollution at a New Zealand Urban Primary School; a Case Study. *Atmos. Pollut. Res.* **2019**, *10*, 435–444. [CrossRef]
2. Korsavi, S.S.; Montazami, A.; Mumovic, D. Indoor Air Quality (IAQ) in Naturally-Ventilated Primary Schools in the UK: Occupant-Related Factors. *Build. Environ.* **2020**, *180*, 106992. [CrossRef]
3. Nunes, R.A.O.; Branco, P.T.B.S.; Alvim-Ferraz, M.C.M.; Martins, F.G.; Sousa, S.I.V. Gaseous Pollutants on Rural and Urban Nursery Schools in Northern Portugal. *Environ. Pollut.* **2016**, *208*, 2–15. [CrossRef] [PubMed]

4. Salvi, S. Health Effects of Ambient Air Pollution in Children. *Paediatr. Respir. Rev.* **2007**, *8*, 275–280. [CrossRef] [PubMed]
5. Zhang, H.; Srinivasan, R. A Systematic Review of Air Quality Sensors, Guidelines, and Measurement Studies for Indoor Air Quality Management. *Sustainability* **2020**, *12*, 9045. [CrossRef]
6. Simoni, M.; Annesi-Maesano, I.; Sigsgaard, T.; Norback, D.; Wieslander, G.; Nystad, W.; Canciani, M.; Sestini, P.; Viegi, G. School Air Quality Related to Dry Cough, Rhinitis and Nasal Patency in Children. *Eur. Respir. J.* **2010**, *35*, 742–749. [CrossRef]
7. Szabados, M.; Csákó, Z.; Kotlík, B.; Kazmarová, H.; Kozajda, A.; Jutraž, A.; Kukec, A.; Otorepec, P.; Dongiovanni, A.; Di Maggio, A.; et al. Indoor air quality and the associated health risk in primary school buildings in Central Europe-the InAirQ study. *Indoor Air* **2021**, *31*, 989–1003. [CrossRef]
8. Lolli, F.; Marinello, S.; Coruzzolo, A.M.; Butturi, M.A. Post-Occupancy Evaluation's (POE) Applications for Improving Indoor Environment Quality (IEQ). *Toxics* **2022**, *10*, 626. [CrossRef]
9. Meir, I.A.; Garb, Y.; Jiao, D.; Cicelsky, A. Post-Occupancy Evaluation: An Inevitable Step Toward Sustainability. *Adv. Build. Energy Res.* **2009**, *3*, 189–219. [CrossRef]
10. Page, M.J.; McKenzie, J.E.; Bossuyt, P.M.; Boutron, I.; Hoffmann, T.C.; Mulrow, C.D.; Shamseer, L.; Tetzlaff, J.M.; Akl, E.A.; Brennan, S.E.; et al. The PRISMA 2020 Statement: An Updated Guideline for Reporting Systematic Reviews. *Syst. Rev.* **2021**, *10*, 89. [CrossRef]
11. Yusoff, M.S.B. ABC of Content Validation and Content Validity Index Calculation. *Educ. Med. J.* **2019**, *11*, 49–54. [CrossRef]
12. Yusoff, M.S.B. ABC of Response Process Validation and Face Validity Index Calculation. *Educ. Med. J.* **2019**, *11*, 55–61. [CrossRef]
13. Polit, D.F.; Beck, C.T. The Content Validity Index: Are You Sure You Know What's Being Reported? Critique and Recommendations. *Res. Nurs. Health* **2006**, *29*, 489–497. [CrossRef]
14. Grant, J.S.; Davis, L.L. Selection and Use of Content Experts for Instrument Development. *Res. Nurs. Health* **1997**, *20*, 269–274. [CrossRef]
15. Hambleton, R.K.; Swaminathan, H.; Algina, J.; Coulson, D.B. Criterion-Referenced Testing and Measurement: A Review of Technical Issues and Developments. *Rev. Educ. Res.* **1978**, *48*, 1–47. [CrossRef]
16. Statistical Office of the Republic of Slovenia. Population-Slovenian Regions and Municipalities in Figures. Available online: https://www.stat.si/obcine/sl/Theme/Index/PrebivalstvoGostota (accessed on 25 July 2022). (In Slovenian).
17. Yang, J.; Nam, I.; Yun, H.; Kim, J.; Oh, H.-J.; Lee, D.; Jeon, S.-M.; Yoo, S.-H.; Sohn, J.-R. Characteristics of Indoor Air Quality at Urban Elementary Schools in Seoul, Korea: Assessment of Effect of Surrounding Environments. *Atmos. Pollut. Res.* **2015**, *6*, 1113–1122. [CrossRef]
18. Rivas, I.; Viana, M.; Moreno, T.; Bouso, L.; Pandolfi, M.; Alvarez-Pedrerol, M.; Forns, J.; Alastuey, A.; Sunyer, J.; Querol, X. Outdoor Infiltration and Indoor Contribution of UFP and BC, OC, Secondary Inorganic Ions and Metals in PM2.5 in Schools. *Atmos. Environ.* **2015**, *106*, 129–138. [CrossRef]
19. Vu, D.C.; Ho, T.L.; Vo, P.H.; Bayati, M.; Davis, A.N.; Gulseven, Z.; Carlo, G.; Palermo, F.; McElroy, J.A.; Nagel, S.C.; et al. Assessment of Indoor Volatile Organic Compounds in Head Start Child Care Facilities. *Atmos. Environ.* **2019**, *215*, 116900. [CrossRef]
20. Ćurguz, Z.; Stojanovska, Z.; Žunić, Z.S.; Kolarž, P.; Ischikawa, T.; Omori, Y.; Mishra, R.; Sapra, B.K.; Vaupotič, J.; Ujić, P.; et al. Long-Term Measurements of Radon, Thoron and Their Airborne Progeny in 25 Schools in Republic of Srpska. *J. Environ. Radioact.* **2015**, *148*, 163–169. [CrossRef]
21. Branco, P.T.B.S.; Nunes, R.A.O.; Alvim-Ferraz, M.C.M.; Martins, F.G.; Sousa, S.I.V. Children's Exposure to Indoor Air in Urban Nurseries–Part II: Gaseous Pollutants' Assessment. *Environ. Res.* **2015**, *142*, 662–670. [CrossRef] [PubMed]
22. Reche, C.; Viana, M.; Rivas, I.; Bouso, L.; Àlvarez-Pedrerol, M.; Alastuey, A.; Sunyer, J.; Querol, X. Outdoor and Indoor UFP in Primary Schools across Barcelona. *Sci. Total Environ.* **2014**, *493*, 943–953. [CrossRef] [PubMed]
23. Rim, D.; Gall, E.T.; Kim, J.B.; Bae, G.-N. Particulate Matter in Urban Nursery Schools: A Case Study of Seoul, Korea during Winter Months. *Build. Environ.* **2017**, *119*, 1–10. [CrossRef]
24. Reche, C.; Rivas, I.; Pandolfi, M.; Viana, M.; Bouso, L.; Àlvarez-Pedrerol, M.; Alastuey, A.; Sunyer, J.; Querol, X. Real-Time Indoor and Outdoor Measurements of Black Carbon at Primary Schools. *Atmos. Environ.* **2015**, *120*, 417–426. [CrossRef]
25. Moreno, T.; Rivas, I.; Bouso, L.; Viana, M.; Jones, T.; Àlvarez-Pedrerol, M.; Alastuey, A.; Sunyer, J.; Querol, X. Variations in School Playground and Classroom Atmospheric Particulate Chemistry. *Atmos. Environ.* **2014**, *91*, 162–171. [CrossRef]
26. Buonanno, G.; Fuoco, F.C.; Morawska, L.; Stabile, L. Airborne Particle Concentrations at Schools Measured at Different Spatial Scales. *Atmos. Environ.* **2013**, *67*, 38–45. [CrossRef]
27. Portela, N.B.; Teixeira, E.C.; Agudelo-Castañeda, D.M.; Civeira, M.S.; Silva, L.F.O.; Vigo, A.; Kumar, P. Indoor-Outdoor Relationships of Airborne Nanoparticles, BC and VOCs at Rural and Urban Preschools. *Environ. Pollut.* **2021**, *268*, 115751. [CrossRef]
28. Nunes, R.A.O.; Branco, P.T.B.S.; Alvim-Ferraz, M.C.M.; Martins, F.G.; Sousa, S.I.V. Particulate Matter in Rural and Urban Nursery Schools in Portugal. *Environ. Pollut.* **2015**, *202*, 7–16. [CrossRef]
29. Becerra, J.A.; Lizana, J.; Gil, M.; Barrios-Padura, A.; Blondeau, P.; Chacartegui, R. Identification of Potential Indoor Air Pollutants in Schools. *J. Clean. Prod.* **2020**, *242*, 118420. [CrossRef]

30. Villanueva, F.; Tapia, A.; Lara, S.; Amo-Salas, M. Indoor and Outdoor Air Concentrations of Volatile Organic Compounds and NO_2 in Schools of Urban, Industrial and Rural Areas in Central-Southern Spain. *Sci. Total Environ.* **2018**, *622–623*, 222–235. [CrossRef]
31. Majd, E.; McCormack, M.; Davis, M.; Curriero, F.; Berman, J.; Connolly, F.; Leaf, P.; Rule, A.; Green, T.; Clemons-Erby, D.; et al. Indoor Air Quality in Inner-City Schools and Its Associations with Building Characteristics and Environmental Factors. *Environ. Res.* **2019**, *170*, 83–91. [CrossRef]
32. Canha, N.; Almeida, S.M.; Freitas, M.C.; Trancoso, M.; Sousa, A.; Mouro, F.; Wolterbeek, H.T. Particulate Matter Analysis in Indoor Environments of Urban and Rural Primary Schools Using Passive Sampling Methodology. *Atmos. Environ.* **2014**, *83*, 21–34. [CrossRef]
33. Ward, T.J.; Palmer, C.P.; Hooper, K.; Bergauff, M.; Noonan, C.W. The Impact of a Community–Wide Woodstove Changeout Intervention on Air Quality within Two Schools. *Atmos. Pollut. Res.* **2013**, *4*, 238–244. [CrossRef]
34. Slezakova, K.; de Oliveira Fernandes, E.; Pereira, M.C. Assessment of Ultrafine Particles in Primary Schools: Emphasis on Different Indoor Microenvironments. *Environ. Pollut.* **2019**, *246*, 885–895. [CrossRef] [PubMed]
35. Amato, F.; Rivas, I.; Viana, M.; Moreno, T.; Bouso, L.; Reche, C.; Àlvarez-Pedrerol, M.; Alastuey, A.; Sunyer, J.; Querol, X. Sources of Indoor and Outdoor PM2.5 Concentrations in Primary Schools. *Sci. Total Environ.* **2014**, *490*, 757–765. [CrossRef]
36. Almeida, S.M.; Canha, N.; Silva, A.; Freitas, M.C.; Pegas, P.; Alves, C.; Evtyugina, M.; Pio, C.A. Children Exposure to Atmospheric Particles in Indoor of Lisbon Primary Schools. *Atmos. Environ.* **2011**, *45*, 7594–7599. [CrossRef]
37. Kalimeri, K.K.; Saraga, D.E.; Lazaridis, V.D.; Legkas, N.A.; Missia, D.A.; Tolis, E.I.; Bartzis, J.G. Indoor Air Quality Investigation of the School Environment and Estimated Health Risks: Two-Season Measurements in Primary Schools in Kozani, Greece. *Atmos. Pollut. Res.* **2016**, *7*, 1128–1142. [CrossRef]
38. Poulhet, G.; Dusanter, S.; Crunaire, S.; Locoge, N.; Gaudion, V.; Merlen, C.; Kaluzny, P.; Coddeville, P. Investigation of Formaldehyde Sources in French Schools Using a Passive Flux Sampler. *Build. Environ.* **2014**, *71*, 111–120. [CrossRef]
39. Branco, P.T.B.S.; Alvim-Ferraz, M.C.M.; Martins, F.G.; Sousa, S.I.V. Quantifying Indoor Air Quality Determinants in Urban and Rural Nursery and Primary Schools. *Environ. Res.* **2019**, *176*, 108534. [CrossRef] [PubMed]
40. Oliveira, M.; Slezakova, K.; Madureira, J.; de Oliveira Fernandes, E.; Delerue-Matos, C.; Morais, S.; do Carmo Pereira, M. Polycyclic Aromatic Hydrocarbons in Primary School Environments: Levels and Potential Risks. *Sci. Total Environ.* **2017**, *575*, 1156–1167. [CrossRef]
41. Mishra, N.; Bartsch, J.; Ayoko, G.A.; Salthammer, T.; Morawska, L. Volatile Organic Compounds: Characteristics, Distribution and Sources in Urban Schools. *Atmos. Environ.* **2015**, *106*, 485–491. [CrossRef]
42. de Blas, M.; Navazo, M.; Alonso, L.; Durana, N.; Gomez, M.C.; Iza, J. Simultaneous Indoor and Outdoor On-Line Hourly Monitoring of Atmospheric Volatile Organic Compounds in an Urban Building. The Role of inside and Outside Sources. *Sci. Total Environ.* **2012**, *426*, 327–335. [CrossRef] [PubMed]
43. Godoi, R.H.M.; Godoi, A.F.L.; Gonçalves Junior, S.J.; Paralovo, S.L.; Borillo, G.C.; Gonçalves Gregório Barbosa, C.; Arantes, M.G.; Charello, R.C.; Rosário Filho, N.A.; Grassi, M.T.; et al. Healthy Environment—Indoor Air Quality of Brazilian Elementary Schools Nearby Petrochemical Industry. *Sci. Total Environ.* **2013**, *463–464*, 639–646. [CrossRef] [PubMed]
44. Tran, D.T.; Alleman, L.Y.; Coddeville, P.; Galloo, J.-C. Indoor–Outdoor Behavior and Sources of Size-Resolved Airborne Particles in French Classrooms. *Build. Environ.* **2014**, *81*, 183–191. [CrossRef]
45. Viana, M.; Rivas, I.; Querol, X.; Alastuey, A.; Álvarez-Pedrerol, M.; Bouso, L.; Sioutas, C.; Sunyer, J. Partitioning of Trace Elements and Metals between Quasi-Ultrafine, Accumulation and Coarse Aerosols in Indoor and Outdoor Air in Schools. *Atmos. Environ.* **2015**, *106*, 392–401. [CrossRef]
46. Mainka, A.; Brągoszewska, E.; Kozielska, B.; Pastuszka, J.S.; Zajusz-Zubek, E. Indoor Air Quality in Urban Nursery Schools in Gliwice, Poland: Analysis of the Case Study. *Atmos. Pollut. Res.* **2015**, *6*, 1098–1104. [CrossRef]
47. Li, K.; Shen, J.; Zhang, X.; Chen, L.; White, S.; Yan, M.; Han, L.; Yang, W.; Wang, X.; Azzi, M. Variations and Characteristics of Particulate Matter, Black Carbon and Volatile Organic Compounds in Primary School Classrooms. *J. Clean. Prod.* **2020**, *252*, 119804. [CrossRef]
48. Laiman, R.; He, C.; Mazaheri, M.; Clifford, S.; Salimi, F.; Crilley, L.R.; Megat Mokhtar, M.A.; Morawska, L. Characteristics of Ultrafine Particle Sources and Deposition Rates in Primary School Classrooms. *Atmos. Environ.* **2014**, *94*, 28–35. [CrossRef]
49. Elbayoumi, M.; Ramli, N.A.; Md Yusof, N.F.F.; Madhoun, W.A. The Effect of Seasonal Variation on Indoor and Outdoor Carbon Monoxide Concentrations in Eastern Mediterranean Climate. *Atmos. Pollut. Res.* **2014**, *5*, 315–324. [CrossRef]
50. Madureira, J.; Paciência, I.; Rufo, J.; Severo, M.; Ramos, E.; Barros, H.; de Oliveira Fernandes, E. Source Apportionment of CO2, PM10 and VOCs Levels and Health Risk Assessment in Naturally Ventilated Primary Schools in Porto, Portugal. *Build. Environ.* **2016**, *96*, 198–205. [CrossRef]
51. Al-Hemoud, A.; Al-Awadi, L.; Al-Rashidi, M.; Rahman, K.A.; Al-Khayat, A.; Behbehani, W. Comparison of Indoor Air Quality in Schools: Urban vs. Industrial "oil & Gas" Zones in Kuwait. *Build. Environ.* **2017**, *122*, 50–60. [CrossRef]
52. *ANSI/ASHRAE Standard 62.1*; Ventilation for Acceptable Indoor Air Quality. The American Society of Heating, Refrigerating and Air-conditioning Engineers (ASHRAE): Peachtree Corners, GA, USA, 2016.

53. Cavaleiro Rufo, J.; Madureira, J.; Paciência, I.; Aguiar, L.; Teixeira, J.P.; Moreira, A.; de Oliveira Fernandes, E. Indoor Air Quality and Atopic Sensitization in Primary Schools: A follow-up Study. *Porto Biomed. J.* **2016**, *1*, 142–146. [CrossRef] [PubMed]
54. Zhang, L.; Morisaki, H.; Wei, Y.; Li, Z.; Yang, L.; Zhou, Q.; Zhang, X.; Xing, W.; Hu, M.; Shima, M.; et al. Characteristics of Air Pollutants inside and Outside a Primary School Classroom in Beijing and Respiratory Health Impact on Children. *Environ. Pollut.* **2019**, *255*, 113147. [CrossRef] [PubMed]

Disclaimer/Publisher's Note: The statements, opinions and data contained in all publications are solely those of the individual author(s) and contributor(s) and not of MDPI and/or the editor(s). MDPI and/or the editor(s) disclaim responsibility for any injury to people or property resulting from any ideas, methods, instructions or products referred to in the content.

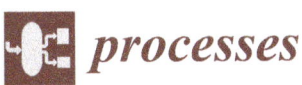

Article

Spread of SARS-CoV-2 Infections in Educational Settings by Level of Education, Taking into Account the Predominant Virus Variant

An Galičič *, Natalija Kranjec, Jan Rožanec, Ivana Obid, Eva Grilc, Branko Gabrovec and Mario Fafangel

National Institute of Public Health, Trubarjeva cesta 2, SI-1000 Ljubljana, Slovenia
* Correspondence: an.galicic@nijz.si

Abstract: The COVID-19 pandemic has negatively affected educational settings (ES) in Slovenia. To effectively limit the emergence and spread of SARS-CoV-2 infections in ES, it is important to identify the pathways of introduction and transmission of infection. This study aims to analyse the spread of infections in ES according to the level of education, taking into account the predominant variant of the virus in Slovenia in order to advise on public health action. We calculated the incidence rate of infection by age group, according to the level of the ES. Additionally, we analysed data on the reported outbreak criteria in ES. In Slovenia, SARS-CoV-2 infections in children and adolescents (1–18 years) accounted for 16.8% of all confirmed infections. The incidence and leading outbreak criteria differed according to the level of the ES and predominant SARS-CoV-2 variant. The occurrence of cases in ≥3 different "bubbles" was the most common outbreak criteria (59%). A high number of employee-imported outbreaks was observed in pre-school settings (44%). As countries move away from widespread nonpharmaceutical interventions, the focus should be on vaccination promotion among teaching staff in pre-school settings and systemic solutions, such as self-testing and ventilation, to enable safe educational environments.

Keywords: COVID-19; surveillance; outbreaks; educational settings; children

1. Introduction

In Slovenia, after the declaration of the COVID-19 epidemic at the beginning of March 2020, educational settings (ES) were closed and distance education introduced. Children and adolescents started returning to ES gradually in May 2020, where they finished the school year. The 2020/21 school year also started in ES, but only remained there until mid-October, when ES gradually closed. At the end of January 2021, ES began to gradually reopen, and classes were held according to different models [1,2] during the ongoing pandemic (Table 1). During the course of the pandemic, preventive and hygienic measures were recommended (e.g., formation of permanent groups, ventilation), and over time the use of protective masks became mandatory for teaching staff and adolescents in secondary school, and then became mandatory for children in primary school, but not for pre-school children. The measure of employee testing and self-testing also became mandatory for children in primary schools.

Several studies have reported low transmission of SARS-CoV-2 infections in ES in Australia [3], Ireland [4], Germany [5], North Carolina, USA [6], Italy [7], Canada [8] and Norway [9]. In Veneto, Italy, during the period January–June 2021, 69% of ES-related infections produced no secondary cases, 24% produced one or two cases, and 7% produced more than two cases [10]. However, individual studies have also reported major outbreaks of COVID-19 in ES in Israel [11], Utah, USA [12], Poland [13] and California, USA [14]. In such analyses, it is important to consider the predominant SARS-CoV-2 variant during the study period, as SARS-CoV-2 variants have different levels of infectivity, with the Omicron variant (B.1.1.529) having the highest infectivity [15].

Table 1. Openness of educational settings in Slovenia during the COVID-19 pandemic (March 2020–January 2022).

Year	Level of Education	Jan	Feb	Mar	Apr	May	Jun	Jul	Aug	Sep	Oct	Nov	Dec
2020	Pre-school setting												
	Primary school												
	Secondary school												
2021	Pre-school setting												
	Primary school												
	Secondary school												
2022	Pre-school setting												
	Primary school												
	Secondary school												

Legend: green—open educational settings, orange—partially open educational settings (individual levels/alternately/regional), red—closed educational settings, grey—summer holidays, white—nonobservation period.

The closure of ES has a detrimental effect on the physical and mental health of children and adolescents, as well as on their educational performance and development of social skills [16,17]. The European Centre for Disease Prevention and Control (ECDC) has identified school closures during the pandemic as a measure of last resort to prevent the spread of SARS-CoV-2 infections, but also noted the importance of monitoring the occurrence of infections in ES [18]. In Slovenia, a monitoring system with an algorithm for responding to infections in ES, and collaboration between ES and the National Institute of Public Health (NIJZ) have been set up to monitor outbreaks of SARS-CoV-2 infections in ES; a similar monitoring system is being used in England [19].

Delivering classes during the spread of SARS-CoV-2 infections requires an awareness that outbreaks of SARS-CoV-2 infections in ES will occur. Knowledge of the prevailing modes of introduction and spread is essential for effective containment of infections in ES, allowing targeted implementation and adaptation of measures. For this purpose, we have prepared an analysis of the spread of SARS-CoV-2 infections in ES according to the level of education, taking into account the predominant SARS-CoV-2 virus variant in Slovenia.

2. Materials and Methods

In this study, the study population consisted of children and adolescents (aged 1–18 years). In order to interpret the data by level of education, the age groups of children and adolescents were adjusted to the age structure of each level of education (Table 2). The levels of education do not include post-secondary or university education.

Table 2. Presentation of age groups of children and adolescents by level of education in the Republic of Slovenia.

Level of Education	Age Group	Population by Age Group on 01.07.2021 [20]	Proportion of Population [21]
Pre-school setting *	1–5 years	100,652	4.78%
Primary school	6–14 years	198,454	9.42%
Secondary school	15–18 years	75,787	3.60%

* In the 2021/22 school year, 85,957 children were included in pre-school setting, which represents 85.4% of all children aged from 1 to 5.

The observation period in the study represents the time after the establishment of the outbreak monitoring system in ES during which the delivery of classes in the premises of ES took place during the COVID-19 pandemic, from 26 January 2021 to 24 June 2021 and from 1 September 2021 to 18 January 2022. The periods of dominance of the individual SARS-CoV-2 virus variants in Slovenia were taken into account in the study. The period of dominance of a virus variant was defined by reaching 50% prevalence of that variant in the population. A more detailed time definition of the period is shown in Table 3.

Table 3. Periods of classes in educational premises and the prevalence of each SARS-CoV-2 variant in Slovenia.

Time Period	Delivery of Classes in Educational Settings	Predominant SARS-CoV-2 Variant ** [22]
26 January 2021–28 March 2021	YES	Wuhan variant (B.1.258.17)
29 March 2021–24 June 2021	YES	Alpha variant (B.1.1.7)
25 June 2021–4 July 2021	NO	Alpha variant (B.1.1.7)
5 July 2021–31 August 2021	NO	Delta variant (B.1.617.2)
1 September 2021–2 January 2022	YES	Delta variant (B.1.617.2)
03 January 2022–18 January 2022	YES	Omicron variant (B.1.1.529)

** The period of dominance of a virus variant was defined by reaching 50% prevalence of that variant in the population.

2.1. Confirmed Cases of SARS-CoV-2 Infections among Children, Adolescents and the General Population in Slovenia

Data on confirmed cases of SARS-CoV-2 infection in Slovenia were obtained from the official register of communicable diseases, maintained by the NIJZ, based on age at the time of official confirmation of infection.

We performed a descriptive analysis of data from the epidemiological monitoring system for SARS-CoV-2 infections in Slovenia. We calculated incidence rates of SARS-CoV-2 infections by age groups of children, adolescents, the rest of the population and the general population of Slovenia. Data on the population by defined age groups were obtained from the Statistical Office of the Republic of Slovenia Si-STAT database, as of 1 July 2021 [20]. In this part of the analysis, we have extended the data analysis to the period from the occurrence of the first case of infection in Slovenia, 4 March 2020, until 18 January 2022, with a focus on the periods of delivery of classes in ES.

2.2. COVID-19 Outbreaks in Educational Settings

We performed a descriptive data analysis on the fulfilled criteria that triggered SARS-CoV-2 infection outbreaks in ES. Data on the fulfilled criteria for SARS-CoV-2 outbreaks in ES were obtained from the system for monitoring outbreaks in ES, which is used by the managers of ES for reporting in accordance with the instructions of the Ministry of Education, Science and Sport and NIJZ algorithm. The monitoring system is comprehensive in terms of legal obligations and addresses all ES in Slovenia. Reporting was carried out in accordance with the NIJZ guidelines [23]. ES reported a worsening epidemiological situation to the epidemiological department when at least one of the following criteria was met: (c1) $\geq$ 15% of children/adolescents from the "bubble" had a confirmed infection within a 14-day period; (c2) $\geq$ 10% of the ES teaching staff had a confirmed infection within a 14-day period; or (c3) confirmed cases occurred in $\geq$ 3 different "bubbles". In the event that several criteria were simultaneously met at the time of the outbreak, all criteria met were considered in the analysis. In total, 12% of pre-school settings (48/412), 41% of primary schools (184/454) and 28% of secondary schools (43/155) reported to the ES outbreaks monitoring system.

3. Results

3.1. Confirmed SARS-CoV-2 Infection Cases in Children, Adolescents and the General Population in Slovenia

From the confirmation of the first COVID-19 case in Slovenia until 18 January 2022, a total of 559,469 COVID-19 cases were confirmed. Of these, 9911 were confirmed in the 1–5 age group, 57,983 in the 6–14 age group and 26,077 in the 15–18 age group. The incidence rate of COVID-19 cases per 100,000 population by age group of children, adolescents and the rest of the population according to the predominant SARS-CoV-2 variant and openness of ES in Slovenia is shown in Table 4. Figure 1 shows the monthly incidence rate per 100,000 population by age group for children, adolescents and the general population of

Slovenia. The figure shows the observed periods of the predominant SARS-CoV-2 virus variant during the open period of ES.

Table 4. Incidence rate of confirmed COVID-19 cases per 100,000 population by age group according to the period of predominance of variant SARS-CoV-2 and the openness of educational settings in Slovenia.

	Time Period	1–5 Years	6–14 Years	15–18 Years	Others
Period before the establishment of an outbreak monitoring system in educational settings	4 March 2020–25 January 2021	7481	12,910	41,683	88,613
Wuhan variant	26 January 2021–28 March 2021	8067	18,261	27,287	26,940
Alpha variant	29 March 2021–24 June 2021	6786	21,587	33,832	21,154
Summer school holidays	25 June 2021–31 August 2021	1470	3447	19,383	4881
Delta variant	1 September 2021–2 January 2022	51,097	155,704	143,851	88,121
Omicron variant	3 January 2022–18 January 2022	23,566	80,265	78,048	39,037

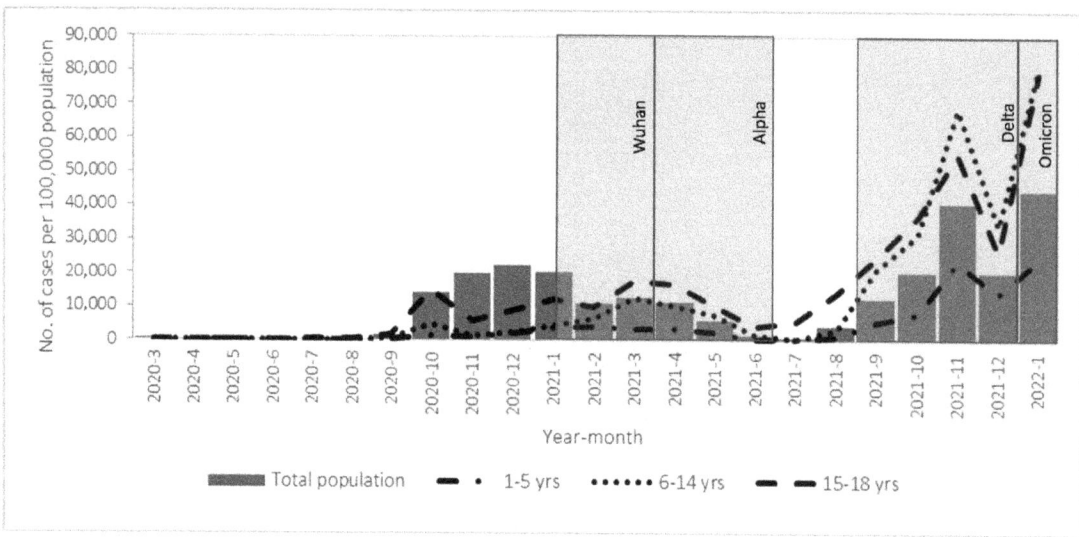

Figure 1. Monthly incidence rate of SARS-CoV-2 cases per 100,000 population by age group and total population in Slovenia, period 4 March 2020–18 January 2022. The periods of the predominant variant of the SARS-CoV-2 virus during the period of open ES are marked in the shaded fields.

3.2. COVID-19 Outbreaks in Educational Settings

During the observed period, 527 outbreaks were reported, of which 117 were in preschool settings, 319 in primary schools and 91 in secondary schools. The most common cause for the outbreak was the criterion that ≥ 3 different "bubbles" had confirmed cases (59%), followed by $\geq 15\%$ of children/adolescents in the "bubble" had a confirmed infection within a 14-day period (25%) and $\geq 10\%$ of teaching staff in ES had a confirmed infection within a 14-day period (16%). The representation of each criterion at each level of ES according to the predominant SARS-CoV-2 variant in Slovenia is shown in Table 5 and Figure 2.

Table 5. Representation of the fulfilled COVID-19 outbreak criteria in educational settings in Slovenia in the period from 26 January 2021 to 18 January 2022, taking into account the periods of predominance of each SARS-CoV-2 variant in Slovenia.

	Pre-School Settings				Primary Schools				Secondary Schools			
	c1	c2	c3	Sum	c1	c2	c3	sum	c1	c2	c3	Sum
Wuhan variant	5	19	15	39	12	10	30	52	3	0	7	10
Alpha variant	2	13	7	22	15	6	35	56	7	0	12	19
Delta variant	9	28	24	61	67	3	121	191	14	2	39	55
Omicron variant	1	10	13	24	19	7	58	84	6	3	20	29

Legend: c1—≥15% of children/adolescents in bubble (fixed children's groups) had a confirmed infection; c2—≥10% of employees had a confirmed infection; c3—confirmed cases occurred in ≥3 bubbles.

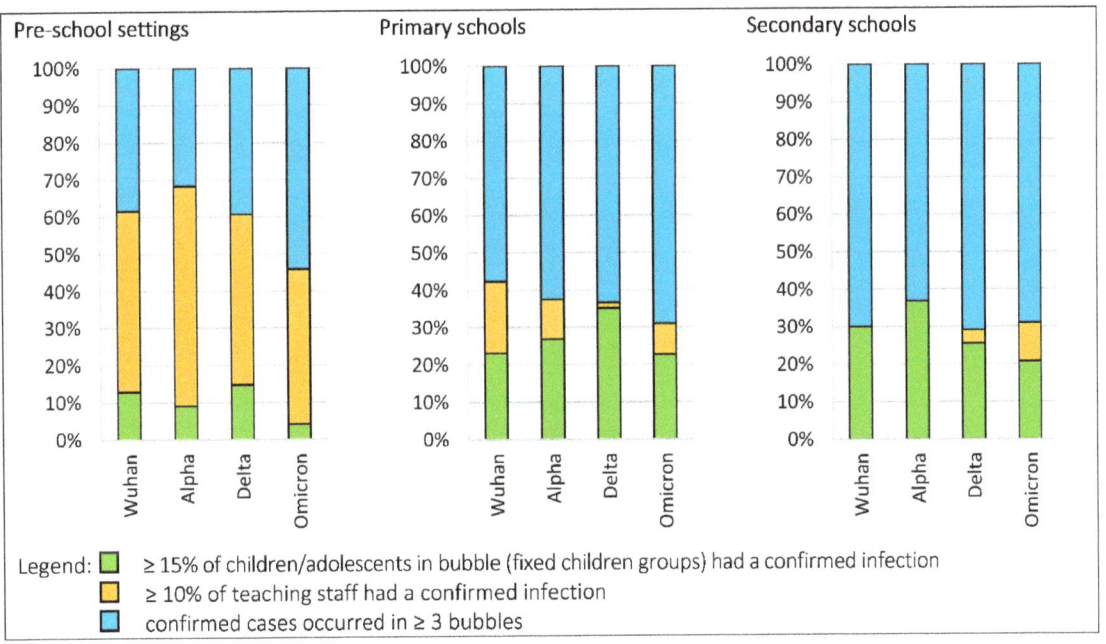

Figure 2. Representation of the fulfilled COVID-19 outbreak criteria in educational settings in Slovenia in the period from 26 January 2021 to 18 January 2022, taking into account the periods of prevalence of each SARS-CoV-2 variant in Slovenia.

4. Discussion

In Slovenia, in the period from the first COVID-19 case on 4 March 2020 to 18 January 2022, 16.8% of SARS-CoV-2 infection cases were confirmed in the age group of children and adolescents (1–18 years). During the first wave and through the summer of 2020, the number of infections among children and adolescents was low, then the number of infections started to rise at the start of the school year, until the closure of society and the consequent closure of schools at the end of October 2020. Until the gradual reopening of schools in the spring of 2021, the infection rates of children and adolescents at each level of education did not exceed those of the general population. After the gradual reopening of schools in the spring of 2021, the number of infections among children and adolescents first increased slightly and then started to decrease until the start of school in September 2021. During this period, the infection rate among children aged 6–15 years was similar to the infection rate in the general population, while the infection rate in the 15–18 age group exceeded the infection rate in the general population, especially in the months of summer 2021. The large number of COVID-19 outbreaks on graduation trips attended by adolescents aged 17 and 18 years may also have contributed to the increase in infections [23]. In autumn 2021, after the start of the new school year and when the Delta variant was predominant, the number of cases among children and adolescents started to rapidly increase. The infection rates in the 6–14 and 15–18 age groups were consistently higher than in the general population. In October 2021, the infection rate in the 6–14 age group exceeded the infection rate in the 15–18 age group for the first time, and this continued until the end of our observation period in January 2022. In the beginning of 2022, when the Omicron variant prevailed, the number of confirmed cases among children and adolescents increased, but the infection rates for the 6–14 and 15–18 age groups remained higher than the infection rates in the general population. Over the entire observation period, the infection rate in the 1–5 age group was the lowest among all three groups of children and adolescents, and lower than the infection rate in the general population.

The COVID-19 vaccination rate among children and adolescents in Slovenia is low. In the 6–14 age group, until the predominance of the Omicron variant, vaccination coverage under the basic scheme did not reach 10%. Among adolescents aged 15–18 years, vaccination coverage with all doses started to increase during the 2021 summer school holidays and reached 43% coverage during the Omicron variant period. Data on the vaccination prevalence among teaching staff in ES was not available [24]. Vaccination experts in Slovenia recommend basic vaccination for all children and adolescents aged 12 years and older. Primary vaccination for younger children aged 5–11 years is recommended for children with chronic diseases and children aged 5–11 years who are in contact with persons at higher risk of severe COVID-19 disease and cannot be effectively protected by vaccination. People aged 18 and older are recommended to receive one additional vaccination dosage [25].

When the SARS-CoV-2 infection is introduced into ES, it can spread between members of the same "bubble" or among employees (e.g., due to socializing in common areas). With higher local transmission, the infection can be simultaneously introduced by different persons, generating further infections. The results of our research showed that during the observed period at all levels of education, the most common cause of outbreaks in ES was the occurrence of infection in ≥ 3 different "bubbles" in the ES, which means the simultaneous introduction of infection into the ES by different persons. The least common cause of the outbreak in ES varied according to the level of education; in pre-school settings, it was the occurrence of infection in $\geq 15\%$ of "bubble" members, and in primary and secondary schools, it was the occurrence of infection in $\geq 10\%$ of teaching staff. The results show that the proportion varied according to the level of education and the predominant SARS-CoV-2 variant.

In pre-school settings, the prevalence of infection in $\geq 10\%$ of the teaching staff was the leading cause during the Wuhan, Alpha and Delta variants, and the prevalence of infection in ≥ 3 different "bubbles" in ES was the leading cause during the Omicron variant. Regardless of the predominant variant, the least common cause of the outbreak in the pre-school settings was the occurrence of infection in $\geq 15\%$ of the "bubble" members. The important role of teaching staff in the spread of SARS-CoV-2 infection in pre-school settings was also shown by a retrospective study of SARS-CoV-2 outbreaks in November and December 2020 in pre-school settings in Berlin (Germany), which concluded that the spread of SARS-CoV-2 in the pre-school environment occurred mainly through teaching staff, while children transmitted the infections mainly to the home environment [26]. A possible reason for the higher representation of the fulfilled criterion for the spread of infections among teaching staff in pre-school settings compared with the other ES is that there are more teaching staff in each department who, due to the nature of their work, have more close contacts with children. It may also indicate that pre-school teaching staff have more contacts with other employees outside the department.

In primary schools, during the entire observed period, the most common cause of an outbreak in ES was the occurrence of infection in ≥ 3 different "bubbles", with the highest proportion in the period of predominance of the Omicron variant and the lowest proportion in the period of predominance of the Wuhan variant. The least common cause of an outbreak in primary schools was infection in $\geq 10\%$ of teaching staff with the highest proportion in the Wuhan variant predominant period and the lowest proportion in the Delta variant predominant period.

In secondary schools, just as in primary schools, the most common cause of an outbreak in ES throughout the observation period was the occurrence of infection in ≥ 3 different "bubbles" in ES. The proportion of this cause ranged between 60% and 70%, regardless of the virus variant. The rarest cause of the outbreak in secondary schools was infection in $\geq 10\%$ of the teaching staff, which was not recorded during the period of predominance of the Wuhan and Delta variants. During the period of dominance of the Delta variant, the share of this cause was less than 4%, which almost tripled in the Omicron period. A seroprevalence survey among adolescents and teaching staff in English secondary schools (UK) in September and December 2020 also suggested a role for local transmission, finding that the incidence rate was not significantly different between adolescents and teaching staff, but was similar to the population incidence rate [27].

Similar to a Spanish study [28], our results show that when analysing outbreaks and transmissions and their causes, it is important to consider the predominant SARS-CoV-2 variant at each time period in the population, as variants of SARS-CoV-2 have different levels of infectivity [15]. This is also shown in a German study [29], which found that at the appearance of the Alpha variant (B.1.1.7), the susceptibility and infectiousness of children aged 1–6 years were significantly higher compared to the pre-Alpha period and may have been approaching those of adults.

The primary importance of ES is the educational development of children and adolescents; furthermore, ES have a positive impact on their physical and mental health and psycho-social development. The extent of the overall positive impact that ES have on the development of children and adolescents was shown during the COVID-19 pandemic and the closure of ES. During this period, a decline in educational and social development, worsening of mental health problems, and negative changes in sleeping patterns, eating habits and screen use were observed [2,16,17,30]. From this perspective, it is necessary to examine the social acceptability of the measure to close ES in relation to its effectiveness in controlling the pandemic.

Data on the fulfilment of the criteria that triggered the infection outbreak in ES, which were analysed in this study, were reported in the monitoring system by the managers of individual ES. Perhaps better-quality data would have been collected if the department of epidemiology had reported to the system after an individual outbreak had been investigated. Nevertheless, we estimate that the data collected are of sufficient quality for analysis, as the ES have a detailed algorithm in place to identify the fulfilment of the criteria in the ES and report to the monitoring system. At the same time, teaching staff in ES were empowered to report through a videoconference presentation and had the possibility of online consultation in case of any questions. An important advantage of this study is the long time period covered, which includes the periods of predominance of the four SARS-CoV-2 variants in Slovenia. We have not found such results in previous studies, so our research will provide important insights for the design of targeted measures at different levels of education, including in the light of the emergence of new variants, that will allow undisturbed delivery of classes in ES, without closures and all the consequences for children's health and development.

The need for targeted measures at different levels of education, indicated from the results of this study, should be incorporated into the COVID-19 management strategy. This strategy, linked with the characteristics of the Omicron variant, is relaxing strict nonpharmaceutical interventions and replacing them with measures focusing on the protection of the most vulnerable populations and systemic solutions associated with the management of a broader spectre of respiratory diseases. In relation to the most vulnerable population groups, our results indicate the need to design measures with the focus on teaching staff in pre-school settings, among which promotion of vaccination against COVID-19 is significant. High vaccination prevalence among teaching staff in pre-school settings could have a significant impact on developing less severe disease symptoms and reduce absenteeism from work, both important to continue undisturbed education at ES during pandemics. Systemic solutions, from this study's results, could be self-testing of primary and secondary school children and adolescents. This would limit infections in a population group with many interactions outside of the ES, and who are responsible for the transmission into the ES. Another systemic solution on the ES infrastructure level is the ability to effectively ventilate closed spaces, as required by the characteristics of COVID-19 transmission [31]. Additionally, it is important to maintain sufficient capacities at national and international levels to monitor SARS-CoV-2 variants for the purpose of rapid adaptation of measures and strategies [32].

5. Conclusions

The first study of its kind to investigate the spread of infection in ES by level of education, taking into account the predominant SARS-CoV-2 variant, showed that the predominant causes and frequency of their occurrence vary according to the level of education, as well as the predominant SARS-CoV-2 variant. In designing further measures to limit the spread of SARS-CoV-2 infections in ES, it is necessary to be aware that the key actions are at the population level and not only in ES; since, as the results show, the most common cause of the spread of infection in ES is the simultaneous introduction of the virus by several persons from different "bubbles". The results also showed that different virus variants affect the way the virus spreads at each level of the ES, as it is linked to the infectivity of the SARS-CoV-2 variant. This is particularly evident at the pre-school level, where interactions are closer. These findings should be taken into account in the event that new variants of SARS-CoV-2 emerge. This would mean further targeting of the recommendations at teaching staff general adherence to the recommendations and self-testing, thereby controlling infections in these population groups with many interactions also outside the ES. Measures recommended by our study are aligned with the strategy, which responds to the characteristics of the Omicron variant, as most countries are moving away from strict nonpharmaceutical interventions and replacing them with a focus on protection of the most vulnerable populations (e.g., vaccination) and systemic solutions enabling safe educational environments linked to the management of a broader spectrum of respiratory diseases (e.g., self-testing and ventilation improvements). This way, it is possible to avoid measures that have a negative impact on the process of education and socialisation in the educational system.

Author Contributions: Conceptualisation, A.G. and M.F.; Methodology, A.G. and N.K.; Formal Analysis, J.R., I.O. and N.K.; Writing—Original Draft Preparation, A.G., J.R., N.K. and I.O.; Writing—Review & Editing, M.F., E.G. and B.G.; Visualisation, N.K. and A.G.; Supervision, M.F. All authors have read and agreed to the published version of the manuscript.

Funding: The study was conducted in Slovenia as part of a NIJZ project. The project title is "Measures to manage the spread of COVID-19 with a focus on vulnerable groups of population". This research is co-financed by the Republic of Slovenia and the European Union under the European Social Fund in the framework of the EU response to the COVID-19 pandemic (Grant No. C2711-21-053701). The content of this article represents the views of the authors only and is their sole responsibility; it cannot be considered to reflect the views of the European Commission or any other body of the European Union. The European Commission does not accept any responsibility for the use that may be made of the information it contains.

Data Availability Statement: Data supporting the findings of this study are available from the corresponding author upon reasonable request.

Acknowledgments: We would like to thank all Slovenian ES (pre-school settings, primary schools and secondary schools) that have been reporting the epidemiological situation in their ES throughout the monitoring period.

Conflicts of Interest: The authors declare no conflict of interest.

References

1. Kustec, S.; Logaj, V.; Krek, M.; Flogie, A.; Truden-Dobrin, P.; Ivanuš-Grmek, M. *Education in the Republic of Slovenia in the Context of COVID-19: Models and Recommendations*, 1st ed.; Logaj, V., Ed.; Ministry of Education, Science and Sport, the National Institute of Education of the Republic of Slovenia: Ljubljana, Slovenia, 2020. (In Slovenian)
2. Kustec, S.; Logaj, V.; Krek, M.; Flogie, A.; Truden-Dobrin, P.; Ivanuš-Grmek, M. *School Year 2021/22 in the Republic of Slovenia in the Context of COVID-19: Models and Recommendations*, 1st ed.; Logaj, V., Ed.; Ministry of Education, Science and Sport, the National Institute of Education of the Republic of Slovenia: Ljubljana, Slovenia, 2021. (In Slovenian)
3. Macartney, K.; Quinn, H.E.; Pillsbury, A.J.; Koirala, A.; Deng, L.; Winkler, N.; Katelaris, A.L.; O'Sullivan, M.V.N.; Dalton, C.; Wood, N.; et al. Transmission of SARS-CoV-2 in Australian Educational Settings: A Prospective Cohort Study. *Lancet Child Adolesc. Health* **2020**, *4*, 807–816. [CrossRef]
4. Heavey, L.; Casey, G.; Kelly, C.; Kelly, D.; McDarby, G. No Evidence of Secondary Transmission of COVID-19 from Children Attending School in Ireland, 2020. *Euro Surveill.* **2020**, *25*, 29–32. [CrossRef] [PubMed]
5. Ehrhardt, J.; Ekinci, A.; Krehl, H.; Meincke, M.; Finci, I.; Klein, J.; Geisel, B.; Wagner-Wiening, C.; Eichner, M.; Brockmann, S.O. Transmission of SARS-CoV-2 in Children Aged 0 to 19 Years in Childcare Facilities and Schools after Their Reopening in May 2020, Baden-Württemberg, Germany. *Euro Surveill.* **2020**, *25*, 8–11. [CrossRef] [PubMed]
6. Zimmerman, K.O.; Akinboyo, I.C.; Brookhart, M.A.; Boutzoukas, A.E.; McGann, K.A.; Smith, M.J.; Maradiaga Panayotti, G.; Armstrong, S.C.; Bristow, H.; Parker, D.; et al. Incidence and Secondary Transmission of SARS-CoV-2 Infections in Schools. *Pediatrics* **2021**, *147*, e2020048090. [CrossRef] [PubMed]
7. Gandini, S.; Rainisio, M.; Iannuzzo, M.L.; Bellerba, F.; Cecconi, F.; Scorrano, L. A Cross-Sectional and Prospective Cohort Study of the Role of Schools in the SARS-CoV-2 Second Wave in Italy. *Lancet Reg. Health–Eur.* **2021**, *5*, 100092. [CrossRef] [PubMed]
8. Bark, D.; Dhillon, N.; St-Jean, M.; Kinniburgh, B.; McKee, G.; Choi, A. SARS-CoV-2 Transmission in Kindergarten to Grade 12 Schools in the Vancouver Coastal Health Region: A Descriptive Epidemiologic Study. *CMAJ Open* **2021**, *9*, E810–E817. [CrossRef] [PubMed]
9. Brandal, L.T.; Ofitserova, T.S.; Meijerink, H.; Rykkvin, R.; Lund, H.M.; Hungnes, O.; Greve-Isdahl, M.; Bragstad, K.; Nygård, K.; Winje, B.A. Minimal Transmission of SARS-CoV-2 from Paediatric COVID-19 Cases in Primary Schools, Norway, August to November 2020. *Euro Surveill.* **2021**, *26*, 2–7. [CrossRef] [PubMed]
10. Tonon, M.; Da Re, F.; Zampieri, C.; Nicoletti, M.; Caberlotto, R.; De Siena, F.P.; Lattavo, G.; Minnicelli, A.; Zardetto, A.; Sforzi, B.; et al. Surveillance of Outbreaks of SARS-CoV-2 Infections at School in the Veneto Region: Methods and Results of the Public Health Response during the Second and Third Waves of the Pandemic between January and June 2021. *Int. J. Environ. Res. Public Health* **2021**, *18*, 12165. [CrossRef]
11. Stein-Zamir, C.; Abramson, N.; Shoob, H.; Libal, E.; Bitan, M.; Cardash, T.; Cayam, R.; Miskin, I. A Large COVID-19 Outbreak in a High School 10 Days after Schools' Reopening, Israel, May 2020. *Euro Surveill.* **2020**, *25*, 2–6. [CrossRef] [PubMed]
12. Lopez, A.S.; Hill, M.; Antezano, J.; Vilven, D.; Rutner, T.; Bogdanow, L.; Claflin, C.; Kracalik, I.T.; Fields, V.L.; Dunn, A.; et al. Transmission Dynamics of COVID-19 Outbreaks Associated with Child Care Facilities—Salt Lake City, Utah, April–July 2020. *Morb. Mortal. Wkly. Rep.* **2020**, *69*, 1319–1323. [CrossRef] [PubMed]
13. Okarska-Napierała, M.; Mańdziuk, J.; Kuchar, E. SARS-CoV-2 Cluster in Nursery, Poland. *Emerg. Infect. Dis.* **2021**, *27*, 317–319. [CrossRef] [PubMed]
14. Lam-Hine, T.; McCurdy, S.A.; Santora, L.; Duncan, J.; Corbett-Detig, R.; Kapusinszky, B.; Willis, M. Outbreak Associated with SARS-CoV-2 B.1.617.2 (Delta) Variant in an Elementary School—Marin County, California, May–June 2021. *Morb. Mortal. Wkly. Rep.* **2021**, *70*, 1214–1219. [CrossRef] [PubMed]
15. Galán, J.C.; Cantón, R. New Variants in SARS-CoV-2: What Are We Learning from the Omicron Variant? *Arch. Bronconeumol.* **2022**, *58*, 3–5. (In Spanish) [CrossRef] [PubMed]
16. Fantini, M.P.; Reno, C.; Biserni, G.B.; Savoia, E.; Lanari, M. COVID-19 and the Re-Opening of Schools: A Policy Maker's Dilemma. *Ital. J. Pediatrics* **2020**, *46*, 79. [CrossRef]
17. Viner, R.; Russell, S.; Saulle, R.; Croker, H.; Stansfield, C.; Packer, J.; Nicholls, D.; Goddings, A.-L.; Bonell, C.; Hudson, L.; et al. School Closures during Social Lockdown and Mental Health, Health Behaviors, and Well-Being Among Children and Adolescents during the First COVID-19 Wave: A Systematic Review. *JAMA Pediatrics* **2022**, *176*, 400–409. [CrossRef] [PubMed]
18. European Centre for Disease Prevention and Control. COVID-19 in Children (1–18 Years) and the Role of School Settings in COVID-19 Transmission—First Update. 2020. Available online: https://www.ecdc.europa.eu/en/publications-data/children-and-school-settings-COVID-19-transmission (accessed on 3 May 2022).

19. Public Health England. COVID-19 Education Settings Resource Pack. Interim Guidance. For Early Years/Nurseries, Childminders, Primary Schools, Secondary Schools and SEND Settings. London: London Coronavirus Response Centre, Public Health England. 2021. Available online: https://www.egfl.org.uk/sites/default/files/LCRC%20schools%20resource%20pack%20V2 0%2027042021.pdf (accessed on 4 June 2021).
20. Statistical Office of the Republic of Slovenia. Database Si-STAT: Population by: Age, Municipality, Halfyear, 2021H2. Published: 5 January 2022, Id.Table: 05C4003S. Available online: https://pxweb.stat.si/SiStatData/pxweb/sl/Data/-/05C4003S.px (accessed on 20 July 2022). (In Slovenian).
21. Statistical Office of the Republic of Slovenia. Database Si-STAT: Children Included in Kindergarten by: Gender, Municipality, School Year. Published: 21 June 2022, id.table: 0952531S. Available online: https://pxweb.stat.si/SiStatData/pxweb/sl/Data/-/0952531S.px (accessed on 20 July 2022). (In Slovenian).
22. National Laboratory for Health, Environment and Food. Tracking SARS-CoV-2 Variants at the National Laboratory for Health, Environment and Food in Collaboration with the Clinical Institute for Special Laboratory Diagnostics at the Paediatric Clinic of the University Clinical Centre Ljubljana. 2022. Available online: https://www.nlzoh.si/wp-content/uploads/2022/03/Porocilo-st-56-sekvenciranje-NLZOH-in-KISLD_28-3-2022.pdf (accessed on 31 March 2022). (In Slovenian).
23. National Institute of Public Health. Emergence of SARS-CoV-2 Infections among Graduation Trip Participants—Krf. 2021. Available online: https://www.nijz.si/sl/pojav-okuzb-s-sars-cov-2-med-udelezenci-maturantskega-izleta-krf (accessed on 31 March 2022). (In Slovenian)
24. National Institute of Public Health. Vaccination Coverage against COVID-19 in Slovenia. 2022. Available online: https://app.powerbi.com/view?r=eyJrIjoiYWQ3NGE1NTMtZWJkMi00NzZmLWFiNDItZDc5YjU5MGRkOGMyIiwidCI6ImFkMjQ1ZGFlLTQ0YTAtNGQ5NC04OTY3LTVjNjk5MGFmYTQ2MyIsImMiOjl9 (accessed on 28 July 2022). (In Slovenian)
25. National Institute of Public Health. Guidelines and Recommendations for Vaccination against COVID-19. 2022. Available online: https://www.nijz.si/sl/cepljenje-proti-COVID-19-za-strokovno-javnost (accessed on 28 July 2022). (In Slovenian)
26. Ruf, S.; Hommes, F.; van Loon, W.; Seybold, J.; Kurth, T.; Mall, M.A.; Mockenhaupt, F.P.; Theuring, S. A Retrospective Outbreak Investigation of a COVID-19 Case Cluster in a Berlin Kindergarten, November 2020. *Int. J. Environ. Res. Public Health* **2021**, *19*, 36. [CrossRef] [PubMed]
27. Ladhani, S.N.; Ireland, G.; Baawuah, F.; Beckmann, J.; Okike, I.O.; Ahmad, S.; Garstang, J.; Brent, A.J.; Brent, B.; Walker, J.; et al. SARS-CoV-2 Infection, Antibody Positivity and Seroconversion Rates in Staff and Students following Full Reopening of Secondary Schools in England: A Prospective Cohort Study, September–December 2020. *eClinicalMedicine* **2021**, *37*, 100948. [CrossRef] [PubMed]
28. Gamboa Moreno, E.; Garitano Gutiérrez, I.; Portuondo Jiménez, J.; Cabrera Rodríguez, A.; Aldeguer Corbi, J.; Tapia Alonso, N.; Arrospide, A.; Picón Santamaría, A. Low transmission of SARS-CoV-2 at school settings: A population-based study in the Basque Country. *Rev. Esp. Salud Publica* **2021**, *95*, e202112196. (In Spanish) [PubMed]
29. Loenenbach, A.; Markus, I.; Lehfeld, A.-S.; An der Heiden, M.; Haas, W.; Kiegele, M.; Ponzi, A.; Unger-Goldinger, B.; Weidenauer, C.; Schlosser, H.; et al. SARS-CoV-2 Variant B.1.1.7 Susceptibility and Infectiousness of Children and Adults Deduced from Investigations of Childcare Centre Outbreaks, Germany, 2021. *Euro Surveill.* **2021**, *26*, 2–5. [CrossRef] [PubMed]
30. Beck, M. Experiences with Non-Pharmaceutical Interventions and Student Mental Health and Wellbeing during COIVD-19. Master's Thesis, Norwegian University of Science and Technology, Trondheim, Norway, May 2022. Available online: https://ntnuopen.ntnu.no/ntnu-xmlui/handle/11250/3005184 (accessed on 28 July 2022).
31. Federation of European Heating, Ventilation and Air Conditioning Associations. REHVA COVID-19 Guidance Document: How to Operate HVAC and Other Building Service Systems to Prevent the Spread of the Coronavirus (SARS-CoV-2) Disease (COVID-19) in Workplaces. 2021. Available online: https://www.rehva.eu/fileadmin/user_upload/REHVA_COVID-19_guidance_document_V4.1_15042021.pdf (accessed on 8 September 2022).
32. World Health Organization. Statement on the Twelfth Meeting of the International Health Regulations (2005) Emergency Committee Regarding the Coronavirus Disease (COVID-19) Pandemic. 2022. Available online: https://www.who.int/news/item/12-07-2022-statement-on-the-twelfth-meeting-of-the-international-health-regulations-(2005)-emergency-committee-regarding-the-coronavirus-disease-(COVID-19)-pandemic (accessed on 12 July 2022).

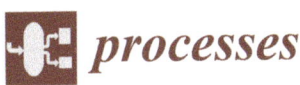

Article

Ecological Environmental Effects and Their Driving Factors of Land Use/Cover Change: The Case Study of Baiyangdian Basin, China

Boyu Xia [1,2,*] and Linchang Zheng [1,2,*]

1. School of Economics, Hebei University, Baoding 071000, China
2. Research Center for Resource Utilization and Environmental Protection, Hebei University, Baoding 071000, China
* Correspondence: xiaboyu@stumail.hbu.edu.cn (B.X.); zhenglinchang@126.com (L.Z.)

Abstract: Due to the combined effects of the natural environment, climate change and human activities, profound changes have occurred in terms of the eco-environmental effects of land use/cover change (LUCC) in the Baiyangdian basin. Therefore, based on land remote sensing monitoring data from 2000 to 2020, the Eco-environmental Quality Index (EQI) was introduced in this study to measure the eco-environmental effects of land use change in the Baiyangdian basin. Subsequently, the GeoDetector model was applied to detect the formation mechanism of the eco-environmental effects in the Baiyangdian basin from 2000 to 2020. The results of the study showed that cropland, woodland and grassland were the most widely distributed land use types in the Baiyangdian basin. The area of cropland declined the most and was mostly converted to construction land. The EQI increased slightly during the study period. The eco-environment of the mountainous areas in the western part of the basin and in Baiyangdian Lake was better than that of other areas. Land use intensity had a significantly stronger influence on the quality of the eco-environment than other factors. The interaction between the influencing factors was mainly a non-linear enhancement and a two-factor enhancement, with non-linear enhancement dominating.

Keywords: Baiyangdian basin; land use/cover change; eco-environmental quality index; spatio-temporal pattern; GeoDetector; factor detector; interaction detector

1. Introduction

Ecological and environmental problems are one of the most important global issues faced by mankind today. Natural disasters such as sea level rises [1] and extreme weather phenomena [2] caused by global ecological problems such as the greenhouse effect and the sharp decline in forest resources are seriously threatening the survival and development of mankind [3]. As the most prominent landscape marker of the Earth's surface system, the study of land use/cover change (LUCC) is an important element of global climate and environmental research, which plays an important role in global environmental change [4]. Since 1992, LUCC has been the focus of global environmental change and sustainability research, such as that of the International Institute for Applied Systems Analysis (IIASA), the International Geosphere–Biosphere Program (IGBP) and the International Human Dimensions Program on Global Environmental Change (IHDP) [5,6]. Previous studies on LUCC have focused on the spatial and temporal patterns as well as the evolution of LUCC [7], the driving forces and driving mechanisms of LUCC [8], the modelling and sustainable use of LUCC [9] and the ecological and environmental effects of LUCC [10], the first three studies of which were relatively more mature. Research on the eco-environmental effects of LUCC and its formation mechanisms has received increasing attention in recent years due to the significant environmental impact of human activities, including land use, land development and economic growth [11].

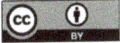

An accurate understanding of the eco-environmental effects, processes and formation mechanisms of regional LUCC is an important way to improve the eco-environment of the region. By influencing the structure and function of natural elements such as soil, climate, hydrology and biodiversity through ecological processes including energy exchange, water cycling, soil erosion and accumulation, as well as crop production, LUCC ultimately results in changes in the environment and ecosystems [12–14]. In recent years, with the development of satellite remote sensing technology, breakthroughs have been made in the measurement methods and indicators of the eco-environmental effects of LUCC. The most obvious manifestation is that some new methods and indicators have been applied to the study of the eco-environmental effects of LUCC. For example, the normalized difference vegetation index (NDVI) [15,16], enhanced vegetation index (EVI) [17] and other indicators can be used to evaluate changes in regional eco-environments by monitoring the amount of vegetation. In addition, the use of LUCC data interpreted from remote sensing imagery to study the eco-environmental effects of LUCC has become a mainstream academic practice. The emergence of new indicators such as the ecosystem services value (ESV) [18], the new remote-sensing-based ecological index (RSEI) [19] and the eco-environmental quality index (EQI) [20] has largely filled the gap in academic research. Among them, EQI is widely used in ecological research because it can better reflect the relationship between land use and the ecological environment [21].

In recent years, studies on the eco-environmental effects of LUCC have been characterized by the following features. The focus of research has gradually expanded from the eco-environmental effects of single factors such as water bodies, forests and carbon to the overall eco-environmental effects of the region [22,23]; the study objects are mainly in cities, and most of the studies focus on the impact of urbanization or human activities on the regional eco-environment, ignoring natural factors as a prerequisite for the formation and evolution of the regional eco-environment [11,24]. In addition, ecological environmental change is the result of complex interactions between multiple factors, i.e., the interactions between drivers have a strong spatial heterogeneity on ecological environmental change, but previous studies have not provided a comprehensive explanation for this complex interaction [25]. The GeoDetector method is a spatial statistical method that can not only detect the explanatory power of the main driving factors but also express the interactions between different driving factors [26]. The method has a higher explanatory efficiency than other spatial heterogeneity detection tools [23] and has been widely used in research on public health [27], socio-economics [28] and urban thermal environments [29].

As the largest freshwater lake in North China, Baiyangdian Lake provides an important supporting role for regional biodiversity and eco-environmental protection. In recent years, with the implementation of regional planning, the establishment of the Xiong'an New Area and the layout of new industries, the land cover in the Baiyangdian basin has changed dramatically [30]. These changes have also profoundly altered the spatial pattern of EQI in the Baiyangdian basin. It is important to monitor changes in the EQI of the Baiyangdian basin and identify the spatial heterogeneity and driving mechanisms of EQI in order to understand the regional ecological environment, the rational use of land resources, the restoration and management of the ecological environment and ecosystem service functions. The main objectives of this study included: (1) a comprehensive analysis of the land use and its characteristics of the Baiyangdian basin from 2000 to 2020; (2) an evaluation of the EQI changes caused by land use change; and (3) an exploration of the spatial and temporal patterns and formation mechanisms of EQI.

2. Materials and Methods
2.1. Study Area

Baiyangdian Lake, located in the North China Plain, is a lake in the southern branch of the Daqing River system and is one of the most important ecological water bodies in the Xiong'an New Area. With a total area of 366 km^2 and an average water storage of 1.32 billion cubic meters, Baiyangdian Lake is the largest lake in Hebei Province and is known as the kidney of North China and the pearl of North China [31]. The Baiyangdian basin spans four provinces, namely Beijing, Tianjin, Hebei and Shanxi, and is located between 113°20′–116°54′ E and 38°05′–40°04′ N. The basin covers an area of approximately 33,096.57 km² (Figure 1). Its topography slopes from northwest to southeast, forming three major landform units: mountains (hills), plains and wetlands. In terms of climate, the Baiyangdian basin belongs to a temperate continental monsoon climate zone, with four distinct seasons and simultaneous rain and heat. Precipitation in the basin is unevenly distributed spatiotemporally, with an annual average of about 640 mm. A total of 80% of the precipitation is concentrated in July, August and September with large inter-annual variations. Spatially, precipitation decreases from the mountains to the plains. The average annual temperature of the basin ranges from 7.3 to 12.7 °C and decreases from the plains in the southeast to the mountains in the northwest [32].

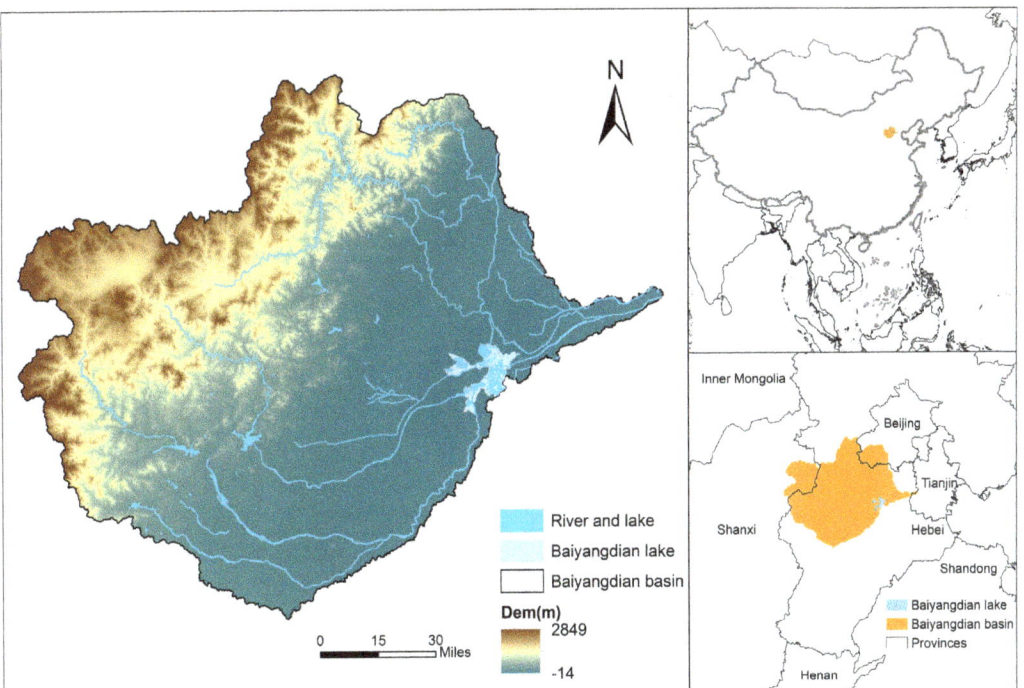

Figure 1. Location of the study area and its topographic features.

2.2. Methods

2.2.1. Direction of Land Use Change

This study used the land use transfer matrix to construct an index to quantify the transfer direction of each land use type in the Baiyangdian basin. The land use transfer matrix is a visual representation of the area transferred in and out of a land type from the start year to the end year over a period of change as well as the direction of change for each land type and is widely used in LUCC studies. The calculation is as follows:

$$S_{ij} = \begin{bmatrix} S_{11} & S_{12} & S_{13} & \cdots & S_{1n} \\ S_{21} & S_{22} & S_{23} & \cdots & S_{2n} \\ \vdots & \vdots & \vdots & \ddots & \vdots \\ S_{n1} & S_{n2} & S_{n3} & \cdots & S_{nn} \end{bmatrix} \quad (1)$$

where S is the area of the transferred land type; i and j are the beginning and end periods, respectively; n is the number of land use types; the number of rows indicates the part of the land use type in period i that changed to the land use type in period j; and the diagonal part indicates the part of the same land type that did not change from period i to period j. The land use net change area (NC) clearly reflects the direction of land use change over the study period and is expressed as follows:

$$NC = \begin{cases} S_{ij} - S_{ji}, S_{ij} \geq S_{ji} \\ S_{ji} - S_{ij}, S_{ij} < S_{ji} \end{cases} \qquad (2)$$

where S_{ij} is the area of land type j changed to land type i; S_{ji} is the area of land type i changed to land type j; and NC denotes the net area of change between land type i and land type j.

2.2.2. Land Use Intensity Index

The land use intensity index mainly reflects the breadth and depth of land use in a given region, but it also reflects the extent to which socio-economic factors interfere with the natural complex of the land. The land use intensity analysis method proposed by Xianghong et al. [33] classifies land use types according to the degree of influence of social factors and assigns a graded index to each land use type separately. The calculation is as follows:

$$L = 100 \times \sum_{i=1}^{n} A_i \times C_i \qquad (3)$$

where L is the land use intensity comprehensive index in a certain region; A_i is the grade index of land use type i; C_i is the area percentage of land use type i; and n is the number of land use types. According to the degree of influence of human activities on each land use type, a value of 4 is assigned to construction land, 3 to cropland, 2 to woodland, water and grassland areas, and 1 to unused land.

2.2.3. Eco-Environmental Quality Index

The eco-environmental quality index (EQI) expresses the overall characteristics of eco-environmental quality in a region by constructing a quantitative relationship between LUCC and eco-environmental quality. According to the needs of this study, the Baiyangdian basin was divided into 1465 eco-environmental units using a 5 km × 5 km square grid. As the secondary land use classification system has a high resolution and reflects obvious differences in ecological functions, this study used the secondary classification system to assess the eco-environmental quality of each eco-environmental unit in the Baiyangdian basin with reference to relevant studies at home and abroad [28]. The reference EQI background values for each land use type were determined by expert scoring and hierarchical analysis taking into account previous studies [24]. The calculation is as follows:

$$EQI_t = \frac{(\sum_{i=1}^{n} LUA_{i,t} \times EV_i)}{\sum_{i=1}^{n} LUA_{i,t}}. \qquad (4)$$

where EQI_t denotes the eco-environmental quality index in period t; EV_i denotes the background value of eco-environmental quality corresponding to land use type i (Table 1); $LUA_{i,t}$ represents the area of land use type i in period t; and n denotes the number of land use types in a certain region.

Table 1. Land use classification and eco-environmental indicators.

Level 1 Land Use Types		Level 2 Land Use Types		Background Value of Eco-Environmental Quality
Code	Primary Land Use Types	Code	Secondary Land Use Types	
1	Cropland	11	Paddy land	0.30
		12	Dry land	0.25
2	Woodland	21	Forestland	0.95
		22	Shrub forest	0.65
		23	Sparse forestland	0.45
		24	Other forestland	0.40
3	Grassland	31	High-cover grassland	0.75
		32	Medium-cover grassland	0.45
		32	Low-cover grassland	0.20
4	Water area	41	River canal	0.55
		42	Lake	0.75
		43	Reservoir pit	0.55
		46	Bottom land	0.55
5	Construction land	51	Urban land	0.20
		52	Rural settlement	0.20
		53	Other construction land	0.15
6	Unused land	61	Sand	0.01
		63	Saline-alkali land	0.05
		64	Marshland	0.65
		65	Bare land	0.05
		66	Exposed rock land	0.01

2.2.4. GeoDetector

The GeoDetector model is a new model for detecting the variability of an attribute value of a geographical thing between different regions and the driving factors behind it [34]. GeoDetector is widely used in nature, society, environment and other related fields because of its advantages such as less sample size limitations, no multicollinearity and it being good at handling type volume. GeoDetector consists of four detectors: a factor detector, an interaction detector, an ecological detector and a risk detector. In this study, the factor detector and the interaction detector were used to reveal the effects of different factors and their interactions on the EQI.

The factor detector is used to identify the extent to which factors affect the eco-environmental quality and whether there is significant spatial consistency. The calculation is as follows:

$$q = 1 - \frac{\sum_{h=1}^{L} N_h \sigma_h^2}{N \sigma^2} \quad (5)$$

where q is the impact detecting indicator for the EQI and takes values in the range [0, 1]; N is the number of units across the region; N_h is the number of sample units in layer h; h is the classification of factors affecting EQI; and σ^2 and σ_h^2 are the variances of indicators in the study area and the variances of layer i, respectively.

The interaction detector is used to reflect the impact of the interaction between the 2 influencing factors on the EQI. First, we computed the q-values of the two factors X1 and X2. Then, we superimposed these two factors and computed their q-values q(X1 ∩ X2). Finally, we compared the values of q(X1), q(X2) and q(X1 ∩ X2). The interaction of the two factors will result in one of the following five situations:

(1) Non-linear reduction: q(X1 ∩ X2) < Min(q(X1), q(X2)).
(2) Single-factor non-linear attenuation: Min(q(X1), q(X2)) < q(X1 ∩ X2) < Max(q(X1), q(X2)).
(3) Two-factor enhancement: q(X1 ∩ X2) > Max(q(X1), q(X2)).
(4) Independent: q(X1 ∩ X2) = q(X1) + q(X2).
(5) Non-linear enhancement: q(X1 ∩ X2) > q(X1) + q(X2).

The spatial and temporal pattern of the eco-environmental effect of LUCC in the Baiyangdian basin is formed by the combined effect of many factors. By referring to previous studies and repeated experiments, this paper selected thirteen factors from five aspects: topography, climate, soil and vegetation, human activities and location, to explore the mechanism of the formation of the spatial pattern of the eco-environment in the Baiyangdian basin. Topography is a decisive factor in the formation of the spatial and temporal distribution of the eco-environment. Since the Earth was formed, the structure of its crust and surface form has been changing. Changes in land and sea, mountains and rivers, as well as the birth and death of life, are all the result of changes in the Earth's surface morphology. This paper, therefore, selected topographic relief (X1), slope (X2) and altitude (X3) to detect the influence of topography on the spatial and temporal evolution of the quality of the eco-environment [35,36]. Over historical periods, topography has determined the evolutionary processes and trends in eco-environmental quality. Climate, soil and vegetation, human activities and location are the main drivers of the spatial and temporal evolution of eco-environmental quality over short periods. Climate is the most direct and sensitive factor in the evolution of regional eco-environmental quality, which can influence the evolution of regional eco-environmental quality at any spatial or temporal scale as well as play an important role in the evolution of regional eco-environmental quality. This paper therefore selected precipitation (X4) and temperature (X5) to detect the influence of climate on the spatial and temporal evolution of the eco-environmental quality [26]. Soil and vegetation are the most prominent sign of the surface system of the Earth and have a significant impact on eco-environmental quality. Therefore, in this study, soil type (X6), organic carbon content of soil (X7) and NDVI (X8) were chosen to characterize the influence of soil and vegetation on the spatial and temporal evolution of eco-environmental quality [37]. Human activity is the most dynamic factor influencing the evolution of eco-environmental quality. In this study, land use intensity (X9), population density (X10) and nighttime lighting (X11) were chosen to detect the influence of human activities on eco-environmental quality [21]. Among these indicators, with reference to the research of Cai et al. [38], this study introduced nighttime lighting to indicate the socio-economic level of the Baiyangdian basin. In addition, the distance from roads (X12) and the distance from railways (X13) were also included in the model to explore the influence of accessibility on the spatial heterogeneity of the eco-environment in the Baiyangdian basin [21].

2.3. Data Source

The data required for this study included normalized difference vegetation index (NDVI) data, land use data, soil type data, digital elevation data (DEM), precipitation data, temperature data and nighttime lighting data (Table 2). The NDVI and land use data were for the five periods of 2000, 2005, 2010, 2015 and 2020; the soil type data were 1 km raster data; and the land use data were 30 m raster data. The above data were obtained from the Resource and Environment Science and Data Centre of the Chinese Academy of Sciences (http://www.resdc.cn/, accessed on 1 September 2021). DEM data were obtained from the Geospatial Data Cloud (http://www.gscloud.cn/, accessed on 1 September 2021). Population density data (100 m resolution) were obtained from worldpop (https://www.worldpop.org/, accessed on 1 January 2022). Nighttime lighting data for 2000–2020 were derived from the National Geophysical Data Center (NGDC), part of the National Oceanic and Atmospheric Administration (NOAA) (https://www.ngdc.noaa.gov/eog/download.html, accessed on 1 January 2022). The boundary of the Baiyangdian basin was extracted with reference to the study by Haag et al. [39] and Sliwinski et al. [40].

Table 2. GeoDetector indicator system and unit.

Category	Detecting Factors	Unit
Topography	Topographic relief (X1)	m
	Slope (X2)	°
	Altitude (X3)	m
Climate	Precipitation (X4)	mm
	Temperature (X5)	°C
Soil and vegetation	Soil type (X6)	Dimensionless
	Organic carbon content of soil (X7)	g/kg
	NDVI (X8)	Value
Human activities	Land use intensity (X9)	Value
	Population density (X10)	person/km^2
	Nighttime lighting (X11)	Value
Location	Distance from road (X12)	km
	Distance from railway (X13)	km

3. Results

3.1. Land Use/Cover Change Analysis of the Baiyangdian Basin

Overall, there were more land use types in the Baiyangdian basin during the study period, containing a total of six primary land use types and twenty-one secondary land use types. The mutual transformation between the different types of land use in the Baiyangdian basin from 2000 to 2020 was very clear (Table 3). Cropland was the predominant land use type in the study area. The relatively low altitude and suitable climate have contributed to the development of the agricultural sector in the Baiyangdian basin [26]. However, since 2000, the proportion of cropland in the basin declined from 44.63% to 40.49% in 2020, showing a phenomenon of gradual decline. Woodland was mainly located in the Taihang Mountains of the western part of the basin, and its area increased from 21.09% in 2000 to 21.11% in 2020. This includes an increase of 1.64% in the area of forestland over the study period. Compared to woodland, the proportion of grassland decreased from 23.80% in 2000 to 22.61%, showing a significant downward trend.

Table 3. Land use patterns in the Baiyangdian basin from 2000 to 2020.

	2000		2005		2010		2015		2020	
	Area km^2	Proportion	Area km^2	Proportion	Area km^2	Proportion	Area km^2	Proportion	Area km^2	Proportion
Paddy land	104	0.31%	151	0.46%	162	0.49%	91	0.28%	42	0.13%
Dry land	14,660	44.32%	14,565	44.03%	14,482	43.78%	13,479	40.75%	13,356	40.36%
Forestland	2461	7.44%	2462	7.44%	2464	7.45%	3004	9.08%	3037	9.18%
Shrub forest	3679	11.12%	3678	11.12%	3674	11.11%	3135	9.48%	3146	9.51%
Sparse forestland	672	2.03%	672	2.03%	686	2.07%	690	2.09%	683	2.06%
Other forestland	167	0.50%	178	0.54%	178	0.54%	127	0.38%	124	0.38%
High-cover grassland	2899	8.76%	2900	8.77%	3015	9.11%	2993	9.05%	2959	8.94%
Medium-cover grassland	3732	11.28%	3722	11.25%	3555	10.75%	3487	10.54%	3300	9.97%
Low-cover grassland	1243	3.76%	1237	3.74%	1227	3.71%	1121	3.39%	1241	3.75%
River canal	113	0.34%	113	0.34%	113	0.34%	174	0.53%	174	0.52%
Lake	51	0.15%	48	0.14%	37	0.11%	34	0.10%	68	0.21%
Reservoir pit	97	0.29%	95	0.29%	91	0.27%	107	0.32%	113	0.34%
Bottom land	597	1.80%	536	1.62%	518	1.57%	333	1.01%	380	1.15%
Urban land	390	1.18%	477	1.44%	510	1.54%	752	2.27%	738	2.23%
Rural settlement	2064	6.24%	2071	6.26%	2084	6.30%	2821	8.53%	2926	8.84%
Other construction land	131	0.40%	155	0.47%	261	0.79%	520	1.57%	623	1.88%
Sand	4	0.01%	4	0.01%	4	0.01%	1	0.00%	1	0.00%
Saline-alkali land	0	0.00%	0	0.00%	0	0.00%	1	0.00%	0	0.00%
Marshland	0	0.00%	0	0.00%	0	0.00%	206	0.62%	172	0.52%
Bare land	8	0.03%	8	0.02%	8	0.02%	1	0.00%	1	0.00%
Exposed rock land	10	0.03%	10	0.03%	10	0.03%	0	0.00%	7	0.02%

Water areas were not the dominant land use type in the study area, but water, as a source of life, has an essential function in the eco-environment of the Baiyangdian basin. From 2000 to 2015, due to the large-scale reclamation of the lake for farming by the people in the study area, the water area (excluding bottom land) in the basin showed a gradual decline. After 2015, along with the introduction of the Beijing–Tianjin–Hebei Coordinated Development and the establishment of the Xiong'an New Area, the local government carried out large-scale work on the Baiyangdian basin to return cropland to the lake as well as to provide eco-environmental protection. Until 2020, the proportion of water area in the basin grew to 1.07%, which was the highest level during the study period. Compared to other land use types, the area of construction land increased significantly over the study period, with its proportion of the total area increasing from 7.82% in 2000 to 12.95% in 2020. Among the construction land, both rural settlements and the urban land expanded more significantly, with their proportion increasing from 1.18% and 6.24% in 2000 to 2.23% and 8.84% in 2020, respectively. The expansion of rural settlements and urban land was mainly due to population growth and migration. Between 2000–2020, the population density in the Baiyangdian basin rose from 431 to 500 people per square kilometer. Notably, 2000–2020 was a period of accelerated infrastructure development in China [41]. As a result, the area of other construction land also increased to a greater extent, with its proportion increasing from 0.40% in 2000 to 1.88% in 2020. The unused land in the Baiyangdian basin was dominated by marshland. Prior to 2015, there was no marshland in the study area. However, in 2015, the majority of the bottom land in Baiyangdian Lake was transformed into marshland. As of 2020, marshland accounted for 0.52% of the basin's total area, indicating that water storage in Baiyangdian Lake had increased to a large extent since 2015, roughly coinciding with the return of cropland to the lake.

Table 4 shows the direction of change for each land use type in the Baiyangdian basin from 2000 to 2020 (due to space constraints, this paper only shows the direction of land use change for larger areas). During the study period, the conversion of dry land to construction land was the main direction of land use change in the Baiyangdian basin. From 2000 to 2020, the dry land area in the Baiyangdian basin decreased by a total of 1304.8263 km^2, 1261.5756 km^2 of which was converted to construction land, accounting for 96.67% of its total converted area. The reduction in the dry land area included 755.3776 km^2 converted to rural settlements, 266.3679 km^2 converted to urban land and 266.3679 km^2 converted to other construction land. The expansion of construction land came mainly from the occupation of farmland, with most of the cropland converted to construction land located near cities and villages (Figure 2). The conversion trend of rural settlements to urban land within the study area is notable. From 2000 to 2020, a total of 48.3221 km^2 of rural settlement was transformed into urban land. This indicated that the urban expansion not only involved the occupation of cropland but also that more and more rural areas around cities will gradually be incorporated into the urban sphere with economic development. The conversion of shrub forest to forestland was also evident. During the study period, 473.6854 km^2 of shrub forest was converted to forestland, accounting for 88.97% of the area converted from shrub forest. It indicated that, after a period of prohibition of indiscriminate logging and the protection of forests, the forest area and quality of the Baiyangdian basin improved to a great extent. However, according to the above study, most of the reduced cropland was converted into construction land, suggesting that the local government's policy of returning cropland to woodland was not effectively implemented by the local people. The transfer of grassland and other land types also occurred more frequently during the study period. On the one hand, 117.4426 km^2 of medium-cover grassland was converted to high-cover grassland from 2000 to 2020, indicating that grassland was effectively protected in some areas. On the other hand, 102.8970 km^2 and 80.9788 km^2 of medium-cover grassland was converted to other construction land and low-cover grassland, respectively, indicating that eco-environmental degradation and the encroachment of ecological land by construction land existed in the Baiyangdian basin. In terms of the change from bottom land to marshland, a total of 135.2766 km^2 of bottom land was converted to marshland during the study period, accounting for 62.21% of the reduction in bottom land area, and the conversion was mainly in the vicinity of Baiyangdian Lake (Figure 2). This indicated that the water storage capacity of Baiyangdian Lake increased to a large extent over the study period. It also indicated that the eco-environment of Baiyangdian Lake improved considerably after a period of treatment of the lake and its upstream basin.

Table 4. Direction of land use change in the Baiyangdian basin from 2000 to 2020.

Rank	The Direction of Land Use Change	NC (km^2)
1	Dry land→rural settlement	755.3776
2	Shrub forest→forestland	473.6854
3	Dry land→urban land	266.3679
4	Dry land→other construction land	239.8301
5	Bottom land→marshland	135.2766
6	Medium-cover Grassland→high-cover Grassland	117.4426
7	Medium-cover Grassland→other construction land	102.8970
8	Medium-cover Grassland→low-cover Grassland	80.9788
9	Rural settlement→urban land	48.3221
10	Paddy land→dry land	47.8082

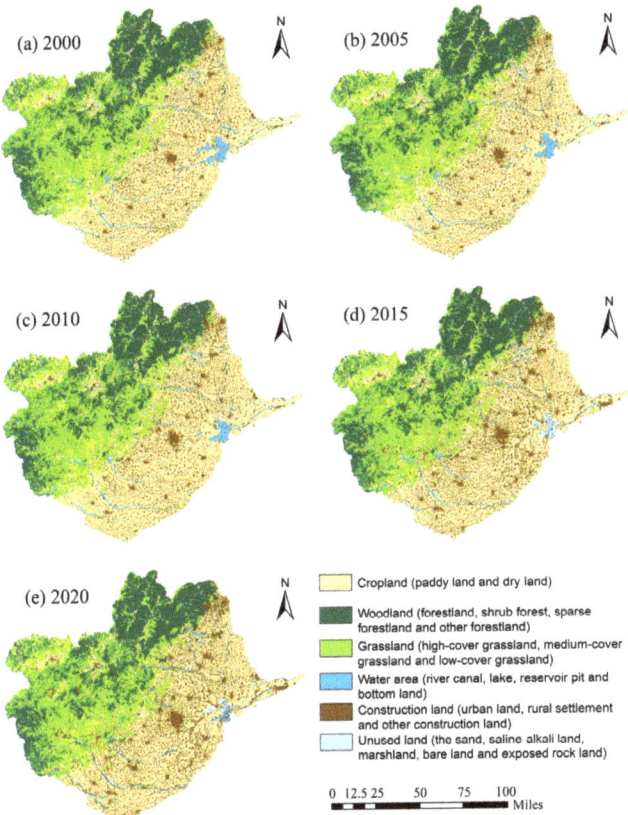

Figure 2. Spatial and temporal distribution of land use types in the Baiyangdian basin from 2000 to 2020.

3.2. Spatial and Temporal Evolutionary Characteristics of the EQI

The results of the Baiyangdian basin EQI measurement between 2000 and 2020 are shown in Figure 3. Since the 21st century, China has made great achievements in terms of urbanization and industrialization. However, this has inevitably led to the encroachment of cropland and ecological land by construction land. The increasingly serious contradiction between man and land has also led to a series of serious ecologically damaging land use activities such as deforestation and the reclamation of lakes into cropland. It is in this context that the EQI of the Baiyangdian basin fell from 0.4199 to 0.4191 between 2000 and 2005. From 2005 to 2010, the EQI of the Baiyangdian basin increased from 0.4191 to 0.4192. The improvement in the quality of the eco-environment was related to the policies that have been implemented by the local government in the Baiyangdian basin, including the Key Shelterbelt Construction Program (KSCP), the Natural Forest Conservation Program (NFCP), the Afforestation Program for Taihang Mountain (APTM) and the Grain to Green Program (GTGP) [42,43]. During this period, the area of sparse forestland and high-cover grassland in the Baiyangdian basin increased by 14.05 km^2 and 115.33 km^2, respectively, which led to an increase in the EQI to some extent. Since 2010, China has gradually stepped into a new normal of economic development. As a result of increased pressure on resources and the environment, as well as increased consumer awareness of environmental protection, China has also become more aware of the importance of environmental protection. All provinces, autonomous regions and municipalities directly under the central government, and this includes the Baiyangdian basin governments at all levels, have actively introduced measures related to ecological restoration. As a result, between 2010 and 2015, the EQI of the Baiyangdian basin improved to a greater extent, with its value increasing from 0.4192 to 0.4225. However, the previously emerged conflict between humans and land has shown an explosive trend in recent years, manifested by a decline in the EQI, whose value dropped from 0.4225 in 2015 to 0.4214 in 2020. This was mainly due to a certain conflict between the restrictions on the red line of cropland in the Baiyangdian basin and urbanization. In conclusion, the EQI of the Baiyangdian basin generally showed a fluctuating upward trend from 2000 to 2020. However, the decline in the EQI in recent years indicates that the contradiction between humans and land in the Baiyangdian basin is becoming more pronounced. How to manage the balance between cropland, construction land and ecological land in the future is an urgent issue for local governments in the Baiyangdian basin.

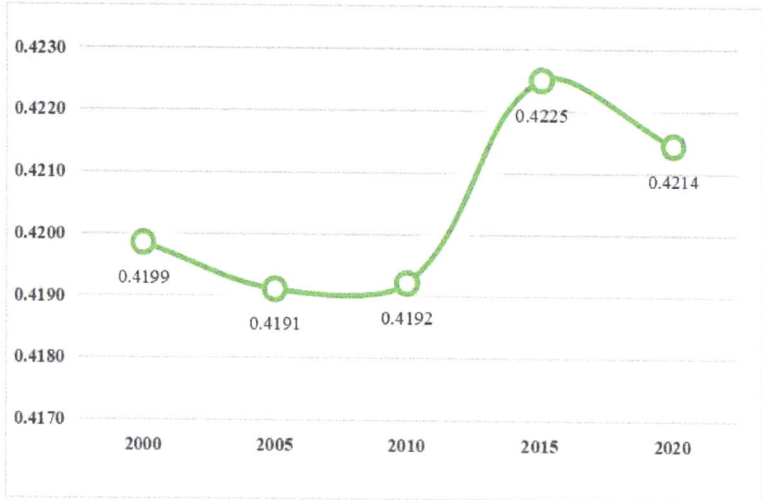

Figure 3. The EQI of the Baiyangdian basin from 2000 to 2020.

The spatial and temporal pattern of the EQI in the Baiyangdian basin is shown in Figure 4. The results of the study showed that the spatial and temporal patterns of eco-environmental quality in the Baiyangdian basin remained generally stable during the study period. The EQI showed a trend of being higher in the northwest and lower in the southeast, indicating that the eco-environmental quality of the Taihang Mountains in the western part of the study area was generally better than that of the North China Plain in the eastern part of the study area. The North China Plain, where the eastern part of the Baiyangdian basin is located, is a population and economic agglomeration in northern China. Socio-economic development and population agglomeration were the main reasons for the poorer eco-environmental quality in the eastern part of the basin. Baiyangdian Lake is a hotspot of eco-environmental quality in the North China Plain, and it plays an integral role in the ecological regulation function of the core area of the Beijing–Tianjin–Hebei urban agglomeration as well as the Baiyangdian basin. From 2000 to 2020, the EQI of Baiyangdian Lake showed a fluctuating upward trend, indicating an improvement in the quality of the eco-environment near Baiyangdian Lake. The Taihang Mountains, where the northwestern part of the basin is located, is an area with high values of the EQI. The main characteristics of the Taihang Mountains in the western part of the basin are higher altitude, complex natural conditions, lower average temperatures and more luxuriant vegetation cover, hence its higher EQI. Moreover, the EQI of the Taihang Mountains in the western part of the basin continued to rise gradually over the study period.

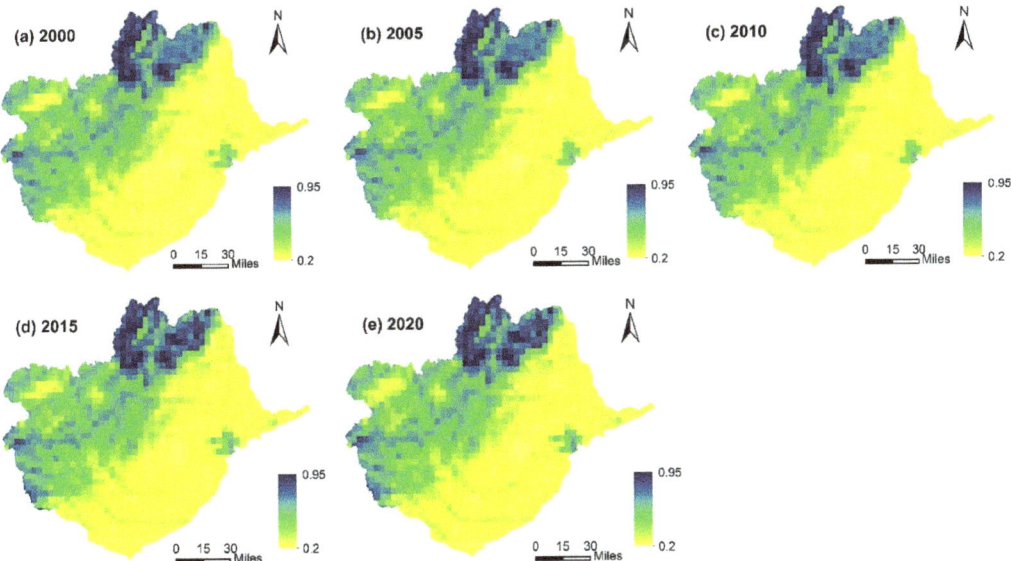

Figure 4. Spatial and temporal distribution of EQI in the Baiyangdian basin from 2000 to 2020.

3.3. Driving Factors for the Spatial and Temporal Evolution of EQI

3.3.1. Detection and Analysis of Impact Factors

With reference to the specific situation of the Baiyangdian basin, this study used the GeoDetector model to detect the spatial and temporal patterns of land use eco-environmental quality in the basin (Figure 5). At a certain level of a significance test, a larger q-value for an indicator indicates a greater influence of that indicator on the spatial and temporal evolution of the EQI. All the influencing factors from 2000–2020 passed the significance test at the 1% level. At the 1% significance level, the combined influence of the driving factors in the Baiyangdian basin from 2000 to 2020 were ranked as follows: land use intensity > altitude > topographic relief > slope > temperature > population > nighttime lighting > soil type > organic carbon content of soil > distance from road > distance from railway > NDVI > precipitation. From 2000 to 2020, the influence of land use intensity on the EQI of the Baiyangdian basin was significantly stronger than the other factors, and it was the most important driving factor in the spatial and temporal evolution of eco-environmental quality. Specifically, the influence of topographic factors, including topographic relief, slope and altitude, on the quality of the eco-environment showed a fluctuating downward trend during the study period. The impact of temperature on the eco-environmental quality of the Baiyangdian basin showed a fluctuating downward trend. Compared to other influencing factors, soil and vegetation factors had a relatively small impact on the spatial and temporal evolution of the eco-environmental quality of the Baiyangdian basin. In particular, the NDVI was still at a relatively low level, although it showed a slow increase during the study period. In 2020, the q-value for NDVI was only 0.164, which was still low, although it was a significant increase compared to 0.011 in 2000. The q-values for soil type and organic carbon content of soil were also relatively small and remained generally stable over the study period. In terms of human activity factors, the impact of land use intensity on eco-environmental quality was higher than the other two factors, indicating that the eco-environmental quality of the Baiyangdian basin was more susceptible to the impact of human land development activities. The impact of population on the eco-environmental quality of the Baiyangdian basin decreased gradually, while the impact of nighttime lighting increased. Overall, human activities played a significant role in the spatial and temporal evolution of the eco-environmental quality of the Baiyangdian basin. Railways had a higher impact on the EQI than roads; however, location had a smaller impact on the EQI over the study period.

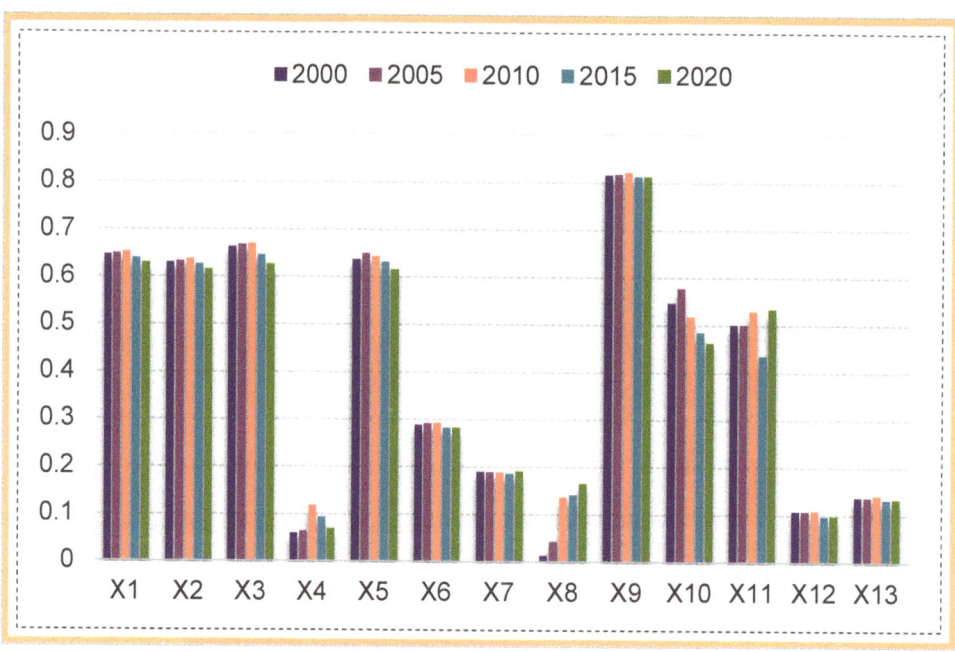

Figure 5. Results of impact factor detection for the spatial and temporal evolution of the EQI.

3.3.2. Detection and Analysis of Interaction Factors

Based on the results of the GeoDetector interaction detector analysis, it can be seen that the influence of the impact factors on the EQI during the period 2000–2020 did not occur in isolation. During the study period, all the interactions between the influencing factors had an enhancing effect on the EQI of the Baiyangdian basin (Figure 6). The two main types of synergistic enhancement were two-factor enhancement and non-linear enhancement, but the former was significantly stronger than the latter in the Baiyangdian basin. Land use intensity, as the factor with the highest q-value, reflected the extent to which human society has exploited the natural complex of the land. The link between the factors and land use intensity was stronger, so the strength of the effect between land use intensity and other factors within the Baiyangdian basin was significantly stronger than the strength of the effect between any two other factors. However, there was more of a two-factor enhancement between land use intensity and the other factors. The number of non-linear enhancements decreased gradually over time. Prior to 2005, the interaction of precipitation and NDVI with other factors was more of a non-linear enhancement. From 2010–2020, only a few of the interactions between the factors were non-linear enhancements, while other interactions between the factors were two-factor enhancements. In conclusion, the interactions between the factors exhibited significant non-linear enhancement and two-factor enhancement effects over the study period. The combined effects of topography, climate, soil and vegetation, location and human activities influenced the spatial and temporal patterns of eco-environmental quality in the Baiyangdian basin.

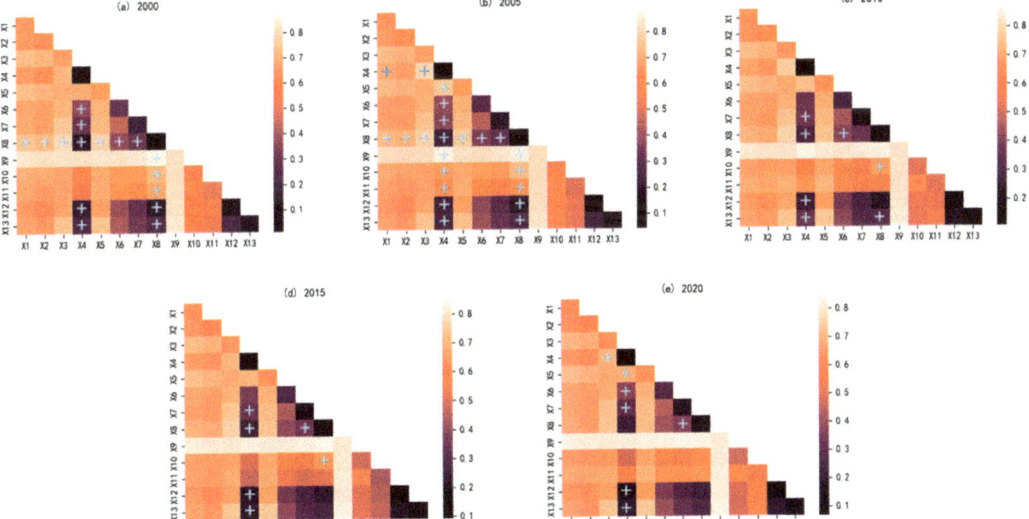

Figure 6. Results of interaction factor detection for the EQI in the Baiyangdian basin. Note: + means that the two detection factors were non-linear enhancement, and no + means that the two detection factors were two-factor enhancement.

4. Discussion

4.1. Comparing with Previous Studies

The eco-environment is the basis for the survival and development of human society, and no civilization can develop in isolation from the natural environment [44]. At the same time, human development can have an impact on the natural environment in return [45]. Since the reform and opening up, China has made tremendous achievements in economic development, which has led to profound changes in land use while also causing a series of eco-environmental problems [24]. Previous studies have shown that with industrialization and urbanization, the eco-environment across China has shown a trend of gradual deterioration [11,28]. In this study, however, the EQI of the Baiyangdian basin increased during the study period. This was mainly due to the low level of urbanization in the Baiyangdian basin, where the problem of conflict between people and land was not as significant compared to hotspot regions. At the same time, the protection of ecological land by local governments in the Baiyangdian basin also played a non-negligible role.

Some scholars have argued that socio-economic factors are the most direct influences on the quality of the ecological environment [46]. However, based on a geographically weighted regression model, Fang et al. concluded that precipitation and the proportion of forestland were the dominant factors influencing the spatial and temporal variation in the value of ecosystem services in the Yangtze and Yellow River basins, meaning that natural factors were the dominant factors leading to the spatial and temporal evolution of the ecological environment [10]. Similar conclusions were reached by Guo et al. in their study of desertification in the Yellow River source area [47]. This paper creatively introduced nighttime lighting (X11) to represent the socio-economic level and incorporated it into the model. Nighttime lighting data is an unbiased, labor-saving type of remote sensing data that has been successfully used in recent years for many aspects such as economic output estimation, the analysis of urbanization processes and energy consumption calculations [48,49]. Different from previous studies, this paper found that the combined effects of topography, climate, soil and vegetation, human activities and location drove the spatial and temporal patterns of eco-environmental quality in the Baiyangdian basin. In comparison, the impact of human activities on the EQI of the Baiyangdian basin was stronger than the impact of topography, climate, soil and vegetation as well as location in this paper, and similar conclusions were reached in the research of Ge et al. [46]. The topography of the basin is complex, so topographic factors such as topographic relief, slope and altitude also had a significant impact on the EQI of the Baiyangdian basin.

4.2. Policy Implications

Exploring the eco-environmental effects and driving factors of LUCC in the Baiyangdian basin is important for scientific research and sustainable regional development [28,50,51]. In 2018, the Chinese government formulated the Baiyangdian eco-environmental management and protection plan, aiming to maintain ecological security and promote sustainable development in northern China [52]. However, how to translate the specific entries of the plan into reality is a problem faced by local governments in the Baiyangdian basin. The results of this study provide an important reference for ecological conservation and restoration in the Baiyangdian basin. Consistent with previous studies, the findings of this paper suggested that ecological environments tended to be poorer in largely populated and economically developed regions [28,53,54]. It showed that in recent decades, people focused more on economic development, industrialization and urbanization rather than on the protection of the eco-environment. Although the eco-environmental quality of the Baiyangdian basin has improved, the EQI tended to be lower in urban areas. In addition, as the urban areas expanded, this impact was gradually spread to the periphery of the urban areas. Therefore, the eco-environmental problems associated with urban expansion should be fully considered. Land use intensity was an important factor affecting the EQI of the Baiyangdian basin. Therefore, the rationality of land use type conversion should be emphasized in the construction of the Beijing–Tianjin–Hebei urban agglomeration and the Xiong'an New Area. In addition, the natural ecosystem should be protected, and measures should be taken in accordance with local conditions. Efforts should be made to rebuild the ecosystem in Baiyangdian Lake and the Taihang Mountains in the western part of the basin by limiting or avoiding human activities that lead to negative developments in the ecosystem. At the same time, the self-healing function of the ecosystem should be fully utilized. Finally, in terms of cropland, local governments should earnestly implement the policy of compensating the balance of land acquisition, strictly abide by the red line of cropland protection and ensure the efficient use of cropland resources in the Baiyangdian basin based on eco-environmental restoration [55].

4.3. Limitations and Future Directions

There were still some limitations in this study. (1) The existing methods for evaluating eco-environmental quality are lacking in perfection. The EQI of LUCC cannot fully represent the overall eco-environmental quality. Eco-environmental quality is a complex concept, and the broad definition of eco-environmental quality should also take into account factors such as biodiversity and the atmosphere. As far as the EQI of LUCC itself is concerned, there is still room for perfection. The ecosystem is a natural complex, and features ranging from a large basin to a small urban park can be described as an ecosystem. Urban land can still be subdivided into land types such as parks and green belts to evaluate the quality of the ecological environment in different areas of a city. A comprehensive discussion of the above issues was beyond the scope of this study due to the limitations of the data sources, but these factors are crucial to exploring micro-level studies of eco-environmental quality. Therefore, further research is needed in the future to make the EQI more realistic and to better evaluate the impact of different scales and different land use classification systems on ecological and environmental quality assessment results. (2) In terms of influencing factors, although nighttime lighting can reflect the road density of a region to some extent, road density should also be taken into account in future studies, considering the integrity of the detection factor system. Furthermore, the interactions between different influencing factors are very complex. Due to methodological limitations, only the strength of the interaction between the two factors was investigated in this paper. The interactions between more than two factors and the driving mechanisms of the interactions between the influencing factors need to be further refined in subsequent studies.

5. Conclusions

This paper investigated the spatial and temporal distribution patterns of eco-environmental quality in the Baiyangdian basin based on LUCC data and EQI from 2000 to 2020. Based on the GeoDetector model, ten detecting factors were then selected from four aspects, topography, climate, soil and vegetation, human activities and location, to explore and analyze the spatial and temporal evolution mechanisms of eco-environmental quality in the Baiyangdian basin. The spatial and temporal distribution patterns of eco-environmental quality in the Baiyangdian basin and their influencing factors were effectively revealed. The specific results of the study were as follows:

(1) The spatial and temporal land cover changes in the Baiyangdian basin from 2000 to 2020 were complex. During the study period, the area of cropland in the Baiyangdian basin decreased gradually, but the dominance of cropland was difficult to shake. The area of woodland and grassland remained stable in general, and the area of forestland and high-cover grassland increased. In terms of water area, the proportion of water area gradually decreased before 2010, and after 2010, the proportion of both water area and marshland showed an increasing trend. The evolution of the water area roughly coincided with the reclamation of the lake into cropland in the early years and the return of cropland to the lake in the later years. The proportion of construction land was lower, but the expansion of construction land was the fastest during the study period. In terms of the direction of land cover change, dry land had the largest area of conversion outward, and most of the dry land was converted into urban land, rural settlements and other construction land. This indicated that as the scope of human activities has increased, the conflict between people and land has become an urgent problem in the Baiyangdian basin. The change from shrub forest to forestland was also evident. Also evident was the change from bottom land to marshland and from medium- to high-cover grassland. However, there still existed a shift from medium-cover grassland to low-cover grassland and from medium-cover grassland to other construction land in the Baiyangdian basin during the study period. This indicated that some areas in the Baiyangdian basin are still experiencing some eco-environmental degradation and encroachment by human activities on ecological land during the study period. The transformation of rural settlement into urban land is noteworthy. Although the area transferred from rural settlement to urban land was only 48.3221 km^2, this represents the future direction of land use change to a certain extent, which is to alleviate the contradiction between people and land while at the

(2) Overall, the EQI in the Baiyangdian basin showed significant spatial and temporal heterogeneity over the study period. From 2000 to 2020, the EQI of the Baiyangdian basin showed a fluctuating upward trend. Specifically, the EQI of the Baiyangdian basin declined slowly before 2005. From 2005 to 2015, the EQI of the Baiyangdian basin increased significantly. After 2015, the EQI of the Baiyangdian basin showed a small decline. Spatially, the eco-environmental quality index of the Baiyangdian basin had the characteristic of gradually decreasing from northwest to southeast. The EQI of the Taihang Mountains in the western part of the study area was higher than that of the North China Plain in the east, mainly due to the fact that the North China Plain is a population and economic agglomeration in northern China. The concentration of population and economy can easily cause the deterioration of the ecological environment. Baiyangdian Lake, located in the central part of the North China Plain, had a higher EQI and was the hotspot of the EQI in the eastern part of the whole basin.

(3) The results of the factor detector from 2000 to 2020 showed that the impact of land use intensity on the eco-environmental quality was significantly higher than that of the other detecting factors in the Baiyangdian basin. The spatial and temporal evolution of the eco-environmental quality of the Baiyangdian basin was significantly influenced by human activities, whose impact remained generally stable. The influence of topography on the spatial and temporal evolution of eco-environmental quality was relatively strong, but its influence tended to fluctuate downwards during the study period. Climate, soil and vegetation as well as location had some influence on the spatial and temporal evolution of the eco-environmental quality of the Baiyangdian basin, but their influence was weaker compared to topography and human activities. The strength of the interaction between the influencing factors was greater than that of a single factor. The types of effects were mainly non-linear enhancement and two-factor enhancement.

Author Contributions: B.X. wrote this paper; supervision, B.X. and L.Z.; funding acquisition, L.Z. All authors have read and agreed to the published version of the manuscript.

Funding: This work was funded by the National Social Science Fund of China (Grant No. 20ATJ004) and the Humanities and Social Science major Project of Hebei Education Department (Grant No. ZD201811).

Institutional Review Board Statement: Not applicable.

Informed Consent Statement: Not applicable.

Data Availability Statement: Details in Section 2.3 Data Source.

Conflicts of Interest: The authors declare no conflict of interest.

References

1. Koerper, J.; Hoeschel, I.; Lowe, J.A.; Hewitt, C.D.; Salas y Melia, D.; Roeckner, E.; Huebener, H.; Royer, J.-F.; Dufresne, J.-L.; Pardaens, A.; et al. The Effects of Aggressive Mitigation on Steric Sea Level Rise and Sea Ice Changes. *Clim. Dyn.* **2013**, *40*, 531–550. [CrossRef]
2. Liu, L.; Wen, Y.; Liang, Y.; Zhang, F.; Yang, T. Extreme Weather Impacts on Inland Waterways Transport of Yangtze River. *Atmosphere* **2019**, *10*, 133. [CrossRef]
3. Arrow, K.; Bolin, B.; Costanza, R.; Dasgupta, P.; Folke, C.; Holling, C.S.; Jansson, B.-O.; Levin, S.; Mäler, K.-G.; Perrings, C.; et al. Economic Growth, Carrying Capacity, and the Environment. *Ecol. Econ.* **1995**, *15*, 91–95. [CrossRef]
4. Vitousek, P. Beyond Global Warming: Ecology and Global Change. *Ecology* **1994**, *75*, 1903–1910. [CrossRef]
5. Yi, L.; Zhang, Z.; Zhao, X.; Liu, B.; Wang, X.; Wen, Q.; Zuo, L.; Liu, F.; Xu, J.; Hu, S. Have Changes to Unused Land in China Improved or Exacerbated Its Environmental Quality in the Past Three Decades? *Sustainability* **2016**, *8*, 184. [CrossRef]

6. Zhang, Z.; Wang, X.; Zhao, X.; Liu, B.; Yi, L.; Zuo, L.; Wen, Q.; Liu, F.; Xu, J.; Hu, S. A 2010 Update of National Land Use/Cover Database of China at 1:100000 Scale Using Medium Spatial Resolution Satellite Images. *Remote Sens. Environ.* **2014**, *149*, 142–154. [CrossRef]
7. Dewan, A.M.; Yamaguchi, Y. Land Use and Land Cover Change in Greater Dhaka, Bangladesh: Using Remote Sensing to Promote Sustainable Urbanization. *Appl. Geogr.* **2009**, *29*, 390–401. [CrossRef]
8. Lambin, E.F.; Turner, B.L.; Geist, H.J.; Agbola, S.B.; Angelsen, A.; Bruce, J.W.; Coomes, O.T.; Dirzo, R.; Fischer, G.; Folke, C.; et al. The Causes of Land-Use and Land-Cover Change: Moving beyond the Myths. *Glob. Environ. Chang.* **2001**, *11*, 261–269. [CrossRef]
9. Tan, R.; Liu, Y.; Zhou, K.; Jiao, L.; Tang, W. A Game-Theory Based Agent-Cellular Model for Use in Urban Growth Simulation: A Case Study of the Rapidly Urbanizing Wuhan Area of Central China. *Comput. Environ. Urban Syst.* **2015**, *49*, 15–29. [CrossRef]
10. Fang, L.; Wang, L.; Chen, W.; Sun, J.; Cao, Q.; Wang, S.; Wang, L. Identifying the Impacts of Natural and Human Factors on Ecosystem Service in the Yangtze and Yellow River Basins. *J. Clean. Prod.* **2021**, *314*, 127995. [CrossRef]
11. Du, X.; Huang, Z. Ecological and Environmental Effects of Land Use Change in Rapid Urbanization: The Case of Hangzhou, China. *Ecol. Indic.* **2017**, *81*, 243–251. [CrossRef]
12. Chase, T.N.; Pielke, R.A., Sr.; Kittel, T.G.F.; Nemani, R.R.; Running, S.W. Simulated Impacts of Historical Land Cover Changes on Global Climate in Northern Winter. *Clim. Dyn.* **2000**, *16*, 93–105. [CrossRef]
13. Houghton, R.A.; Hackler, J.L.; Lawrence, K.T. The U.S. Carbon Budget: Contributions from Land-Use Change. *Science* **1999**, *285*, 574–578. [CrossRef]
14. Sala, O.E.; Chapin, F.S.; Armesto, J.J.; Berlow, E.; Bloomfield, J.; Dirzo, R.; Huber-Sanwald, E.; Huenneke, L.F.; Jackson, R.B.; Kinzig, A.; et al. Global Biodiversity Scenarios for the Year 2100. *Science* **2000**, *287*, 1770–1774. [CrossRef]
15. Li, Y.; Cao, Z.; Long, H.; Liu, Y.; Li, W. Dynamic Analysis of Ecological Environment Combined with Land Cover and NDVI Changes and Implications for Sustainable Urban–Rural Development: The Case of Mu Us Sandy Land, China. *J. Clean. Prod.* **2017**, *142*, 697–715. [CrossRef]
16. Moreira, A.; Bremm, C.; Fontana, D.C.; Kuplich, T.M. Seasonal Dynamics of Vegetation Indices as a Criterion for Grouping Grassland Typologies. *Sci. Agric.* **2019**, *76*, 24–32. [CrossRef]
17. Kumari, N.; Srivastava, A.; Dumka, U.C. A Long-Term Spatiotemporal Analysis of Vegetation Greenness over the Himalayan Region Using Google Earth Engine. *Climate* **2021**, *9*, 109. [CrossRef]
18. Chen, S.; Feng, Y.; Tong, X.; Liu, S.; Xie, H.; Gao, C.; Lei, Z. Modeling ESV Losses Caused by Urban Expansion Using Cellular Automata and Geographically Weighted Regression. *Sci. Total Environ.* **2020**, *712*, 136509. [CrossRef]
19. Jiang, F.; Zhang, Y.; Li, J.; Sun, Z. Research on Remote Sensing Ecological Environmental Assessment Method Optimized by Regional Scale. *Environ. Sci. Pollut. Res.* **2021**, *28*, 68174–68187. [CrossRef]
20. Peng, J.; Xu, Y.; Cai, Y.; Xiao, H. Climatic and Anthropogenic Drivers of Land Use/Cover Change in Fragile Karst Areas of Southwest China since the Early 1970s: A Case Study on the Maotiaohe Watershed. *Environ. Earth Sci.* **2011**, *64*, 2107–2118. [CrossRef]
21. Xu, Y.; Li, P.; Pan, J.; Zhang, Y.; Dang, X.; Cao, X.; Cui, J.; Yang, Z. Eco-Environmental Effects and Spatial Heterogeneity of "Production-Ecology-Living" Land Use Transformation: A Case Study for Ningxia, China. *Sustainability* **2022**, *14*, 9659. [CrossRef]
22. Abera, W.; Tamene, L.; Abegaz, A.; Hailu, H.; Piikki, K.; Söderström, M.; Girvetz, E.; Sommer, R. Estimating Spatially Distributed SOC Sequestration Potentials of Sustainable Land Management Practices in Ethiopia. *J. Environ. Manag.* **2021**, *286*, 112191. [CrossRef] [PubMed]
23. Yang, Z.; Fang, H.; Xue, X. Sustainable Efficiency and CO_2 Reduction Potential of China's Construction Industry: Application of a Three-Stage Virtual Frontier SBM-DEA Model. *J. Asian Archit. Build. Eng.* **2021**, *21*, 604–617. [CrossRef]
24. Liu, Y.; Huang, X.; Yang, H.; Zhong, T. Environmental Effects of Land-Use/Cover Change Caused by Urbanization and Policies in Southwest China Karst Area—A Case Study of Guiyang. *Habitat Int.* **2014**, *44*, 339–348. [CrossRef]
25. Ren, Y.; Lü, Y.; Fu, B.; Comber, A.; Li, T.; Hu, J. Driving Factors of Land Change in China's Loess Plateau: Quantification Using Geographically Weighted Regression and Management Implications. *Remote Sens.* **2020**, *12*, 453. [CrossRef]
26. Liu, Y.; Wu, K.; Cao, H. Land-Use Change and Its Driving Factors in Henan Province from 1995 to 2015. *Arab. J. Geosci.* **2022**, *15*, 247. [CrossRef]
27. Wang, J.-F.; Hu, Y. Environmental Health Risk Detection with GeogDetector. *Environ. Modell. Softw.* **2012**, *33*, 114–115. [CrossRef]
28. Hu, P.; Li, F.; Sun, X.; Liu, Y.; Chen, X.; Hu, D. Assessment of Land-Use/Cover Changes and Its Ecological Effect in Rapidly Urbanized Areas—Taking Pearl River Delta Urban Agglomeration as a Case. *Sustainability* **2021**, *13*, 5075. [CrossRef]
29. Zhao, X.; Liu, J.; Bu, Y. Quantitative Analysis of Spatial Heterogeneity and Driving Forces of the Thermal Environment in Urban Built-up Areas: A Case Study in Xi'an, China. *Sustainability* **2021**, *13*, 1870. [CrossRef]
30. Luo, X.; Tong, X.; Pan, H. Integrating Multiresolution and Multitemporal Sentinel-2 Imagery for Land-Cover Mapping in the Xiongan New Area, China. *IEEE Trans. Geosci. Remote Sens.* **2021**, *59*, 1029–1040. [CrossRef]
31. Li, Y.; Lv, J.; Li, L. Coordinated Development of Water Environment Protection and Water Ecological Carbon Sink in Baiyangdian Lake. *Processes* **2021**, *9*, 2066. [CrossRef]
32. Li, J.; Fang, Z.; Zhang, J.; Huang, Q.; He, C. Mapping Basin-Scale Supply-Demand Dynamics of Flood Regulation Service-A Case Study in the Baiyangdian Lake Basin, China. *Ecol. Indic.* **2022**, *139*, 108902. [CrossRef]
33. Xianghong, D.; Xiyong, H.; Yuandong, W.; Li, W. Spatial-Temporal Characteristics of Land Use Intensity of Coastal Zone in China During 2000-2010. *Chin. Geogr. Sci.* **2015**, *25*, 51–61. [CrossRef]

34. Wang, J.; Li, X.-H.; Christakos, G.; Liao, Y.-L.; Zhang, T.; Gu, X.; Zheng, X.-Y. Geographical Detectors-Based Health Risk Assessment and Its Application in the Neural Tube Defects Study of the Heshun Region, China. *Int. J. Geogr. Inf. Sci.* **2010**, *24*, 107–127. [CrossRef]
35. Li, Z.; Liu, W.; Zheng, F. The Land Use Changes and Its Relationship with Topographic Factors in the Jing River Catchment on the Loess Plateau of China. *SpringerPlus* **2013**, *2*, S3. [CrossRef]
36. Lin, J.; Chen, W.; Qi, X.; Hou, H. Risk Assessment and Its Influencing Factors Analysis of Geological Hazards in Typical Mountain Environment. *J. Clean. Prod.* **2021**, *309*, 127077. [CrossRef]
37. Wang, J.-F.; Wang, Y.; Zhang, J.; Christakos, G.; Sun, J.-L.; Liu, X.; Lu, L.; Fu, X.-Q.; Shi, Y.-Q.; Li, X.-M. Spatiotemporal Transmission and Determinants of Typhoid and Paratyphoid Fever in Hongta District, Yunnan Province, China. *PLoS Neglect. Trop. Dis.* **2013**, *7*, e2112. [CrossRef]
38. Cai, B.; Shao, Z.; Fang, S.; Huang, X.; Huq, M.E.; Tang, Y.; Li, Y.; Zhuang, Q. Finer-Scale Spatiotemporal Coupling Coordination Model between Socioeconomic Activity and Eco-Environment: A Case Study of Beijing, China. *Ecol. Indic.* **2021**, *131*, 108165. [CrossRef]
39. Haag, S.; Shakibajahromi, B.; Shokoufandeh, A. A New Rapid Watershed Delineation Algorithm for 2D Flow Direction Grids. *Environ. Model. Softw.* **2018**, *109*, 420–428. [CrossRef]
40. Sliwinski, D.; Konieczna, A.; Roman, K. Geostatistical Resampling of LiDAR-Derived DEM in Wide Resolution Range for Modelling in SWAT: A Case Study of Zglowiaczka River (Poland). *Remote Sens.* **2022**, *14*, 1281. [CrossRef]
41. Banerjee, A.; Duflo, E.; Qian, N. On the Road: Access to Transportation Infrastructure and Economic Growth in China. *J. Dev. Econ.* **2020**, *145*, 102442. [CrossRef]
42. Xu, Z.; Wei, H.; Fan, W.; Wang, X.; Huang, B.; Lu, N.; Ren, J.; Dong, X. Energy Modeling Simulation of Changes in Ecosystem Services before and after the Implementation of a Grain-for-Green Program on the Loess Plateau-A Case Study of the Zhifanggou Valley in Ansai County, Shaanxi Province, China. *Ecosyst. Serv.* **2018**, *31*, 32–43. [CrossRef]
43. Zhou, T.; Shen, W.; Qiu, X.; Chang, H.; Yang, H.; Yang, W. Impact Evaluation of a Payments for Ecosystem Services Program on Vegetation Quantity and Quality Restoration in Inner Mongolia. *J. Environ. Manag.* **2022**, *303*, 114113. [CrossRef] [PubMed]
44. Yang, Y.; Cai, Z. Ecological Security Assessment of the Guanzhong Plain Urban Agglomeration Based on an Adapted Ecological Footprint Model. *J. Clean. Prod.* **2020**, *260*, 120973. [CrossRef]
45. Costanza, R.; de Groot, R.; Sutton, P.; van der Ploeg, S.; Anderson, S.J.; Kubiszewski, I.; Farber, S.; Turner, R.K. Changes in the Global Value of Ecosystem Services. *Glob. Environ. Chang.* **2014**, *26*, 152–158. [CrossRef]
46. Ge, F.; Tang, G.; Zhong, M.; Zhang, Y.; Xiao, J.; Li, J.; Ge, F. Assessment of Ecosystem Health and Its Key Determinants in the Middle Reaches of the Yangtze River Urban Agglomeration, China. *Int. J. Environ. Res. Public Health* **2022**, *19*, 771. [CrossRef]
47. Guo, B.; Wei, C.; Yu, Y.; Liu, Y.; Li, J.; Meng, C.; Cai, Y. The Dominant Influencing Factors of Desertification Changes in the Source Region of Yellow River: Climate Change or Human Activity? *Sci. Total Environ.* **2022**, *813*, 152512. [CrossRef]
48. Keola, S.; Andersson, M.; Hall, O. Monitoring Economic Development from Space: Using Nighttime Light and Land Cover Data to Measure Economic Growth. *World Dev.* **2015**, *66*, 322–334. [CrossRef]
49. Lv, Q.; Liu, H.; Wang, J.; Liu, H.; Shang, Y. Multiscale Analysis on Spatiotemporal Dynamics of Energy Consumption CO2 Emissions in China: Utilizing the Integrated of DMSP-OLS and NPP-VIIRS Nighttime Light Datasets. *Sci. Total Environ.* **2020**, *703*, 134394. [CrossRef]
50. Kang, P.; Chen, W.; Hou, Y.; Li, Y. Linking Ecosystem Services and Ecosystem Health to Ecological Risk Assessment: A Case Study of the Beijing-Tianjin-Hebei Urban Agglomeration. *Sci. Total Environ.* **2018**, *636*, 1442–1454. [CrossRef]
51. Tang, D.; Liu, X.; Zou, X. An Improved Method for Integrated Ecosystem Health Assessments Based on the Structure and Function of Coastal Ecosystems: A Case Study of the Jiangsu Coastal Area, China. *Ecol. Indic.* **2018**, *84*, 82–95. [CrossRef]
52. Zhao, Y.; Wang, S.; Zhang, F.; Shen, Q.; Li, J.; Yang, F. Remote Sensing-Based Analysis of Spatial and Temporal Water Colour Variations in Baiyangdian Lake after the Establishment of the Xiong'an New Area. *Remote Sens.* **2021**, *13*, 1729. [CrossRef]
53. Peng, J.; Liu, Y.; Wu, J.; Lv, H.; Hu, X. Linking Ecosystem Services and Landscape Patterns to Assess Urban Ecosystem Health: A Case Study in Shenzhen City, China. *Landsc. Urban Plan.* **2015**, *143*, 56–68. [CrossRef]
54. Xiao, R.; Yu, X.; Shi, R.; Zhang, Z.; Yu, W.; Li, Y.; Chen, G.; Gao, J. Ecosystem Health Monitoring in the Shanghai-Hangzhou Bay Metropolitan Area: A Hidden Markov Modeling Approach. *Environ. Int.* **2019**, *133*, 105170. [CrossRef]
55. Sklenicka, P. Classification of Farmland Ownership Fragmentation as a Cause of Land Degradation: A Review on Typology, Consequences, and Remedies. *Land Use Policy* **2016**, *57*, 694–701. [CrossRef]
56. Cao, S.; Yu, N.; Wu, Y.; Wang, Z.; Mi, J. The Educational Level of Rural Labor, Population Urbanization, and Sustainable Economic Growth in China. *Sustainability* **2020**, *12*, 4860. [CrossRef]

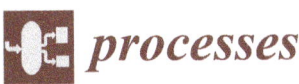

Article

Application of Beetle Colony Optimization Based on Improvement of Rebellious Growth Characteristics in PM$_{2.5}$ Concentration Prediction

Yizhun Zhang [1] and Qisheng Yan [2,*]

1 School of Earth Sciences, East China University of Technology, Nanchang 330013, China
2 School of Science, East China University of Technology, Nanchang 330013, China
* Correspondence: 199760023@ecut.edu.cn

Abstract: Aiming at the shortcomings of the beetle swarm algorithm, namely its low accuracy, easy fall into local optima, and slow convergence speed, a rebellious growth personality–beetle swarm optimization (RGP–BSO) model based on rebellious growth personality is proposed. Firstly, the growth and rebellious characters were added to the beetle swarm optimization algorithm to dynamically adjust the beetle's judgment of the optimal position. Secondly, the adaptive iterative selection strategy is introduced to balance the beetles' global search and local search capabilities, preventing the algorithm from falling into a locally optimal solution. Finally, two dynamic factors are introduced to promote the maturity of the character and further improve the algorithm's optimization ability and convergence accuracy. The twelve standard test function simulation experiments show that RGP–BSO has a faster convergence speed and higher accuracy than other optimization algorithms. In the practical problem of PM$_{2.5}$ concentration prediction, the ELM model optimized by RGP–BSO has more prominent accuracy and stability and has obvious advantages.

Keywords: growth character; rebellious character; beetle swarm optimization; test function; local optimum; character decision

1. Introduction

Optimization plays a crucial role in the efficient operation of almost all real-world systems [1]. The core basis of the optimization process is to achieve trade-offs between multiple conflicting criteria for a given decision problem, with the primary purpose of minimizing computational effort to determine feasible trade-off points [2]. Wolpert, in 1997, proposed the theory that there is no free lunch, i.e., there cannot be one algorithm that will be most efficient for every problem to be solved [3]. Therefore, various optimization algorithms have been proposed and applied in different research fields in the past ten years.

Optimization algorithms mainly include two categories: gradient-based methods and metaheuristics. For continuous and linear problems, gradient-based methods can be used. For example, Zhadan uses the original dual Newton method to consider the linear semidefinite programming problem [4]; Vijayalakshmi used stochastic gradient descent to optimize the ANN model to predict the energy capacity ACs [5]. For more complex issues, metaheuristics are favored for their stability, flexibility, and better ability to jump out of local optima [6], such as the seagull optimization algorithm [7], particle swarm optimization algorithm [8], gray wolf optimization algorithm [9], and whale optimization algorithm [10].

Because of the great potential of metaheuristics in solving complex problems, Jiang developed an optimization algorithm called beetle antennae search (BAS). The algorithm was inspired by the beetle experiment at Cornell University [11]. The long beetle senses the difference in the smell of things according to the antennae's fibers, draws the odor intensity map of the surrounding environment, and finds the direction of the odor according to the map [12]. Its most significant advantage is that the complexity involved is low, and the number of individuals is only one, which can solve the problem in a shorter time. However, the iterative result of the BAS algorithm is very dependent on the initial position of the beetle, and the number of individuals is only one, resulting in low efficiency and effectiveness of the optimization. Inspired by the swarm algorithm, Wang improved the BAS algorithm and expanded the individual into a swarm to become the beetle swarm optimization (BSO) algorithm [13]. Although the BSO algorithm solves the problem of low optimization effectiveness of the BAS algorithm, there are still problems of local optima and poor population diversity in iterations [14].

This paper proposes a beetle swarm optimization algorithm based on rebellious growth personality (RGP–BSO). First, we increase the rebellious character to improve the global search ability of the beetle herd and increase the growth character to enhance the power of the beetle herd to converge to the optimal value. Secondly, the ability of global search and local search of beetles is balanced through a personality selection strategy. Finally, two dynamic factors are introduced to promote the maturity of the character and further improve the convergence ability and accuracy of the algorithm. Using twelve benchmark functions to conduct simulation experiments, the algorithm of RGP–BSO has an extensive performance advantage compared with other optimization algorithms. The model's performance is evaluated using MAPE, RMSE, and MAE in a practical problem of $PM_{2.5}$ concentration prediction to explore the effectiveness of the RGP–BSO optimization algorithm on $PM_{2.5}$ concentration prediction. The ELM model optimized by RGP–BSO has outstanding accuracy and stability with apparent advantages. With appropriate computational resources, high-quality solutions can be obtained, providing theoretical and methodological support for human travel patterns, governmental decision making, etc., and providing data support for the RGP–BSO optimization algorithm to perform better in practical applications.

2. Beetle Swarm Optimization Algorithm

The beetle swarm algorithm is inspired by the particle swarm algorithm and improved by the beetle search algorithm. The updated formula of the beetle swarm algorithm is [13]:

$$X_i^{k+1} = X_i^k + \lambda V_i^k + (1-\lambda) Y_i^k \tag{1}$$

In the formula: i is the ith beetle, k is the number of iterations, and X_i^k is the position of the ith beetle in the kth iteration. V_i^k is the velocity of the ith beetle at the kth iteration. Y_i^k is the increase in the moving position of the ith beetle at the kth iteration, constant $\lambda \in [0, 1]$. The speed update formula of the beetle swarm follows the speed update formula of the particle swarm optimization algorithm. The update of the position of the beetle is based on the search algorithm of the beetle, and the procedure is as follows:

$$V_i^{k+1} = \omega V_i^k + c_1 r_1 (P_i^k - X_i^k) + c_2 r_2 (G^k - X_i^k) \tag{2}$$

$$Y_i^{k+1} = \delta^k * V_i^k \vec{b} * sign(f(x_r) - f(x_l)) \tag{3}$$

In the formula: c_1 and c_2 are two positive numbers. r_1 and r_2 are two random numbers in the range [0,1]. ω is the adaptive inertia weight. P_i^k is the best position experienced by the ith beetle after k iterations. G^k is the global best position of the beetle herd at the kth iteration. δ^k is the step size of the beetle at the kth iteration. $sign$ is a symbolic function that determines whether the search direction after the beetle is the left whisker or the right whisker. $f(x_r)$ is the fitness function, i.e., the solution of the solution function at the position of x_r. x_r and x_l are the positions of the right and left whiskers of the beetle, respectively. $\vec{b}$ is the random orientation of the beetle after the beetle moves. The calculation method is as follows:

$$\vec{b} = \frac{rnd(s,1)}{\|rnd(s,1)\|} \tag{4}$$

$$x_r^{k+1} = x_r^k + V_i^k * d/2 \tag{5}$$

$$x_l^{k+1} = x_l^k - V_i^k * d/2 \tag{6}$$

In the formula: *rnd* represents the random function, and s is the dimension of the problem to be optimized. d represents the distance between the two antennas. To sum up, it can be seen that the Tianniu swarm algorithm is easy to fall into local optima when optimizing, and the ability to jump out of local optima is weak.

3. Improved Beetle Swarm Optimization Algorithm

Aiming at the problem the beetle herd algorithm—it has low precision and can easily fall into local optima—this paper proposes the beetle herd optimization algorithm with rebellious growth character (RGP–BSO).

3.1. Rebellious Growth Character

Inspired by the short flight ability of the beetle, the improved beetle swarm optimization algorithm is used to solve the problem wherein the beetle herd is prone to fall into local optima. When a beetle moves, it will actively share the location it has experienced with the group, which is used as the basis for updating the optimal site of the group. When a beetle moves, it may have a rebellious character. It will not focus more on the global optimal point and its individual optimal point but may envy the optimal point passed by other beetles in the population. Then, it uses the flying ability to randomly fly to the particular optimal moment of a certain beetle in the population. Then, the updated formula for the position of the left and right whiskers is as follows:

$$x_r^{k+1} = P_{rN}^k + V_i^k * d/2 \tag{7}$$

$$x_l^{k+1} = P_{lN}^k - V_i^k * d/2 \tag{8}$$

In the formula: N is a random number, and P_{rN}^k is the individual optimal point experienced by the right whisker of the random Nth beetle in the kth iteration. P_{rN}^k means that when the position of the right whisker of the beetle is updated, the position that he participates in after the update is no longer his optimal position. Instead, the optimal position is that of the original individual randomly selected individual N in the herd, and the original beetle flies to the optimal position of individual N after a short flight. P_{lN}^k is the personal optimal point shared by the left whisker of the random Nth beetle in the kth iteration. The formula for growing rebellious character is as follows:

The rebellious character position movement formula is:

$$X_i^{k+1} = X_i^k + \lambda_1 V_i^k + (1-\lambda_1)Y_i^k \tag{9}$$

The formula for the position movement of the growth character is:

$$X_i^{k+1} = X_i^k + (1-\lambda_2)V_i^k + \lambda_2 Y_i^k \tag{10}$$

λ_1 and λ_2 are adaptive weights, and the value ranges of λ_1 and λ_2 are both [0, 0.5]. The primary role of V is to converge to the global optimum, while the role of Y is to jump out of the local optimum and improve the global search ability. In the rebellious character, to ensure the power of the algorithm to jump out of the local optimum, it is necessary to ensure that Y is always maintained at the corresponding ratio. In the growth character, to keep the ability to converge to the optimum, it is essential to ensure that V is maintained in a particular proportion. After many experiments, it is proved that the algorithm performs best when both λ_1 and λ_2 are kept at [0, 0.5]. As the number of iterations increases, the values of λ_1 and λ_2 become lower and lower until they reach 0. With a decrease in λ_1 and λ_2, the proportion of V in the rebellious character will gradually decrease, and the Y ratio will increase progressively. The global search ability of the rebellious character will become stronger and stronger. The proportion of V in the growth personality will gradually increase, the ratio of Y will gradually decrease, and the movement trend of the growth character will tend progressively to the global best and converge to the global best.

3.2. Dynamic Factors of Personality Maturity

In order to make the character mature, the characteristics and abilities of each character in the later stage of the iteration are gradually enhanced. We accommodate solution details for problems that change with iterations. An adaptive inertia weight reduction strategy is introduced, and the formula is as follows:

$$\lambda = \lambda_{max} - \frac{\lambda_{max} - \lambda_{min}}{K} * k \quad (11)$$

In the formula: the λ_{max} constant is 0.5, the λ_{min} constant is 0, K is the total number of iterations, and k is the current iteration number. When λ_{max} is set to 0.5 and λ_{min} is set to 0, the value range of λ is [0, 0.5]. We substitute λ into λ_1 of Formula (9) to gradually improve the global search ability of rebellious characters. Substituting λ into λ_2 of Formula (10) is used to progressively enhance the growth character's optimization precision.

3.3. Personality Choice Strategies

Each particle faces the problem in different ways in the swarm optimization algorithm. When only sticking to one method, it is easy to miss the optimal solution, increase the optimization time, and reduce the convergence speed. This paper introduces a personality selection strategy to allow each beetle to choose its optimization method in different positions and iterations.

When solving the maximum value problem:

$$\begin{cases} X_i^{k+1} = X_i^k + \lambda_1 V_i^k + (1-\lambda_1) Y_i^k, f(X_i^k) \leq f_{average}^k \\ X_i^{k+1} = X_i^k + (1-\lambda_2) V_i^k + \lambda_2 Y_i^k, f(X_i^k) \geq f_{average}^k \end{cases} \quad (12)$$

When solving the minimum problem:

$$\begin{cases} X_i^{k+1} = X_i^k + \lambda_1 V_i^k + (1-\lambda_1) Y_i^k, f(X_i^k) \geq f_{average}^k \\ X_i^{k+1} = X_i^k + (1-\lambda_2) V_i^k + \lambda_2 Y_i^k, f(X_i^k) \leq f_{average}^k \end{cases} \quad (13)$$

In the formula: $f(X_i^k)$ is the fitness value of the ith beetle in the kth generation. $f_{average}^k$ is the average fitness value of the beetle herd in k iterations. We solve for the minimum value, as an example, when the fitness value of the beetle in the kth iteration is greater than the average fitness value. We prove that when the position of the beetle is not good, the beetle chooses a rebellious character, increasing the weight of individual best positions and the probability of flying into random beetles. When the fitness value of the kth iteration is less than the average fitness value, it proves that the position of the beetle is acceptable, and the beetle chooses the growth character, focusing on the global optimum and the individual optimum.

3.4. Algorithm Process

The specific flow chart of the RGP–BSO algorithm is shown in Figure 1. The steps of the RGP–BSO algorithm are as follows:

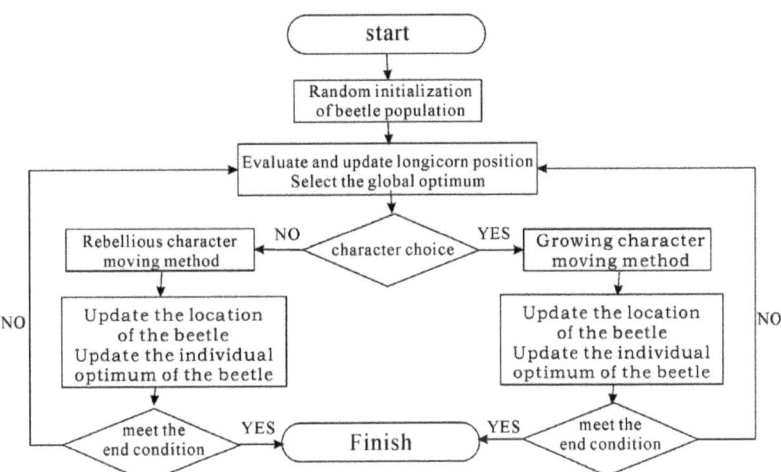

Figure 1. Algorithm flow chart.

Step 1: Initialize the parameters of the beetle herd, including population number, number of iterations, initial position, initial speed, inertia weight, etc. Step 2: Evaluate the status of each beetle, select the globally optimal function, and calculate the average fitness of the beetle population. Step 3: According to Formula (12) or Formula (13), the fitness of each beetle is judged, and the appropriate character is selected. Step 4: According to the two characters of Formulas (9) and (10), update the position of the beetle and update the individual optima. Step 5: Determine whether the number of iterations k satisfies the end condition. If so, output the optimal global value. Otherwise, repeat Steps 2 to 5.

4. Simulation Experiment and Analysis

4.1. Experiment Setup

In order to verify the optimized performance of the RGP–BSO algorithm this paper, particle swarm optimization (PSO) [15], differential evolution (DE) [16], beetle antennae search (BAS) [17], beetle swarm optimization (BSO) [18], sparrow search algorithm (SSA) [19], and cuckoo Search (CS) [20], six algorithms in total, are compared on 12 typical benchmark functions. This comparison is performed to evaluate the algorithm optimization accuracy and convergence speed.

The 12 selected test functions are shown in Table 1. The search range and optimal value of the function are shown in the table. In order to ensure the accuracy of the experiment, the population size of all optimization algorithms is set to 50 and the maximum number of iterations is 100. After several experiments, we have demonstrated that the average performance of each optimization algorithm is more stable when the population size is set to 50. When the number of iterations is set to 100, each optimization algorithm converges to the global optimum or a local optimum, and too many iterations only increase the redundancy time of the operation. Therefore, to ensure the fairness of the experiment, we set the population to 50 and the number of iterations to 100. The simulation software used in this paper is Matlab2018.

Table 1. Test function.

Numbering	Function Name	Function Image	Domain of Definition	Optimal Value
f1	Ackley		$[-5, 5]$	0
f2	Bukin		$[-10, 10]$	0
f3	Cigar		$[-5, 5]$	0
f4	Cross-in-tray		$[-10, 10]$	-2.06261
f5	Drop-wave		$[-5, 5]$	-1
f6	Griewank		$[-600, 600]$	0
f7	Holdertable		$[-10, 10]$	-19.2085

Table 1. Cont.

Numbering	Function Name	Function Image	Domain of Definition	Optimal Value
f8	Levy		[−10,10]	0
f9	Nocon_rastrigin		[−10, 10]	0
f10	Rastrigin		[−5, 5]	0
f11	Shubert		[−10, 10]	−186.7309
f12	Weierstrass		[−1, 1]	0

4.2. Algorithm Performance Analysis

The comparison of algorithm performance indicators is shown in Table 2. In the 12 test functions, each group of algorithms is executed 30 times and the optimal value (Best), the mean value (Mean), and the standard deviation (Std) of the 30 executions are obtained. The data in the analysis table can be obtained. The RGP–BSO algorithm shows strong optimization ability and convergence accuracy on both unimodal and multimodal functions, which corrects the problem of the BSO algorithm falling into local optima easily.

Table 2. Algorithm optimization performance comparison.

Function	Test Indicators	PSO	BAS	BSO	RGP–BSO	DE	SSA	CS
f1	Best	0.00×10^0	8.46×10^{-4}	7.56×10^{-4}	0.00×10^0	1.55×10^{-6}	0.00×10^0	5.46×10^{-4}
	Mean	2.54×10^{-9}	4.02×10^{-3}	9.61×10^{-3}	0.00×10^0	2.68×10^{-5}	0.00×10^0	7.58×10^{-2}
	Std	2.19×10^{-9}	2.13×10^{-3}	6.47×10^{-3}	0.00×10^0	2.25×10^{-5}	0.00×10^0	1.09×10^{-1}
f2	Best	6.72×10^{-2}	2.70×10^{-1}	1.45×10^{-1}	1.00×10^{-1}	5.00×10^{-2}	1.00×10^{-1}	1.09×10^1
	Mean	1.00×10^{-1}	1.29×10^0	3.12×10^{-1}	1.00×10^{-1}	7.53×10^{-1}	1.00×10^{-1}	4.19×10^1
	Std	1.82×10^{-2}	5.98×10^{-1}	1.40×10^{-1}	4.23×10^{-17}	9.70×10^{-1}	4.23×10^{-17}	4.17×10^1
f3	Best	0.00×10^0	1.32×10^{-3}	9.77×10^{-6}	0.00×10^0	3.66×10^{-11}	0.00×10^0	8.85×10^{-2}
	Mean	8.75×10^{-15}	6.41×10^0	1.32×10^{-2}	0.00×10^0	1.03×10^{-8}	0.00×10^0	1.61×10^2
	Std	1.65×10^{-14}	5.83×10^0	1.96×10^{-2}	0.00×10^0	1.23×10^{-8}	0.00×10^0	3.60×10^2
f4	Best	-2.06×10^0	-2.06×10^0	-2.06×10^0	-2.06×10^0	-2.06×10^0	-2.06×10^0	-2.06×10^0
	Mean	-2.06×10^0	-1.92×10^0	-2.06×10^0	-2.06×10^0	-2.06×10^0	-2.06×10^0	-2.06×10^0
	Std	1.03×10^{-15}	1.01×10^{-1}	4.98×10^{-6}	1.05×10^{-15}	2.52×10^{-5}	1.66×10^{-7}	4.28×10^{-4}
f5	Best	-1.00×10^0	-9.36×10^{-1}	-9.99×10^{-1}	-1.00×10^0	-9.93×10^{-1}	-1.00×10^0	-1.00×10^0
	Mean	-1.00×10^0	-6.44×10^{-1}	-9.70×10^{-1}	-1.00×10^0	-9.38×10^{-1}	-1.00×10^0	-9.01×10^{-1}
	Std	2.05×10^{-13}	2.47×10^{-1}	2.69×10^{-2}	0.00×10^0	1.43×10^{-2}	0.00×10^0	9.43×10^{-2}
f6	Best	0.00×10^0	2.60×10^{-10}	1.22×10^{-14}	0.00×10^0	0.00×10^0	0.00×10^0	1.32×10^{-10}
	Mean	0.00×10^0	1.41×10^{-1}	8.45×10^{-1}	0.00×10^0	0.00×10^0	0.00×10^0	9.86×10^{-5}
	Std	0.00×10^0	1.34×10^{-1}	1.55×10^{-9}	0.00×10^0	0.00×10^0	0.00×10^0	1.67×10^{-4}
f7	Best	-1.92×10^1	-1.92×10^1	-1.92×10^1	-1.92×10^1	-1.92×10^1	-1.92×10^1	-1.51×10^1
	Mean	-1.55×10^1	-6.32×10^0	-1.89×10^1	-1.92×10^1	-1.91×10^1	-1.76×10^1	-1.51×10^1
	Std	4.60×10^0	4.97×10^0	1.50×10^0	1.99×10^{-8}	3.73×10^{-1}	1.46×10^0	5.42×10^{-15}
f8	Best	0.00×10^0	6.02×10^{-8}	1.33×10^{-7}	0.00×10^0	1.35×10^{-13}	3.94×10^{-10}	3.44×10^{-9}
	Mean	9.74×10^{-19}	5.53×10^{-6}	5.00×10^{-6}	0.00×10^0	5.37×10^{-11}	8.49×10^{-7}	7.18×10^{-4}
	Std	1.18×10^{-18}	1.12×10^0	6.18×10^{-6}	1.11×10^{-47}	6.70×10^{-11}	1.96×10^{-6}	1.81×10^{-3}
f9	Best	0.00×10^0	7.19×10^{-4}	7.53×10^{-4}	0.00×10^0	2.31×10^{-6}	0.00×10^0	6.92×10^{-7}
	Mean	1.33×10^{-1}	5.13×10^0	3.53×10^{-1}	0.00×10^0	4.86×10^{-3}	0.00×10^0	7.53×10^{-1}
	Std	3.46×10^{-1}	4.68×10^0	4.01×10^{-1}	0.00×10^0	1.71×10^{-2}	0.00×10^0	8.86×10^{-1}
f10	Best	0.00×10^0	9.95×10^{-1}	8.55×10^{-4}	0.00×10^0	3.10×10^{-7}	0.00×10^0	1.45×10^{-4}
	Mean	9.95×10^{-2}	6.13×10^0	6.43×10^{-2}	0.00×10^0	1.87×10^{-2}	0.00×10^0	5.72×10^{-1}
	Std	3.04×10^{-1}	4.88×10^0	1.88×10^{-1}	0.00×10^0	3.79×10^{-4}	0.00×10^0	8.28×10^{-1}
f11	Best	-1.87×10^2	-1.87×10^2	-1.87×10^2	-1.87×10^2	-1.87×10^2	-1.87×10^2	4.46×10^{-9}
	Mean	-1.87×10^2	-5.50×10^1	-1.86×10^2	-1.87×10^2	-1.87×10^2	-1.71×10^2	1.00×10^0
	Std	6.96×10^{-14}	4.75×10^1	2.82×10^0	2.08×10^{-12}	8.80×10^{-2}	1.88×10^1	2.02×10^0
f12	Best	0.00×10^0	0.00×10^0	0.00×10^0	0.00×10^0	0.00×10^0	0.00×10^0	0.00×10^0
	Mean	2.68×10^{-5}	1.39×10^{-1}	5.06×10^{-2}	0.00×10^0	0.00×10^0	0.00×10^0	0.00×10^0
	Std	4.12×10^{-5}	2.07×10^{-1}	5.28×10^{-2}	0.00×10^0	0.00×10^0	0.00×10^0	0.00×10^0

For the functions f1, f3, f5, f6, f9, f10, and f12, the optimization accuracy of the RGP–BSO algorithm even reached 100%. However, in the f2 function, no algorithms found the global optimal solution of 0. The algorithm with the closest optimization value is the PSO algorithm. However, the standard deviation of the PSO algorithm is large and unstable. Although the optimal value of the RGP–BSO algorithm does not reach the accuracy of the PSO algorithm, the standard deviation is the smallest among the seven algorithms, showing good performance stability. For the function f11, although the optimization reached the optimal value, the standard deviation of the RGP–BSO algorithm is slightly inferior to the PSO algorithm. However, in the optimization comparison of the overall test function, RGP–BSO shows better optimization ability, convergence accuracy, and ability to jump out of local optima.

In order to reflect the convergence speed of the algorithms, the convergence curves of each algorithm for the 12 functions are shown in Figure 2. The convergence speed of the RGP–BSO and SSA algorithms is much higher than other algorithms when the convergence value is 0. However, it can be found that the SSA algorithm quickly falls into the local optimum when the convergence value is not 0, failing to converge to the globally optimum value. The RGP–BSO algorithm ensures the convergence speed, considers the convergence accuracy, and finds the optimal global solution in a concise number of iterations.

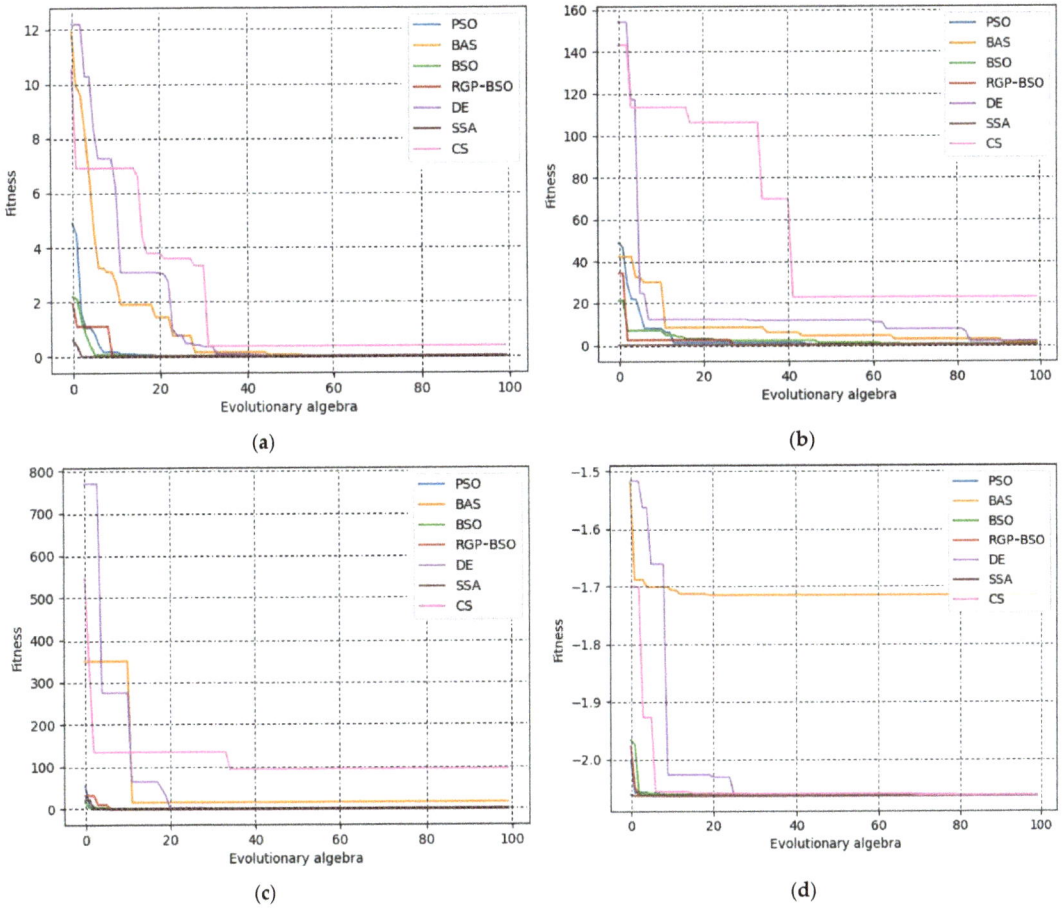

Figure 2. *Cont.*

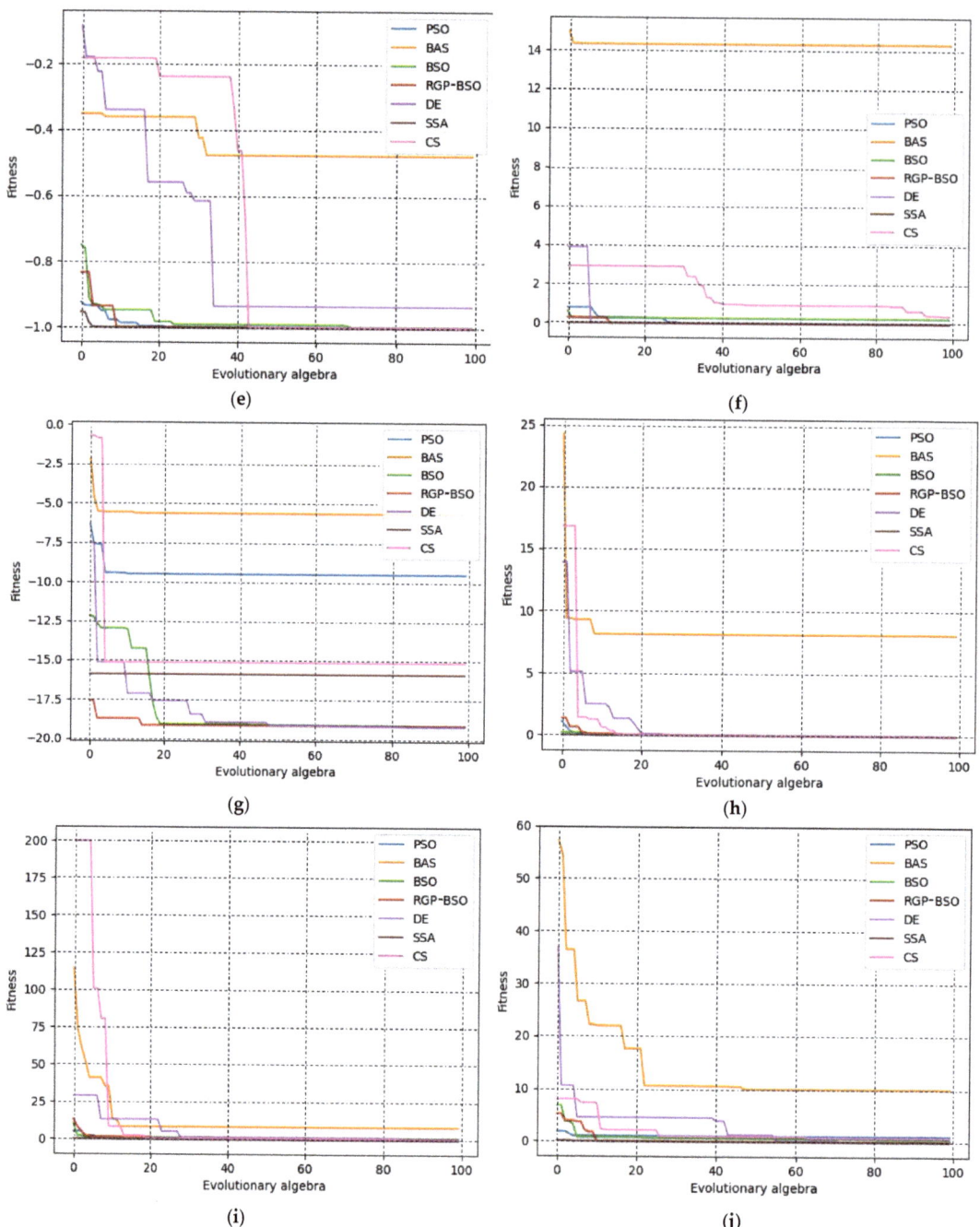

Figure 2. Cont.

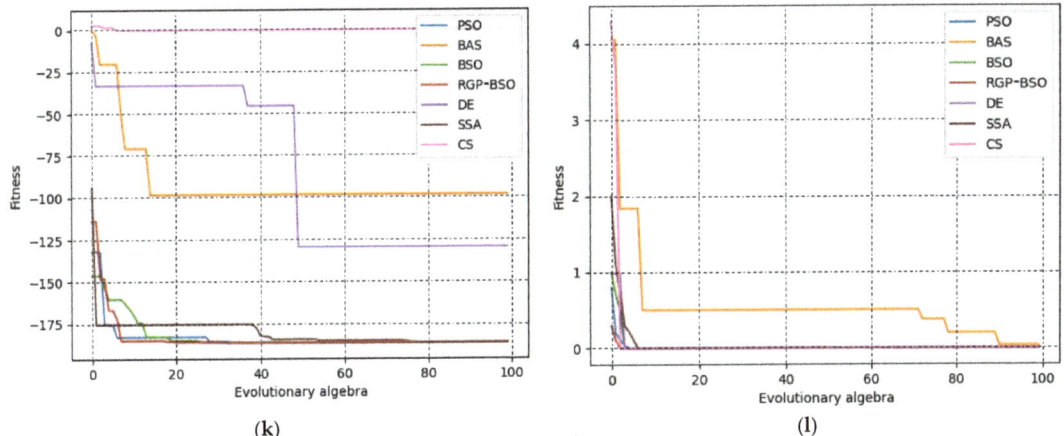

Figure 2. Fitness curve. (**a**) f1 function. (**b**) f2 function. (**c**) f3 function. (**d**) f4 function. (**e**) f5 function. (**f**) f6 function. (**g**) f7 function. (**h**) f8 function. (**i**) f9 function. (**j**) f10 function. (**k**) f11 function. (**l**) f12 function.

5. Construction of RGP–BSO–ELM PM$_{2.5}$ Concentration Prediction Model

In order to further verify the performance of the RGP–BSO optimization algorithm, PSO and BSO are used as comparative optimization algorithms. We optimize the ELM model to predict PM$_{2.5}$ concentration. Most PM$_{2.5}$ concentration predictions only consider time series or space series in the existing research. PM$_{2.5}$ attention is spatially susceptible to external factors such as wind direction, wind speed, relative humidity, and temperature [21]. Temporally, PM$_{2.5}$ concentration is affected by the accumulation of previous PM$_{2.5}$ concentrations [22]. Therefore, Zhang proposed a PM$_{2.5}$ concentration prediction framework based on the K-core idea and label distribution learning. The framework flow chart is shown in Figure 3.

First, the label distribution support vector regression (LDSVR) [23] model was used to calculate the weight of each influencing factor on the PM$_{2.5}$ concentration in the daily data. Secondly, complete ensemble empirical mode decomposition of adaptive noise (CEEMDAN) is used for the modal decomposition of PM$_{2.5}$ concentration factors such as temperature, wind speed, and wind direction. Then, we used the time series forecasting model to predict the data of the influencing factors during the forecast days. Finally, the obtained weight ratio and influencing factor data are used for spatial prediction, and the PM$_{2.5}$ concentration is obtained.

5.1. Research Data

This paper selects Jinan City, Shandong Province, China, as the research area. The data selected are the historical meteorological factors of Jinan in 2019 (CO, NO$_2$, SO$_2$, PM$_{10}$, O$_3$, wind speed, average air pressure, wind direction, average temperature, and relative humidity). The data of the last 35 days are used as the prediction data. The rest of the data are used as the training data.

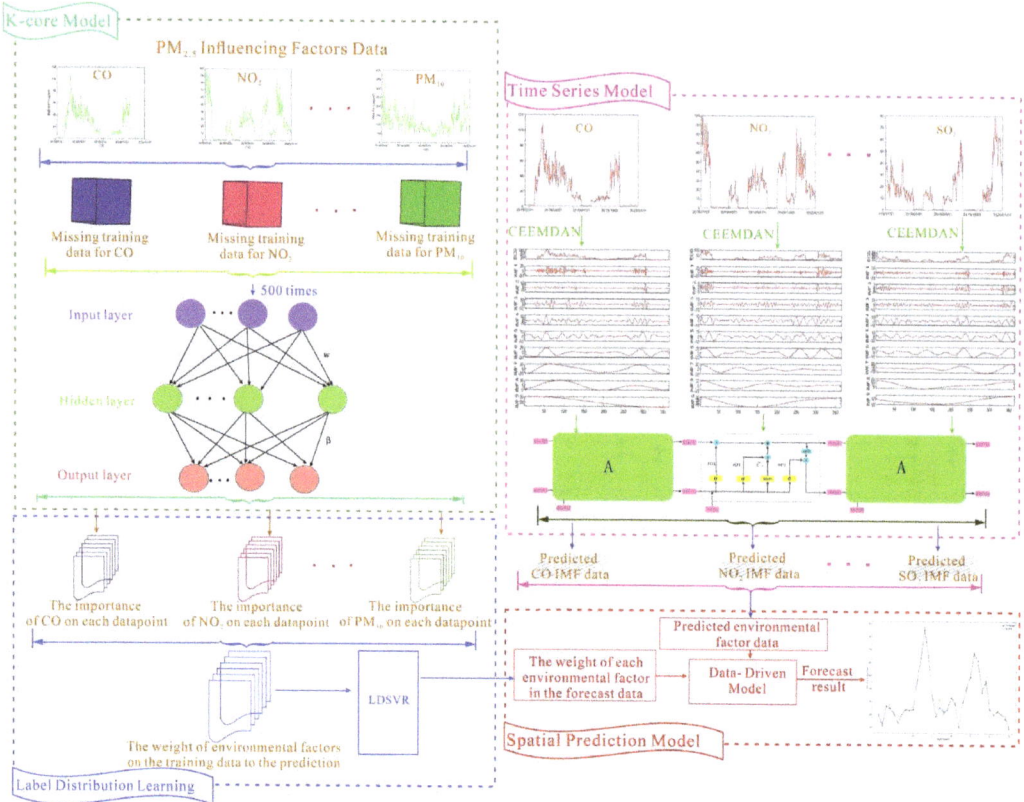

Figure 3. PM$_{2.5}$ forecasting spatiotemporal model frame diagram.

5.2. RGP–BSO–ELM Model Construction

RGP–BSO optimizes the extreme learning machine (ELM) flow chart, as shown in Figure 4. Step 1: Randomize the position and velocity of the beetles, and evaluate the fitness values of all beetles based on the PM$_{2.5}$ training data. Step 2: Evaluate the position of each beetle, select the globally optimal position, and calculate the average fitness of the beetle population. Step 3: According to Formula (12) or Formula (13), the fitness of each beetle is judged, and the appropriate character is selected. Step 4: According to the two characters of Formulas (9) and (10), update the position of the beetle and update the individual optima. Step 5: Determine whether the number of iterations k satisfies the end condition. If so, output the optimal global value. Otherwise, repeat Steps 2 to 5. Step 6: Substitute the parameters of the optimized ELM model into the ELM to construct an RGP–BSO–ELM model to predict the PM$_{2.5}$ concentration.

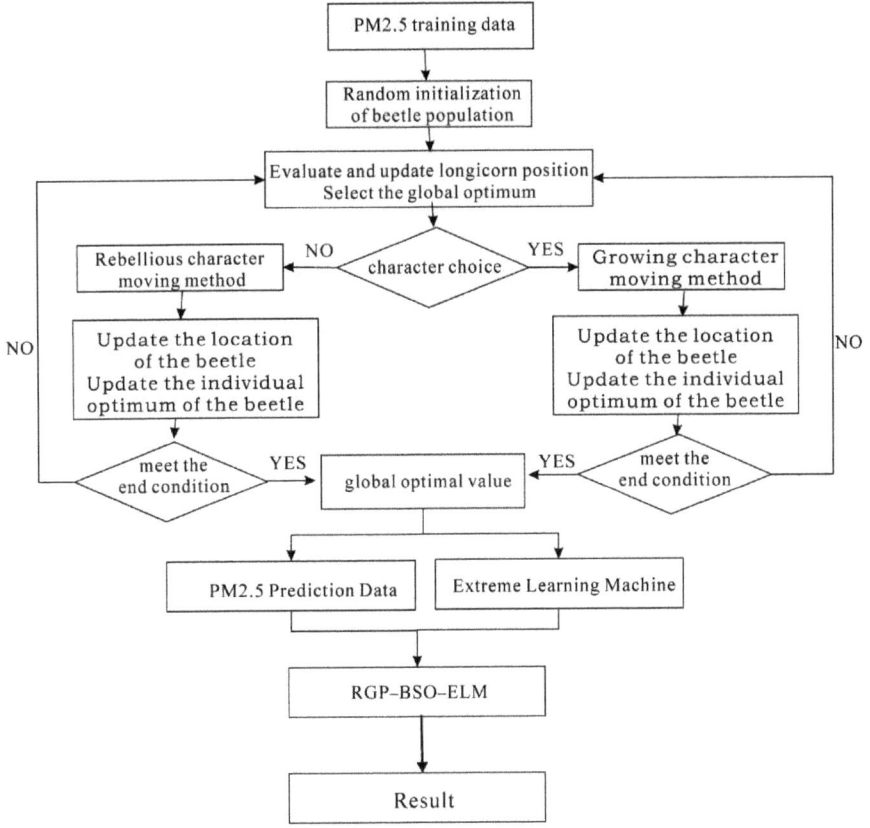

Figure 4. RGP–BSO–ELM Framework Diagram.

5.3. Evaluation Indicators

This paper adopts MAE, MAPE, and RMSE as evaluation indicators. Their calculation formulas are as follows:

$$MAE = \frac{1}{t}\sum_{t=1}^{t}|x_i - \hat{x}_i| \tag{14}$$

$$MAPE = \frac{100}{t}\sum_{i=1}^{t}\left|\frac{x_i - \hat{x}_i}{\hat{x}_i}\right| \tag{15}$$

$$RMSE = \sqrt{\frac{1}{t}\sum_{i=1}^{t}(x_i - \hat{x}_i)^2} \tag{16}$$

where: t is the number of days to predict $PM_{2.5}$ concentration, x_i is the expected value of $PM_{2.5}$ concentration, and $\hat{x}_i$ is the actual value of $PM_{2.5}$ concentration.

5.4. Forecast Result

The prediction results are shown in Figure 5, and the evaluation indicators are shown in Table 3. It can be seen from Figure 5 that the ELM prediction model without an optimization algorithm has significant error. The BSO–ELM, PSO–ELM, and RGP–BSO–ELM models can more accurately predict the changing trend of $PM_{2.5}$ concentration, and the expected results are closer to the actual $PM_{2.5}$ density. From Table 3, the RMSE of the RGP–BSO–ELM model is 2.8236, 2.0408, and 0.3778 smaller than that of ELM, BSO–ELM, and PSO–ELM, respectively. It has been proven that the RGP–BSO–ELM model has better prediction accuracy. At the same time, the RMSE index of RGP–BSO–ELM is the smallest, which demonstrates that the RGP–BSO–ELM model is more stable. The RGP–BSO–ELM model is superior to other models by comprehensive comparison.

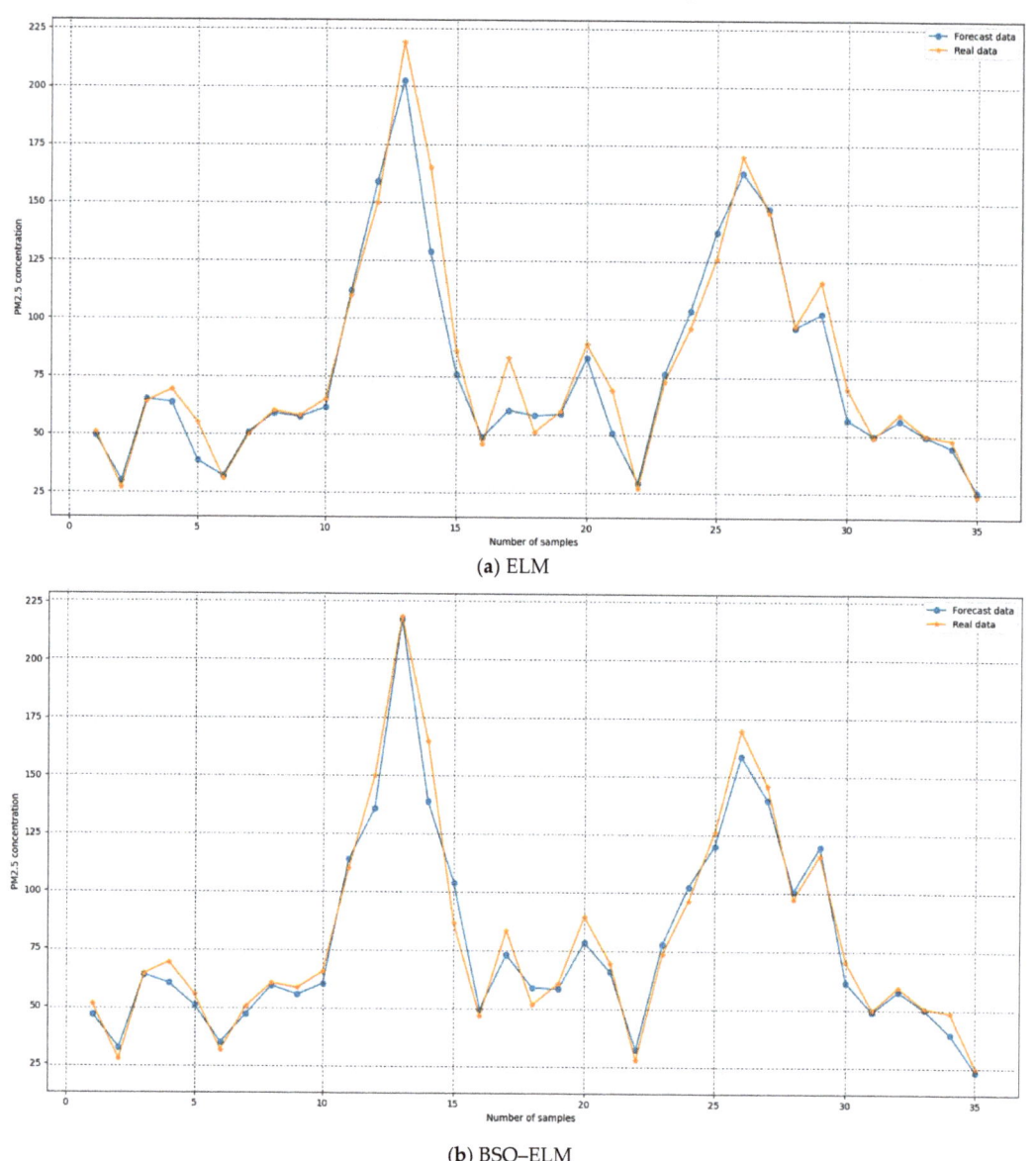

(a) ELM

(b) BSO–ELM

Figure 5. *Cont.*

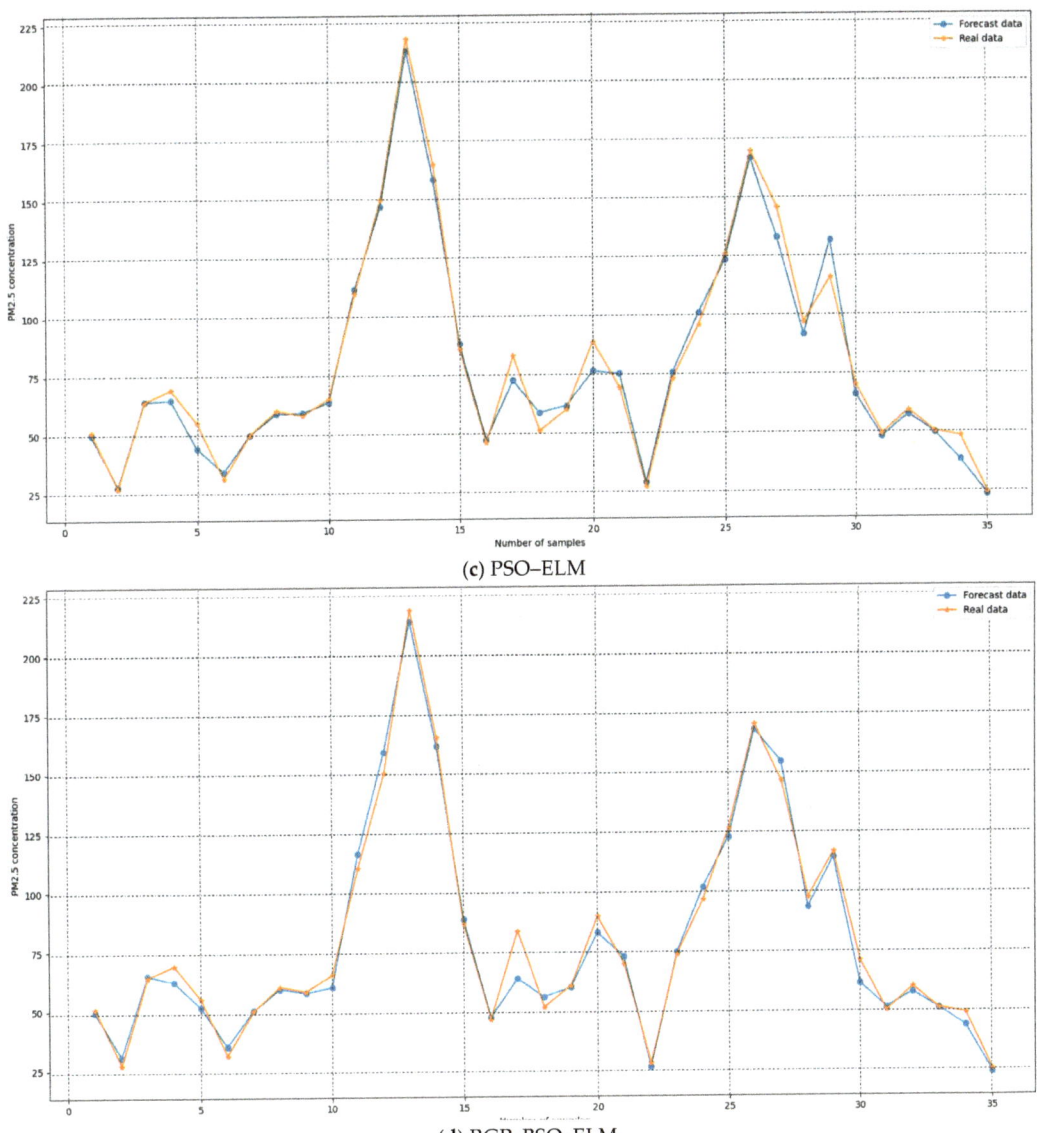

Figure 5. Prediction result graph.

Table 3. Model evaluation index results.

Predictive Model	RMSE	MAE	MAPE
ELM	1.7306	6.7137	0.0814
BSO–ELM	1.3375	5.9309	0.0805
PSO–ELM	1.0035	4.2679	0.0567
RGP–BSO–ELM	0.9137	3.8901	0.0535

6. Conclusions

In order to solve the problems of slow convergence speed, low precision, and quickly falling into the local optima attributed to the BSO algorithm, this paper proposes an RGP–BSO algorithm based on rebellious growth character. The algorithm uses rebellious character and growth character to increase the algorithm's global search ability and local search ability, adjust the understanding of the optimal position of the beetles, and change the weight of the direction of the beetles. A character selection strategy is designed to balance each beetle's global search and local search, making it easier for the beetle herd to jump out of local optima, improving the optimization accuracy of the algorithm. The dynamic factor of character maturity is introduced to promote the maturity of the rebellious character and growth character, improve the characteristics of the beetle herd in the later stage, and further improve the optimization accuracy of the algorithm. We compared six algorithms, namely the PSO, BAS, BSO, SSA, DE, and CS algorithms, in 12 test function simulation experiments. Experiments show that the RGP–BSO algorithm has better convergence speed and optimization accuracy and dramatically improved the ability to jump out of local optima. By modeling the fundamental problem of $PM_{2.5}$ concentration prediction, the RGP–BSO–ELM model has better prediction accuracy, more prominent accuracy and stability, and has obvious advantages.

In future work, we will apply the improved algorithm to other natural scenes and improve the algorithm. It can be seen from Figure 2 that although RGP–BSO has a good convergence speed overall, there are also cases where the convergence speed is slower than DE and SSA algorithms. The goal of our subsequent work is to improve the convergence speed of the algorithm further so that RGP–BSO no longer depends on the selection of the initial population so that the iteration speed can be improved. An additional goal lies in further reducing the running time of the RGP–BSO algorithm so that the algorithm has better time complexity in practical applications to meet complex industrial applications.

Author Contributions: Conceptualization, Y.Z. and Q.Y.; methodology, Y.Z.; software, Y.Z.; validation, Y.Z. and Q.Y.; formal analysis, Y.Z.; investigation, Y.Z.; resources, Y.Z.; data curation, Y.Z.; writing—original draft preparation, Y.Z.; writing—review and editing, Q.Y.; visualization, Y.Z.; supervision, Q.Y.; project administration, Q.Y.; funding acquisition, Q.Y. All authors have read and agreed to the published version of the manuscript.

Funding: The present study was funded by the National Natural Science Foundation of China (No: 71961001).

Institutional Review Board Statement: Not applicable.

Informed Consent Statement: Not applicable.

Data Availability Statement: The data presented in this study are available on request from the corresponding author.

Conflicts of Interest: The authors declare that they have no conflict of interest to report regarding the present study.

References

1. Yang, C.; Luo, J.; Liu, C.; Li, M.; Dai, S.L. Haptics Electromyogrphy Perception and Learning Enhanced Intelligence for Teleoperated Robot. *IEEE Trans. Autom. Sci. Eng.* **2018**, *16*, 1512–1521. [CrossRef]
2. Ghosh, T.; Martinsen, K. A Collaborative Beetle Antennae Search Algorithm Using Memory Based Adaptive Learning. *Appl. Artif. Intell.* **2021**, *35*, 440–475. [CrossRef]
3. Wolpert, D.H.; Macready, W.G. No free lunch theorems for optimization. *IEEE Trans. Evol. Comput.* **1997**, *1*, 67–82. [CrossRef]
4. Zhadan, V.G. Primal–Dual Newton Method with Steepest Descent for the Linear Semidefinite Programming Problem: Newton's System of Equations. *Comput. Math. Math. Phys.* **2022**, *62*, 232–247. [CrossRef]
5. Kaliyamoorthy, V.; Krishnasamy, V.; Kandasamy, N. Prediction of virtual energy storage capacity of the air-conditioner using a stochastic gradient descent based artificial neural network. *Electr. Power Syst. Res.* **2022**, *208*, 107879.
6. Mirjalili, S.; Mirjalili, S.M.; Lewis, A.D. Grey Wolf Optimizer. *Adv. Eng. Softw.* **2014**, *69*, 46–61. [CrossRef]
7. Yu, H.; Qiao, S.; Heidari, A.A.; Bi, C.; Chen, H. Individual Disturbance and Attraction Repulsion Strategy Enhanced Seagull Optimization for Engineering Design. *Mathematics* **2022**, *10*, 276. [CrossRef]

8. Dahbi, E.K.; Elhamadi, T.; Amar, T.N. Optimization of the SIW cavity-backed slots antenna for X-band applications using the Particle Swarm Optimization algorithm. *J. Electromagn. Waves Appl.* **2022**, *36*, 928–939. [CrossRef]
9. Zhang, L.; Gao, T.; Cai, G.; Hai, K.L. Research on electric vehicle charging safety warning model based on back propagation neural network optimized by improved gray wolf algorithm. *J. Energy Storage* **2022**, *49*, 104092. [CrossRef]
10. Yu, D.; Zhang, X.; Tian, G.; Jiang, Z.; Liu, Z.; Qiang, T.; Zhan, C. Disassembly Sequence Planning for Green Remanufacturing Using an Improved Whale Optimisation Algorithm. *Processes* **2022**, *10*, 1998. [CrossRef]
11. Jiang, X.; Li, S. BAS: Beetle Antennae Search Algorithm for Optimization Problems. *Int. J. Robot. Control* **2017**, *1*, 1. [CrossRef]
12. Khan, A.H.; Cao, X.; Li, S.; Katsikis, V.N.; Liao, L. BAS-ADAM: An ADAM Based Approach to Improve the Performance of Beetle Antennae Search Optimizer. *IEEE/CAA J. Autom. Sin.* **2020**, *7*, 461–471. [CrossRef]
13. Wang, T.; Yang, L. Beetle swarm optimization algorithm: Theory and application. *arXiv preprint* **2008**, arXiv:1808.00206. [CrossRef]
14. Wu, D.L.; Qin, T.W. A hybrid deep kernel incremental extreme learning machine based on improved coyote and beetle swarm optimization methods. *Complex Intell. Syst.* **2021**, *7*, 3015–3032. [CrossRef]
15. Chen, Q.; Sun, J.; Palade, V.; Wu, X.; Shi, X. An improved Gaussian distribution based quantum-behaved particle swarm optimization algorithm for engineering shape design problems. *Eng. Optim.* **2022**, *54*, 743–769. [CrossRef]
16. Zheng, L.; Luo, S. Adaptive Differential Evolution Algorithm Based on Fitness Landscape Characteristic. *Mathematics* **2022**, *10*, 1511. [CrossRef]
17. Wang, Z.; Chen, G.; Tan, L. Optimization of stereo calibration parameters for the binocular camera based on improved Beetle Antennae Search algorithm. *J. Phys. Conf. Ser.* **2021**, *2029*, 012095. [CrossRef]
18. Bhagavathi, H.; Rathinavelayatham, S.; Shanmugaiah, K.; Kanagaraj, K.; Elangovan, D. Improved beetle swarm optimization algorithm for energy efficient virtual machine consolidation on cloud environment. *Concurr. Comput. Pract. Exp.* **2022**, *34*, e6828. [CrossRef]
19. Li, J.; Lei, Y.; Yang, S. Mid-long term load forecasting model based on support vector machine optimized by improved sparrow search algorithm. *Energy Rep.* **2022**, *8*, 491–497. [CrossRef]
20. Xiong, Y.; Cheng, J.; Zhang, L. Neighborhood Learning-Based Cuckoo Search Algorithm for Global Optimization. *Int. J. Pattern Recognit. Artif. Intell.* **2022**, *36*, 2251006. [CrossRef]
21. Shen, F.; Zhu, T.; Niu, M. Pro-inflammatory effects of airborne particulate matters in relation to biological and chemical composition. *Chin. Sci. Bull.* **2018**, *63*, 968–978. [CrossRef]
22. Seng, D.; Zhang, Q.; Zhang, X.; Chen, G.; Chen, X. Spatiotemporal prediction of air quality based on LSTM neural network. *Alex. Eng. J.* **2021**, *60*, 2021–2032. [CrossRef]
23. Geng, X.; Hou, P. *Pre-Release Prediction of Crowd Opinion on Movies by Label Distribution Learning*; AAAI Press: Palo Alto, CA, USA, 2015.

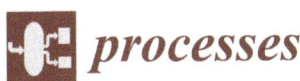

Article

Simulation Analysis of Implementation Effects of Construction Waste Reduction Policies

Qiufei Wang [1,*], Siyu Li [1] and Ye Yang [2]

1. School of Mangement, Shenyang Jianzhu University, Shenyang 110168, China
2. School of Transportation and Geomatics Engineering, Shenyang Jianzhu University, Shenyang 110168, China
* Correspondence: wangqiufei@sjzu.edu.cn

Abstract: The development of the construction industry generates construction waste which could contribute to environmental issues. Construction waste reduction management plays an important role in directly reducing emissions and solving the environmental pollution caused by construction waste. The limited rationality hypothesis and an evolutionary game model are used to construct a simulation model for the effects of environmental policies' influences on the behavior of government and construction enterprises in construction waste reduction activities. Simulation results show that: (1) The government and enterprises evolve in the same direction under the sewage fees system or the subsidy system. The relationship between the initial ratio of the two sides and the position of the saddle point determines the evolution direction of the system. (2) The government could adjust the sewage fees rate, the penalty ratio, and the upper limit of construction waste emission to obtain a superior effect under the sewage fees system. As the subsidy system, the government could adjust the unit subsidy and the upper limit of construction waste emissions by enterprises. (3) The evolution times of the different systems are different. The time required to evolve to a stable state is shorter under the sewage fees system. Under the subsidy system, the time to evolve to a non-reduced state is longer, and the time to evolve to a reduced state is about the same as the time for the government to evolve to a checked state. The time required to evolve to the reduced state is about the same as the time required for the government to evolve to the checked state. This study develops an evolutionary game model between the government and construction enterprises in construction waste reduction activities. This study helps the government analyze the influence of various policies on enterprises' reduction behaviors. The findings could help the government formulate appropriate policies to guide enterprises in waste reduction.

Keywords: construction waste decreasing; evolutionary game; sewage discharge fees; fine; numerical simulation

Citation: Wang, Q.; Li, S.; Yang, Y. Simulation Analysis of Implementation Effects of Construction Waste Reduction Policies. *Processes* **2022**, *10*, 2279. https://doi.org/10.3390/pr10112279

Academic Editor: Rok Fink

Received: 21 September 2022
Accepted: 1 November 2022
Published: 3 November 2022

Publisher's Note: MDPI stays neutral with regard to jurisdictional claims in published maps and institutional affiliations.

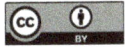

Copyright: © 2022 by the authors. Licensee MDPI, Basel, Switzerland. This article is an open access article distributed under the terms and conditions of the Creative Commons Attribution (CC BY) license (https://creativecommons.org/licenses/by/4.0/).

1. Introduction

Construction waste poses a great risk to the ecological environment due to its growing accumulation problem, and it has become a major obstacle for countries to achieve their sustainable development goals. Considering the importance of construction waste management in environmental sustainability, academia and industry have recognized the importance of reducing the yield of construction waste and improving the efficiency of treatment. The legal effect of the policy to promote the reduction and recycling of waste cannot be underestimated. Many studies show that suitable policies could effectively reduce construction waste emissions (Table 1).

The implementations of specific types of policies were analyzed in many studies. However, construction waste managers often face different policies in practice. Comparing the implementation effects of different policies could provide substantial support to managers.

Simulation models are widely used in various social sciences and economic fields to analyze and compare the implementation effects of different policies. Di W. and Xu Y. et al.

have conducted simulation studies on garbage classification policies [5,6]. Evolutionary game models could be used to analyze the individual impact of different policies.

Table 1. The relevant policy studies.

Type	Conclusion	Author
Incentive policies	Improve the recycling rate of construction waste	Shi et al. [1], 2020
Mandatory policies	Effectively reduce the dumping of illegal construction waste	Seror and Portnov [2], 2020
Combined policies	Improve the recycling rate of resources for construction waste	Andrea D M. [3], 2018
3R principle	Reduce production and increase utilization	Turkyilmaz et al. [4], 2019

2. Materials and Methods

Large amounts of studies have shown that government regulations, related policies, and regulations have a significant impact on the reduction behavior of construction enterprises. The implementation of environmental protection measures could reduce the impact of waste generated by construction projects on the environment, and the government should carry out strict supervision to ensure the implementation of environmental protection measures [7]. The goal of construction companies is to maximize profits, and in the absence of government oversight, the financial factor is the main factor in the adoption of the company's reduction behavior [8]. Managers of construction companies are more focused on the cost, schedule, and quality of projects that determine revenue, rather than waste management [9].

Both the sewage fee system and the subsidy system are economic incentive-based environmental policy instruments based on the Pigou and Coase theorem [10]. The sewage fee system adheres to the polluter-pays principle and imposes a tax on enterprises that emit construction waste. In this way, their operating costs will increase and reduce the cost of government regulation. To protect the environment and conserve resources, the subsidy system encourages enterprises to reduce pollution. Under this system, the enterprises which carry out construction waste reduction will receive financial subsidies (grants, loans, tax breaks, etc.) [11]. Both the subsidy system and the sewage fee system serve the same purpose of equalizing private benefits and private costs for enterprises, and social benefits and social costs, thereby achieving reductions in pollutant emissions and providing incentives for enterprises to adopt pollution control measures. At present, the subsidy system has been widely used in many countries. For example, Italy subsidizes enterprises that perform solid waste recycling and reuse. The government will give priority to companies that optimize construction processes or production procedures to reduce pollution. The German subsidies give priority to small and medium-sized enterprises that have financial difficulties due to pollution control. They also encourage them to introduce new technologies and equipment, optimize their production processes, change their development models, and carry out managerial and technological optimization and innovation.

Many scholars have compared the influence of economic policies and laws and regulations on construction waste reduction activities, respectively. It is affirmed that economic policies could promote the development of construction waste reduction activities. Osmani M. counted the amount of construction waste in the UK and found that the Construction Site Construction Waste Management Plan Regulations established by the government of that country in 2008 did not result in a significant reduction in construction waste emissions. Osmani M. also pointed out that the measures taken in the UK need to be combined with economic incentives to achieve the management of construction waste reduction [12]. Cooper argued that the government taxing enterprises on raw materials and giving them economic incentives have the same impact as the legal system on enterprises. Both of them enable construction enterprises to reduce construction waste emissions at the source and recognize the role of economic instruments in construction waste reduction activities [13]. Duran believed that market-based economic instruments are the best way to achieve construction waste reduction [14].

Some scholars have studied and analyzed the impact of sewage charges and subsidies on construction waste reduction activities. Poon C.S. pointed out that according to the principle of "polluter pays", many countries charge sewage discharge fees in the forms of disposal fees, landfill fees, and other fees for construction waste that needs to be collected or treated. The purpose of sewage charges is to control the discharge of construction waste and realize the reduction management of construction waste [15]. Kularatne R. K. A. conducted a case analysis of solid waste management in Vavuniya City, Sri Lanka, and found that enterprises need a large cost to carry out reduction activities. Thus, many enterprises have stopped reduction activities due to insufficient capital investment in the early stage [16]. The government needs to give financial aid or reward to enterprises that carry out reduction activities to encourage them to continue with reduction activities. Nuria Calvo believes that construction waste reduction involves technological innovation and huge capital investment, so construction enterprises have no incentive to take the initiative to reduce construction waste. The government needs to use market-oriented environmental policy tools such as economic incentives or tax penalties on the basis of law to promote enterprises to reduce construction waste. However, government management departments need to choose appropriate policy tools according to the actual situation [17]. Zhang X summarized the successful experiences of foreign construction waste reduction, introduced and analyzed the three policy tools of the sewage discharge fee, emission reduction subsidy (including tax preference, credit preference, special subsidy, etc.), and landfill fee, and pointed out the specific implementation methods and problems that should be paid attention to [18]. Chen T believed that the current economic policy is infeasible. He also proposed that the government should reward enterprises with outstanding reduction effects for emission reductions, including exemption of pollutant discharge fees and subsidies [19]. According to Wang H, when formulating economic policies, the government needs to take into account the incentives for enterprises to reduce their reduction behavior, as well as the constraints on factors that are not conducive to reduction. That is, when the government gives economic incentives to enterprises to reduce their reduction, it also needs to increase the construction waste charging rate so as to force enterprises to actively seek ways to reduce the amount of construction waste [20].

Government subsidies are an effective policy tool to solve the problem of construction waste [21]. The government could incentivize construction enterprises to attach importance to reducing construction waste through simple economic subsidies. A suitable number of subsidies could allow enterprises to participate in construction waste management [22]. A step-by-step incentive policy is effective, and it makes employees become more active in waste reduction activities [23].

The mere fines or subsidies for the illegal discharging of construction waste have limited in increasing their impact on total resources. Penalties in a single policy that combines fees, fines, and subsidies offer the advantage of working better together [24].

Evolution and the theory of games describe and explain behavior well. Simulation modelling is often used in the analysis and comparison of the implementation effects of different policies. The model could describe policy formulation objectives and activities to predict implementation effects [25]. It is widely used in various social science and economic management studies [26], such as the relationship between policy system change and agricultural structure change [27] and the performance of policy decisions in water resource management plans [28].

In summary, many scholars have conducted in-depth research on construction waste management policies from the aspects of incentive policies, charging policies, and the combination of punishment and compensation, and have achieved fruitful results. However, these studies rarely address the comparison of incentives and penalties for waste reduction and the key factors in companies' efforts to reduce waste. Due to institutional differences in emission reduction policies between different countries and the lack of a clear and consistent understanding, it is not possible to determine which policy works best under which conditions. In order to fill the gap in this research field, an evolutionary game model is used to discuss the impact and key factors of the sewage charging system and subsidy system on the emission reduction behavior of governments and enterprises. It provides a theoretical basis for expanding the management and operation of waste reduction.

Based on the studies, the research gaps are as follows. First, few scholars have discussed the implementation effects and influencing factors of different policies. Based on the 5R theory, this paper compares the impact of the sewage charging system and the subsidy system on construction enterprises in construction waste reduction activities. Moreover, this paper discusses the triggers of construction enterprises' emission reduction behavior, which provides a theoretical basis for policymakers to formulate strategies to promote environmental and economic sustainable development. Second, the evolutionary game model is used to quantify the relationship and influence the degree of related factors. It accurately analyzes the key starting point of enterprise reduction behavior and provides an intuitive macro description of the abstract problem domain. This study helps policymakers gain an in-depth understanding of the key behavioral factors that contribute to the reduction of construction firms and propose targeted strategies accordingly.

3. Results and Discussion

3.1. Building of the Model

The participants' payment matrix is shown in Table 2.

Table 2. Government and corporate payment matrix.

Strategy	Inspection (x)	No Inspection (1 − x)
Reduction (y)	u1, v1	u3, v3
No Reduction (1 − y)	u2, v2	u4, v4

Different strategies of government and enterprise payoff functions are shown in Equations (1)–(4):

$$u_1 = rR - C_g + \theta Q_g,\ v_1 = (1-r)R + R_c - C_c - \theta Q_g \tag{1}$$

$$u_2 = -L_g - C_g + \theta Q + k(Q - Q_g),\ v_2 = -L_c - \theta Q - k(Q - Q_g) \tag{2}$$

$$u_3 = \theta Q_g,\ v_3 = R_c - C_c - \theta Q_g \tag{3}$$

$$u_4 = -L_g + \theta Q_g,\ v_4 = -\theta Q_g \tag{4}$$

3.2. Model Analysis

According to the payment matrix, three conditions are proposed.

Condition 1. $r_R - C_g > 0$. If $u_1 \leq u_3$ is assumed, then (no inspection, no reduction) is the equilibrium point. If it does not meet the above conditions, thus $u_1 > u_3$ must be true, which means $r_R - C_g > 0$.

Condition 2. $(1-r)R + R_c - C_c > -L_c$. Through the same thinking way as condition 1, it could be found that $v_1 > v_2$. In other words, $(1-r)R + R_c - C_c > -L_c$.

Condition 3. $R_c < C_c$. Otherwise, the enterprise will independently reduce construction waste without government inspection, which is unlikely to happen in reality.

The expected returns of government investigations and non-investigation are E_g^1 and E_g^2, and the average government expectation is $\overline{(E_g)}$, which are shown in Equations (5)–(7).

$$E_g^1 = yu_1 + (1-y)u_2 = y(rR - C_R + \theta Q_R) + (1-y)[-L_R - C_R + \theta Q + K(Q - Q_R)] \tag{5}$$

$$E_g^2 = yu_3 + (1-y)u_4 = y\theta Q_g + (1-y)(-L_g + \theta Q_g) \tag{6}$$

$$\overline{(E_g)} = xE_g^1 + (1-x)E_g^2 \tag{7}$$

The replicated dynamic equation for the government is shown in Equation (8):

$$F(x) = dx/dt = x[E_g^1 - \overline{(E_g)}] = x(1-x)\{y[rR - (\theta + k)(Q - Q_R)] - [C_R - (\theta + k)(Q - Q_R)]\} \quad (8)$$

Solving the first derivative of F(x) with respect to x, given by Equation (9):

$$F'(x) = (1 - 2x)\{y[rR - (\theta + k)(Q - Q_g)] - [C_g - (\theta + k)(Q - Q_g)]\} \quad (9)$$

If $dx/dt = 0$, then either $x^* = 0$, $x^* = 1$ or $y^* = [C_g - (\theta + k)(Q - Q_g)]/[rR - (\theta + k)(Q - Q_g)]$. The scope of y^* will be discussed further as followed.

(1) When $y^* \leq 0$, this situation follows condition 1, so $rR > (\theta + k)(Q - Q_g) \geq C_g$. Under it, y is constantly larger than y^*, and the evolutionary stability strategy will be $x = 1$, which corresponds to government inspection;

(2) When $y^* \geq 1$, this situation follows condition 1, so $rR > C_g$, $(\theta + k)(Q - Q_g) > rR > C_g$. Under it, y is constantly smaller than y^*, and the evolutionary stability strategy will be $x = 1$, which corresponds to government inspection;

(3) When $y^* \in (0, 1)$, $rR > C_g > (\theta + k)(Q - Q_g)$. Under these situations, $F(x) = 0$, when $y = y^*$. If $y \neq y^*$, the stability strategy needs to meet the following conditions: $F(x) = 0$ and $F'(x) < 0$. If $y > y^*$, then $F'(0) > 0$ and $F'(1) < 0$, and $x = 1$ is a stable strategy and the government will inspect companies. In the opposite way, when $y < y^*$, then $F'(0) < 0$ and $F'(1) > 0$, and $x = 0$ results in a stable strategy and the government will not inspect companies.

The replicated dynamic equation of the enterprises is shown in Equations (10) and (11):

$$F(y) = dy/dt = y[Ec1 - \overline{(Ec)}] = y(1-y)\{x[(1-r)R + Lc + (\theta + k)(Q - Q_g)] + (R_c - C_c)\} \quad (10)$$

$$F'(y) = (1 - 2y)\{x[(1 - r)R + L_c + (\theta + k)(Q - Q_g)] + (R_c - C_c)\} \quad (11)$$

If $dy/dt = 0$, then either $y^* = 0$, $y^* = 1$, or $x^* = (C_c - R_c)/[(1-r)R + L_c + (\theta + k)(Q - Q_g)]$. The scope of x^* will now be discussed. Condition 3 states that $R_c < C_c$, which requires that x^* must be greater than 0. It creates two cases: $0 < x^* < 1$ and $x^* > 1$.

(1) When $0 < x^* < 1$, $C_c - R_c \leq (1-r)R + L_c + (\theta + k)(Q - Q_g)$. When the probability of government inspection $x = x^*$, $F'(y) = 0$. Then the income of the company will not change regardless of whether the amount of construction waste is decreased or not, so the enterprise will maintain the status quo. If $x > x^*$, then $F'(0) > 0$ and $F'(1) < 0$, and the stability situation is $y = 1$. The enterprises will reduce construction waste because of this. When $x < x^*$, $F'(0) < 0$, and $F'(1) > 0$, $y = 0$ is the stable strategy, and it is unlikely for companies to cut down construction waste emissions;

(2) When $x^* > 1$, $C_c - R_c > (1-r)R + L_c + (\theta + k)(Q - Q_g)$, which is amount to $(1-r)R + R_c - C_c + L_t + (\theta + k)(Q - Q_g) < 0$. However, based on condition 2, $(1-r)R + R_c - C_c + L_c > 0$ and the enterprise will pay higher sewage prices and fines. It means $(\theta + k)(Q - Q_g) < 0$, which is unpractical. Thus, $x^* > 1$ is impossible and the result must be $0 < x^* < 1$;

(3) When $[C_g - (\theta + k)(Q - Q_g)]/[rR - (\theta + k)(Q - Q_g)] \leq 0$ or $[C_g - (\theta + k)(Q - Q_g)]/[rR - (\theta + k)(Q - Q_g)] \geq 1$, the system has four replicated dynamic stable points. The stable point is D (1, 1).

When $0 < [C_g - (\theta + k)(Q - Q_g)]/[rR - (\theta + k)(Q - Q_g)] < 1$, the system has five replicated dynamic stable points, among which the stable points are A (0, 0) and D (1, 1), and the saddle point is E (x^*, y^*). The evolutionary system phase diagram is shown in Figure 1.

Conclusion 1. Governments and companies are evolving in the same direction. In reality, the government does not inspect companies, and companies rarely reduce emissions (Figure 2).

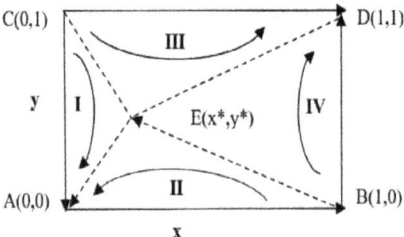

Figure 1. System evolution phase diagram.

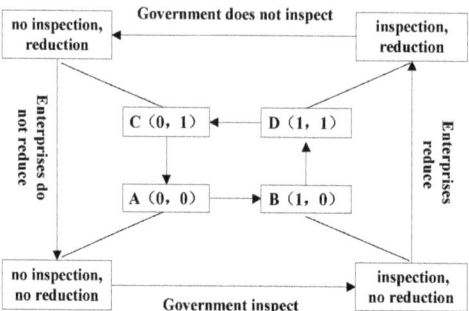

Figure 2. Changes in government and corporate evolution.

Conclusion 2. Whether enterprises choose to reduce their construction waste or not is related to the current inspection probability of the government (Figure 2). Only when the probability of the government inspection, x, at the current stage is greater than $x^* = (C_c - R_c)/[(1 - r) R + L_c + (\theta + k) (Q - Q_g)]$, the enterprise will reduce construction waste. It shows that companies and governments are evolving in the same direction.

Conclusion 3. The loss caused by the government's commitment to the company, L_g, does not affect the company's behavior. The government's loss could be made up through fines. If companies had not been inspected, then they would rarely care about waste reduction or loss.

These studies have shown that there are several factors that may influence the government to inspect companies. These factors include the government's checking costs, C_g, the government's societal interest, rR, and the sum of the sewage prices and fines, $(\theta + k) (Q - Q_g)$. Since R_c, C_c, and L_c barely change, $(1 - r) R$ and $(\theta + k) (Q - Q_g)$ are government-relevant. Regardless of whether or not the government inspects companies for construction waste emissions, companies must pay sewage prices and have to pay fines for excessive construction waste emissions during government inspections. It is more feasible to increase the sewage prices and fines, compared with lowering inspection costs. Therefore, studying the influence of changing both the sewage price rate and the fine ratio together on governments and companies could stress appropriate rates. It also contributes to the publicity of policies.

3.3. Evolutionary Simulations

For further verification of the model and conclusions, and looking for the influence of changes in construction waste charging standards on the behaviors of enterprises, the evolution process was simulated. This will analyze the impact of the combined discharge rate and the proportion of the penalty on evolutionary results. The simulation is studied with the following parameter values: R_c = $4412; C_c = $7353; R = $29,412; r = 0.5; L_c = $4412; $(Q - Q_g)$ = 50(t); C_g = $1471; K = 103($/t); θ = 44($/t); $(\theta + k) (Q - Q_g)$ = $7353, and the initial point of system evolution (x_0, y_0) = (0.3, 0.3).

Two cases are assumed for discussion.

Case 1. When $rR > C_g > (\theta + k)(Q - Q_g)$, or when $(\theta + k) < C_g/(Q - Q_g)$, the system may evolve to (0, 0) or (1, 1). The direction of evolution depends on the initial ratios x_0 and y_0 of government inspection and enterprise reduction. As can be seen from Figure 3, the evolution direction of the government and enterprises is the same. Both may cooperate and evolve to (1, 1) or choose not to cooperate and evolve to (0, 0). The evolutionary direction of the system is related to the initial values of x_0 and y_0. Using the positions of x_0 and y_0 with the data presented in Figure 1, the evolution direction of the system is obtained. Calculations show that when $(\theta + k) = 0.02$, $(\theta + k)(Q - Q_g) = 1$, and $x^* = 1/7$, $y^* = 5/9$, while $x_0 = 0.3$ and $y_0 = 0.3$. Figure 1 shows that the point $(x_0, y_0) = (0.3, 0.3)$ falls in Zone III, and the system evolves to (0, 0). The result is that the government does not inspect, and enterprises do not reduce construction waste. When $(\theta + k) = 0.04, 0.06, 0.08$, and 0.1, the point $(x_0, y_0) = (0.3, 0.3)$ falls in Zone II and the system evolves to (1, 1). The result is that the government inspects companies, and the enterprises reduce their construction waste.

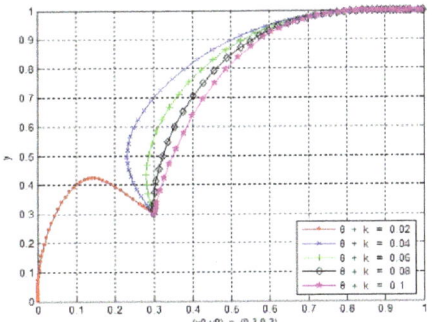

Figure 3. The influence of $(\theta + k)$ changes on the evolution result of the game on both sides of the game.

The sum of the sewage price rate and fine ratio could be understood as a kind of punitive measure for companies. When the sum is low, companies that do not follow policy have been punished. This will not constrain enterprises for a long time. Then, the companies will adopt construction waste-decreasing measures. However, the government's weak punishments may show that the discharge of construction waste is not paid attention to by the government, leading to the final evolution where the government does not inspect, and enterprises do not reduce. When the sum is in a reasonable range, it will put some constraints on companies. The greater the sum, the faster the two parts evolve to cooperate. This means that the government is paying more attention to the construction waste reduction problem, and the government will evolve toward the inspection. This implies that there will also be greater punishment for non-waste-reducing enterprises. Finally, the system will evolve to government inspection and enterprise reduction of construction waste. Figure 4 shows that the inspection probability of the government will be reduced if the sum is too low, and this would gradually evolve to no government inspection. Thus, the value of $(\theta + k)$ has little effect on government behavior. The fees and penalties are determined arbitrarily now, and it is necessary to determine a reasonable rate for them.

Figure 5 shows that enterprises will not evolve to construction waste reduction in a short time if the sum of the sewage rate and the fine ratio are too low. The sum of sewage rate and penalties play a binding role in enterprises, but the low rate has caused the government to lose motivation for inspection. As a result, the government evolves towards no inspection. Figure 5 shows that the value of $(\theta + k)$ exerts little impact on the behavior of enterprises, once it makes the enterprises evolve toward construction waste reduction. Changes in the sum could exert an influence on enterprises' construction waste-reducing activities.

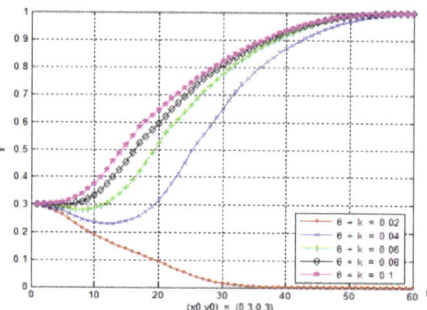

Figure 4. The influence of (θ + k) change on the probability of government inspections, x.

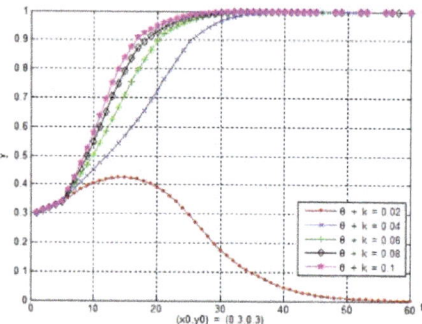

Figure 5. The influence of (θ + k) change on the probability of enterprise construction waste emissions reduction, y.

In conclusion, changes in the sum have an impact on the evolution direction of both governments and enterprises when $rR > C_g > (\theta + k)(Q - Q_g)$.

Case 2. When $(\theta + k)(Q - Q_g) > rR > C_g$ or $rR > (\theta + k)(Q - Q_g) > C_g$, which is the same as when $(\theta + k) > C_g/(Q - Q_g)$, the stable point is only (1, 1).

Figure 6 shows that the system will finally evolve. Figures 7 and 8 show that changes in the sum of the sewage charge rate and fine ratio have no obvious effect on the evolution direction of the government and enterprises, and there is only a small gap between the two parties in their evolution toward cooperation. It could be concluded that the change in the sum has no effect on both sides.

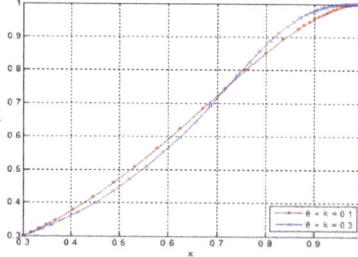

Figure 6. The influence of (θ + k) changes on the evolution result of the game on both sides of the game.

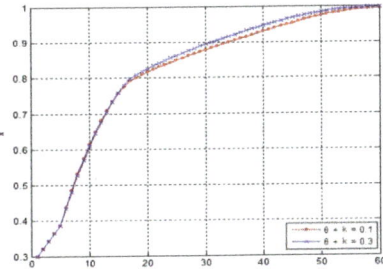

Figure 7. The influence of (θ + k) changes on the probability of government inspections, x.

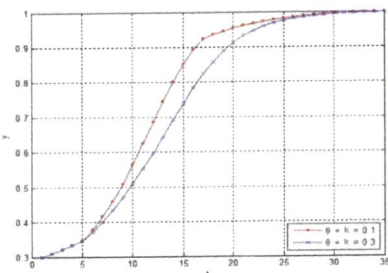

Figure 8. The influence of (θ + k) changes on the probability of enterprise construction waste emissions reduction, y.

3.4. Discussion

(1) Under different policies, the evolution process is different.

The government should formulate relevant policies according to the stage of the cities to guide and promote waste emission reductions [25], instead of blindly imitating advanced cities and directly formulating incentive or mandatory policies. The speed of the evolution of enterprises is higher under the sewage fee system. It shows that enterprises learn faster and adjust faster under the sewage fee system, and the effect of this system on enterprise behaviors is more obvious. When the government carries out the inspection, enterprises could choose the reduction strategy quickly, so as to achieve the reduction target of construction waste in a relatively short time. However, the fast learning and adjustment speed of enterprises also has problems: when the government does not carry out inspections, enterprises could also adjust their strategies quickly. That means that enterprises could easily reach a stable state without reduction as soon as the government relaxes its inspection on enterprises. This requires the government to constantly increase the initial proportion of inspections under the sewage fee system and observe the behavior of enterprises, then make timely adjustments. The system of the sewage fee puts forward high requirements for the government's inspection ability and monitoring ability. Under the subsidy system, governments have more time and opportunities to modify existing policies. Even if the proportion of the government's inspection is too low and leads to the evolution of enterprises in the direction of non-reduction, the government has enough time to detect this trend and make adjustment measures. It provides a long time for the government to revise measures and guide enterprises to take reduction activities. When the government and enterprises evolve in the direction of "inspection and reduction", they have roughly the same evolutionary path and evolution time. When the government is not sure about the capacity of inspection and monitoring, it could use the subsidy system.

(2) There are differences in the influence of relevant factors on firms' emission reduction behavior under different policies.

The main reason for the poor implementation of construction waste reduction policies is that the policymakers ignore the influence of relevant factors on the participants [26,27] and the profit-seeking behavior of the participants [28]. Under the sewage fee system, the government could find the most influential factors and adjust them by adjusting fines, the ratio of sewage fees to fines, the rate of sewage fees, and the cap on construction waste emissions, so that the game system could evolve in the direction of "check and reduce". Under the subsidy system, by adjusting the subsidies given to enterprises and adjusting the cap on their construction waste emissions, the desired effect is not achieved, and the system even evolves in the opposite direction. Increasing the initial inspection ratio by the government is the most effective and safest method, which could promote the construction waste reduction activities of enterprises, and thus achieve the goal of reduction. When enterprises evolve towards construction waste reduction, the government does not adjust the subsidies to enterprises and the cap on construction waste emissions. Because their changes are likely to be counterproductive, they will not achieve the desired "check and reduce" strategy goal.

(3) The reduction policy should be formed based on the development stage of urban reduction.

The sewage fee system is applicable to the development stage of construction waste reduction management. In the development stage of construction waste reduction management, the government's economic incentive policies have taken initial shape, and the market mechanism is relatively mature. Therefore, the government needs to restrict the emission behavior of enterprises through economic means [29]. The government could punish enterprises that do not carry out waste-reduction activities. Then it will increase the excess emission cost of enterprises to encourage them to carry out construction waste reduction activities. In the development stage, the government adopts the regulation fee standard to restrain the emission behavior of enterprises, and the difficulty of work is reduced [30]. The sewage fee system has the nature of punishment, so it is suitable for the development stage of construction waste reduction management. The government could take the following measures to promote enterprises to reduce emissions: First, the government needs to grasp the information of enterprises; second, entrusting a third party to check construction waste discharge; third, we will moderately increase the amount of pollutant discharge fees and fines. The subsidy system applies to the degree stage of construction waste reduction management. When the construction waste reduction management mature period, the sewage fee system has played a deterrent effect. The construction of reduction technologies of the enterprise has become more reasonable, and the management level has been greatly improved. The recycling technology of construction waste and the production technology of recycled building materials have been preliminarily developed. The industrial chain of construction waste reduction has been preliminarily formed [31], instead of focusing on the environmental damage caused by construction waste. Instead, the construction waste reduction industry is regarded as a new industry. The government will no longer punish enterprises that discharge excessive construction waste but invest in enterprises that could achieve reduction and encourage enterprises to carry out technological innovation in the production and application of recycled building materials so that the construction waste reduction industry will become an emerging economic growth point. Therefore, the government needs to adopt subsidy policies to invest in enterprises that could achieve the reduction target of construction waste. It could stimulate the enthusiasm of enterprises to take the initiative to carry out reduction activities. The government could take the following measures to promote emission reduction of enterprises: first, guide construction enterprises to transform into high-tech enterprises; second, take the construction waste reduction of enterprises as the basis for emission reduction subsidies; third, engage in a strict inspection of the emission behavior of enterprises.

4. Conclusions

This study uses the evolutionary game and simulation method to study the incentive effect and influencing factors of the sewage fee system and subsidy system on emission reductions of construction enterprises. The research results show that no matter what system, the evolution direction of governments and enterprises is the same: they either cooperate with each other and actively respond to the reduction policy, or they do not cooperate and passively respond to the policy. Under the sewage fee system, the rate of sewage discharge fee, the penalty rate, and the upper limit of construction waste discharge have important impacts on the enterprises' construction waste reduction activities.

Enterprises learn and adjust quickly. They could make timely changes according to the government's behavior. The government could use this feature to achieve the reduction target by adjusting the influencing factors. The government should also keep an eye on changes in corporate behaviors to prevent the phenomenon of "no inspection, no reduction". The government could guide enterprises to reduce construction waste by raising the sewage fee rate or penalty rate and lowering the ceiling of construction waste discharge. Under the subsidy system, the subsidy per unit and the upper limit of construction waste emissions have important impacts on the enterprises' construction waste reduction activities. Increasing the rate of per-unit subsidy and lowering the ceiling of construction waste emissions could make enterprises evolve in the direction of reduction. However, it will also make the government evolve to the direction of no inspection and finally lead to the uncertain evolutionary results of government and enterprises. Therefore, it is necessary to suitably adjust these two influencing factors.

The government could formulate economic incentive policies for reducing construction waste emissions according to the different stages of urban development. This study provides a new method to study the policy choices of environmental governance. This method could be applied to the policy choices of wastewater treatment, medical waste treatment, and other fields.

Although this study could be helpful for the development of construction waste reduction policies, there are still some limitations. This study does not consider the influence of exogenous factors, such as economic development, political systems, and cultural backgrounds. Therefore, the mode of combining policy instruments with economic instruments and the effect of policy implementation on more behavioral agents will be the focus of future research.

Author Contributions: Conceptualization, methodology, validation, analysis, funding acquisition, Q.W.; writing—original draft preparation, writing—review and editing, S.L.; writing—review and editing, Y.Y. All authors have read and agreed to the published version of the manuscript.

Funding: This research was funded by The Research on the Vulnerability and Governance Mechanism of Urban Waste Resource Symbiosis Network Based on CAS Theory, grant number 18YJC790167. This research was also funded by the Research on the impact of fiscal policy on the participation of enterprises in the ecological governance of the Liao River Basin, grant number lnjc202029.

Data Availability Statement: Not applicable.

Conflicts of Interest: The authors declare no conflict of interest.

References

1. Shi, Y.; Huang, Y.; Xu, J. Technological paradigm-based construction and demolition waste supply chain optimization with carbon policy. *J. Clean. Prod.* **2020**, *277*, 123331. [CrossRef]
2. Seror, N.; Portnov, B.A. Estimating the effectiveness of different environmental law enforcement policies on illegal C&D waste dumping in Israel. *Waste Manag.* **2020**, *102*, 241–248. [CrossRef]
3. Andrea D, M.; Johan, E.; Karel, V.A. Downcycling versus recycling of construction and demolition waste: Combining LCA and LCC to support sustainable policy making. *Waste Manag.* **2018**, *75*, 3–21. [CrossRef]
4. Turkyilimaz, A.; Guney, M.; Karaca, F.; Bagdatkyzy, Z.; Sandybayeva, A.; Sirenova, G. A comprehensive construction and demolition waste management model using PESTEL and 3R for construction companies operating in Central Asia. *Sustainability* **2019**, *11*, 1593. [CrossRef]
5. Di, W.; Wang, R. Modeling and simulation of vehicle path problem in garbage sorting and transportation mode. *Comput. Appl. Softw.* **2021**, *38*, 309–314.
6. Xu, Y.; Li, P.; Li, R. Simulation study on the dynamic mechanism and policy of collaborative governance of waste classification and resource utilization. *Constr. Econ.* **2021**, *42*, 403–407.

7. Kabirifar, K.; Mojtahedi, M.; Wang, C.; Tam, V.W.Y. Construction and demolition waste management contributing factors coupled with reduce, reuse, and recycle strategies for effective waste management: A review. *J. Clean. Prod.* **2020**, *263*, 121265. [CrossRef]
8. Al-Sari, M.I.; Al-Khatib, I.A.; Avraamides, M.; Fatta-Kassinos, D. A study on the attitudes and behavioural influence of construction waste management in Occupied Palestinian Territory. *Waste Manag. Res.* **2012**, *30*, 122–136. [CrossRef]
9. Vieira, C.S.; Pereira, P.M. Use of recycled construction and demolition materials in geotechnical applications: A review. *Resour. Conserv. Recycl.* **2015**, *103*, 192–204. [CrossRef]
10. Mankiw, N.G. *Principles of Economics*; Cengage: Boston, MA, USA, 2011; pp. 430–444.
11. Kelly, D.L. *Subsidies to Industry and the Environment*; National Bureau of Economic Research: Cambridge, MA, USA, 2006; pp. 167–187.
12. Osmani, M. Construction Waste Minimization in the UK: Current pressures for change and approaches. *J. Procedia-Soc. Behav. Sci* **2012**, *40*, 37–40. [CrossRef]
13. Cooper, J.C. Controls and incentives: A framework for the utilisation of bulk wastes. *J. Waste Manag.* **1996**, *16*, 209–213. [CrossRef]
14. Duran, X.; Lenihan, H.; O'Regan, B. A model for assessing the economic viability of construction and demolition waste recycling-the case of Ireland. *J. Resour. Conserv. Recycl.* **2006**, *46*, 302–320. [CrossRef]
15. Poon, C.S.; Yu, A.T.W.; Wong, A.; Yip, R. Quantifying the impact of construction waste charging scheme on construction waste management in Hong Kong. *J. Constr. Eng. Manag.* **2013**, *139*, 466–479. [CrossRef]
16. Kularatne, R.K.A. Erratum to: Case study on municipal solid waste management in Vavuniya township: Practices, issues and viable management options. *J. Constr. Eng. Manag.* **2014**, *17*, 51–62. [CrossRef]
17. Calvo, N.; Varelacandamio, L.; Novocorti, I. A dynamic model for construction and demo-lition (C&D) waste management in Spain: Driving policies based on economic incentives and tax penalties. *J. Sustain.* **2014**, *6*, 416–435.
18. Pan, F.; Xi, B.; Wang, L. Analysis on environmental regulation strategy of local government based on evolutionary game theory. *Syst. Eng.-Theory Pract.* **2015**, *35*, 1393–1404.
19. Milad, Z.; Sungjin, K. Dynamic modeling for life cycle cost analysis of BIM-based construction waste manag. *Sustainability* **2020**, *12*, 2483. [CrossRef]
20. Ma, M.; Tam, V.W.Y.; Le, K.N.; Li, W. Challenges in current construction and demolition waste recycling: A China study. *Waste Manag.* **2020**, *118*, 610–625. [CrossRef]
21. Yusof, N.; Awang, H.; Iranmanesh, M. Determinants and outcomes of environmental practices in Malaysian construction projects. *J. Clean. Prod.* **2017**, *156*, 345–354. [CrossRef]
22. Liu, J.; Yi, Y.; Wang, X. Exploring factors influencing construction waste reduction: A structural equation modeling approach. *J. Clean. Prod.* **2020**, *276*, 123185. [CrossRef]
23. Tam, V.W.Y.; Tam, C.M. Waste reduction through incentives: A case study. *Build. Res. Inf.* **2008**, *36*, 37–43. [CrossRef]
24. Xia, B.; Ding, T.; Xiao, J. Life cycle assessment of concrete structures with reuse and recycling strategies: A novel framework and case study. *Waste Manag.* **2020**, *105*, 268–278. [CrossRef] [PubMed]
25. Smith, J.M.; Price, G.R. The Logic of Animal Conflict. *Nature* **1973**, *246*, 15. [CrossRef]
26. Smith, J.M. Evolution and the theory of games. *Am. Sci.* **1976**, *64*, 41–45.
27. Nowak, M.A.; Sasaki, A.; Taylor, C.; Fudenberg, D. Emergence of cooperation and evolutionary stability in finite populations. *Nature* **2004**, *428*, 646–650. [CrossRef]
28. Yuan, L.; He, W.; Degefu, D.M.; Liao, Z.; Wu, X.; An, M.; Zhang, Z.; Ramsey, T.S. Transboundary water sharing problem; a theoretical analysis using evolutionary game and system dynamics. *J. Hydrol.* **2020**, *582*, 124521. [CrossRef]
29. Yu, S.; Awasthi, A.K.; Ma, W.; Wen, M.; Sarno, L.D.; Wen, C.; Hao, J.L. In support of circular economy to evaluate the effects of policies of construction and demolition waste management in three key cities in Yangtze River Delta. *Sustain. Chem. Pharm.* **2022**, *26*, 100625. [CrossRef]
30. Muhammad, S.A.; Huang, B.; Cui, L. Review of construction and demolition waste manag in China and USA. *J. Environ. Manag.* **2020**, *264*, 110445. [CrossRef]
31. Doron, L. Are economic tools preferable to direct regulatory measures in achieving environmental goals? *Environ. Policy Law* **2020**, *50*, 181–191. [CrossRef]

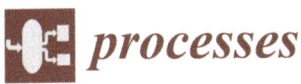

Article

Effect of UV Light and Sodium Hypochlorite on Formation and Destruction of *Pseudomonas fluorescens* Biofilm In Vitro

Melani Sigler Zekanović [1,2], Gabrijela Begić [2], Silvestar Mežnarić [3], Ivana Jelovica Badovinac [4], Romana Krištof [5], Dijana Tomić Linšak [3,6,†] and Ivana Gobin [2,7,*,†]

[1] Ilirija d.d., Tina Ujevica 7, 23210 Biograd na Moru, Croatia
[2] Department of Microbiology and Parasitology, Faculty of Medicine, University of Rijeka, Brace Branchetta 10 20, 51000 Rijeka, Croatia
[3] Department of Environmental Health, Teaching Institute of Public Health, Primorje-Gorski Kotar County, Krešimirova 52a, 51000 Rijeka, Croatia
[4] Faculty of Physics and Centre for Micro- and Nanosciences and Technologies University of Rijeka, Brace Branchetta 10 20, 51000 Rijeka, Croatia
[5] Department of Sanitary Engineering, Faculty of Health Sciences, University of Ljubljana, 1000 Ljubljana, Slovenia
[6] Department for Health Ecology, Faculty of Medicine, University of Rijeka, Brace Branchetta 10 20, 51000 Rijeka, Croatia
[7] Faculty of Health Studies, University of Mostar, 88000 Mostar, Bosnia and Herzegovina
* Correspondence: ivana.gobin@uniri.hr or ivana.gobin@fzs.sum.ba; Tel.: +385-51651265
† These authors contributed equally to this work.

Abstract: *Pseudomonas fluorescens* is one of the first colonizers of bacterial biofilm in water systems and a member of opportunistic premise plumbing pathogens (OPPPs). The aim of this study was to examine the effect of UV light and sodium hypochlorite on the formation and destruction of mature *P. fluorescens* biofilm on ceramic tiles. Planktonic bacteria or bacteria in mature biofilm were exposed to UV light (254 nm) for 5, 20 s. and to 0.4 mg/L sodium hypochlorite for 1 min. Mature biofilm was also exposed to increased concentration of sodium hypochlorite of 2 mg/L for 0.5, 1 and 2 h and combined with UV. Prolonged action of sodium hypochlorite and an increase in its concentration in combination with UV gave the best results in the inhibition of biofilm formation after the pre-treatment and destruction of mature biofilm. The effect of hyperchlorination in combination with UV radiation shows better results after a long exposure time, although even after 120 min there was no completely destroyed biofilm. Furthermore, the mechanism of the effect of combined methods should be explored as well as the importance of mechanical cleaning that is crucial in combating bacterial biofilm in swimming pools.

Keywords: biofilm; disinfection; opportunistic pathogens; *Pseudomonas fluorescens*; UV light

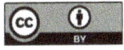

1. Introduction

Water supply systems are inhabited by the group of organisms called opportunistic premise plumbing pathogens (OPPPs) [1]. They are adapted to these systems, and can grow in changing, oligotrophic conditions [2]. OPPPs have similar characteristics, such as disinfectant resistance, biofilm formation, and amoeba digestion resistance. Model OPPPs are *Legionella pneumophila*, *Mycobacterium avium* and *Pseudomonas* spp., a genus for which drinking water is considered a relevant habitat. To these species, we may add *Acinetobacter baumannii*, *Stenotrophomonas maltophila*, *Helicobacter pylori*, *Aeromonas hydrophila*, and *Methylobacterium* spp. [3,4]. OPPPs can cause a range of transmissible and antimicrobial-resistant infections. Because of that there is a need to implement better control measurements and increase awareness [5–7].

Pseudomonas fluorescens is a rod-shaped aerobic, non- fermenting, gram-negative bacterium. It is widely spread in water, soil, plants, and animals [8]. Its presence in water is already well known. It can survive and replicate even in damp places, which relate to water supply sources [9–12], and it has been isolated from still, bottled water [13].

Although not considered a human pathogen, in some cases, especially in immunocompromised patients, it can cause acute diseases or outbreaks of bacteremia [8,9]. It is mostly studied as an environmental or soil bacteria, considering that *Pseudomonas* spp. are widely spread in the environment. But because of its ability to easily form biofilm and potentially cause infections it has been more studied as a growing concern in the food industry or in patients in medical institutions [14–17].

Biofilms are microbial communities in which cells are embedded within self-produced extracellular polymeric substances (EPS) or matrix [18]. The formation of biofilm takes place in several, usually fast phases, and *P. fluorescens* is frequently one of the first colonizers which adhere to the surface with the LapA protein and create microcolonies that will serve as an anchor to other microorganisms in creating a biofilm community. It can act as a "helper" as well, for other species to persist by using a *P. fluorescens* matrix as a shelter [18–20]. *P. fluorescens* are good biofilm producers with a strong EPS production capacity and these biofilms are characterized by an increased resistance to environmental influences and disinfectants [21,22].

Water in distribution systems or in swimming pool systems must be monitored and regulated. Disinfection is the most important process that ensures water safety. Standard doses of disinfectants, based mostly on chlorine, do not destroy OPPPs, and their number in water systems is increasing over time. Chlorine disinfection also creates a more homogeneous bacterial population, dominated by resistant *Pseudomonas* spp. [23–25]. Chemical disinfection of water contributes to the creation of harmful disinfection byproducts. Many of them have adverse health effects [26–28].

To avoid adaptive features of opportunistic pathogens such as resistance to disinfection or formation of biofilms, new technologies are being applied or are combining. Ultraviolet radiation (UV) is a promising technology for reducing OPPPs in water systems [29,30]. It has also been proven that combined disinfection, chlorination, and UV is an effective method to reduce concentrations of toxic byproducts [31–33].

The research into biofilms formed by the OPPPs group of microorganisms is scarce. Those biofilms represent potential source sites from which opportunistic pathogens are released into the aquatic environment. Therefore, in this study we isolated *P. fluorescens* from biofilm on the ceramic tiles of a freshwater swimming pool and examined the effect of the combined method, as well as the individual effect of UV light and sodium hypochlorite on the creation and destruction of already formed, mature *P. fluorescens* biofilm on ceramic tiles in vitro.

2. Materials and Methods

2.1. Bacterial Strains

P. fluorescens used in the in vitro experiment was isolated from mixed biofilm from small ceramic tiles (dimensions 2.5 cm × 2.5 cm), taken out of the freshwater swimming pool. The pool had a double disinfection method implemented, so the water was disinfected with chlorine and UV disinfection. After removal, the tile was washed and added to a tube with 10 mL of sterile water. Bacteria in biofilm were detached by treatment in an ultrasonic bath (Bactosonic, Bandelin, Germany) at 40 kHz for 1 min. Subsequently, ten-time dilutes of the sonicates were planted on a Mueller–Hinton agar (MH, Biolife, Milan, Italy) and after a 48-h incubation, suspected colonies were isolated. *P. fluorescens* was then identified using the API NE system (Biomerieux, Paris, France). Pure bacterial cultures were suspended in an MH broth (Biolife, Milan, Italy) of appropriate concentrations of 10^5 CFU/mL and used in the experiment. For this, the optical density was measured at 600 nm (OD600) (Eppendorf, Bio photometer, model #6131, Hamburg, Germany).

2.2. Mature Biofilm Formation

The method of biofilm formation was described according to the procedure developed by Ivanković et al., and modified [34]. The individual ceramic tiles were mechanically brushed, washed, and then sterilized for 1 h at 180 °C. An agar bacteriological solution (Oxoid, Basingstoke, UK) was prepared according to the manufacturer's instructions and autoclaved at 121 °C/15 min. Three sterile tiles were placed in a Petri dish, with the ceramic surface facing up. After this, the still warm agar solution was poured, making sure that the upper ceramic area of the tiles remained uncovered. Suspensions of *P. fluorescens* in sterile tap water were poured onto the upper side of the tiles that were placed in agar, ensuring that they completely covered their surface, as described. Petri dishes were incubated at 35 °C for 5 days using a rotational shaker (30 rpm). In this way a mature, 5-day old biofilm was formed.

2.3. Pre-Treatments of Planktonic Bacteria with UV Light and Sodium Hypochlorite

In the pre-treatment of the planktonic bacteria, the effect of UV light, sodium hypochlorite, and their combination on the bacterial suspension was tested. The ability of bacteria to form biofilm after treatment was investigated. Bacterial suspensions of 10^5 CFU/mL were prepared as described, transferred to a plastic Petri dish and exposed to UV light at 254 nm (UV lamp-dual wavelength, Muttenz, Switzerland) for 5 s, 20 s, sodium hypochlorite solution 0.4 mg/L for 1 min, and a combination of UV light for 5 s, 20 s and sodium hypochlorite solution 0.4 mg/L for 1 min. A neutralizer was not used. The used UV lamp had two UV tubes for illumination (dual length), one for 254 nm and the other for 366 nm, both with 8 W of power. We only used 254 nm light for our experiment. The lamp was manually installed on two plastic stands so that the microtiter plate with suspension was one centimeter away. Treated bacterial suspension was poured over the ceramic tiles in agar, as described, followed by incubation at 35 °C for 5 days, so that mature biofilm could be formed. After washing unattached bacteria and ultrasound treatment to release bacteria in the biofilm, CFUs were determined by planting tenfold dilutions on MH agar. Treatment was performed in triplicate.

Immediately after treatment, *P. fluorescens* viability was tested (Live/Dead BacLight bacterial viability kit; Invitrogen, Carlsbad, CA, USA), according to the manufacturer's protocol. Briefly, planktonic bacteria were treated as described earlier. Then two nucleic acid stains, propidium iodide (PI) and SYTO-9, were added and incubated for 15 min. The microbiological slides were prepared, and digital images were collected using a fluorescence microscope (Olympus BX51, Tokyo, Japan).

2.4. Mature Biofilm Treatments with UV Light and Sodium Hypochlorite

After incubation for 5 days, the tiles with mature biofilm were transferred to a plastic Petri dish and washed three times in sterile saline solution. After that, the mature biofilm was exposed to various treatments: UV light at 254 nm (UV lamp-dual wavelength, Muttenz, Switzerland) for 5 and 20 s, sodium hypochlorite solution (T.T.T, Sveta Nedjelja, Croatia), 0.4 mg/L for 1 min, and a combination of UV light for 5 or 20 s and sodium hypochlorite solution of 0.4 mg/L for 1 min. The lamp was manually installed on two plastic stands so that the surface of the mature biofilm was only one centimeter away. After this, sodium hypochlorite exposure, 10% sodium thiosulphate solution (Kemika, Zagreb, Croatia), was added to remove the residual sodium hypochlorite. Subsequently, tiles were washed and placed in sterile polypropylene tubes with sterile saline and treated in an ultrasonic bath (BactoSonik—Bandelin, Berlin, Germany) for 1 min/40 kHz. Tenfold serial dilutions were prepared, and samples were inoculated on MH agar. After incubation on 35 °C for 24 h, CFU/mL was determined.

Biofilm was also exposed to increased concentration of sodium hypochlorite of 2 mg/L for 1 min, 0.5, 1 and 2 h and combined with UV light for 5 and 20 s. After treatment, the tiles were processed as previously described and the number of bacteria was determined.

As a control, mature biofilm was grown on the tiles under the same conditions and was not exposed to UV light and sodium hypochlorite. Each experiment was performed three times.

2.5. Scanning Electron Microscopy (SEM)

For the morphological analyses of biofilm on ceramic tiles, the scanning electron microscope Jeol JSM-7800F (JEOL Ltd., Tokyo, Japan) was used. The ability of bacteria to form biofilm after the pretreatment and destruction of mature biofilm was analyzed. Before microscopy, tiles fixation was done with 4% glutaraldehyde and 0.5% paraformaldehyde (Sigma Aldrich, Burlington, MA, USA) prepared at 4 °C in 0.1 M PBS (Sigma-Aldrich, Burlington, MA, USA). Dehydration was carried out in a series of increasing concentrations of ethanol from 50% to 100% (Sigma-Aldrich, Burlington, MA, USA) each for 20 min. Due to the increase in stability and conductivity, samples were sputtered with a gold layer.

2.6. Statistical Analyses

In order to analyze the normality of results and distribution in differently treated experimental groups Shapiro–Wilk test was used. To analyze the effect of different treatments in experimental groups, a nonparametric Mann–Whitney U-test was used for groups without normal distribution, and for groups with normal (Gaussian) distribution statistical significance was tested by a t-test. Results were expressed as means and standard deviation. Comparison with the control group was analyzed using the Wilcoxon signed-rank test. Results were considered statistically significant at $p < 0.05$ and are presented graphically using TIBCO Statistica 14.0, Excel office 365 and Sigmaplot 14.0.

3. Results

3.1. The Effect of UV Light and Sodium Hypochlorite on Biofilm Formation

To examine the influence of UV light (UV) and sodium hypochlorite (Cl) on the ability of *P. fluorescens* to form biofilms, the bacterial suspension was treated with UV for 5 and 20 s and with 0.4 mg/L Cl for 1 min. A combination of Cl and UV was also carried out, under the same described conditions. After 5 days of incubation, bacteria ability to form biofilm was determined (Figure 1).

Results showed that all treatments applied to planktonic bacteria in bacterial suspension significantly inhibited biofilm formation (5 days incubation) compared to the control ($p = 0.002$). The results showed that the number of bacteria in the biofilm depends on the applied treatment. Extending the exposure time of UV from 5 to 20 s significantly inhibited the number of bacteria in the biofilm ($p = 0.02$). Furthermore, the application of one-minute of Cl leads to a significant inhibition compared to UV radiation ($p = 0.001$). This was followed by a more pronounced effect of the combination of 5 s of UV and 1 min of Cl ($p < 0.01$). The most effective pre-treatment was the combination of 20 s of UV and 1-min Cl ($p < 0.001$) where 99.99% inhibition was achieved.

Dead/live staining showed that after applying individual treatments, as well as the UV 5″ + Cl 1′ combined treatment, a significant number of viable cells was present and explained their ability to create biofilm after 5 days. For a UV 20″ + Cl 1′ combined treatment, there was a dominance of dead cells that were colored with red fluorescence, but there were also individual viable cells that were obviously capable of creating biofilm after 5 days of incubation (Figure 2D).

3.2. The Effect of UV Light and Sodium Hypochlorite on Mature Biofilm Destruction

Mature 5-day old biofilm was exposed to UV for 5 and 20 s, and 0.4 mg/L Cl for 1 min. A combination of UV and Cl was performed under the same described conditions. We compared the effect of individual treatments to untreated mature biofilm as a control. Treatments were also compared mutually (Figure 3.).

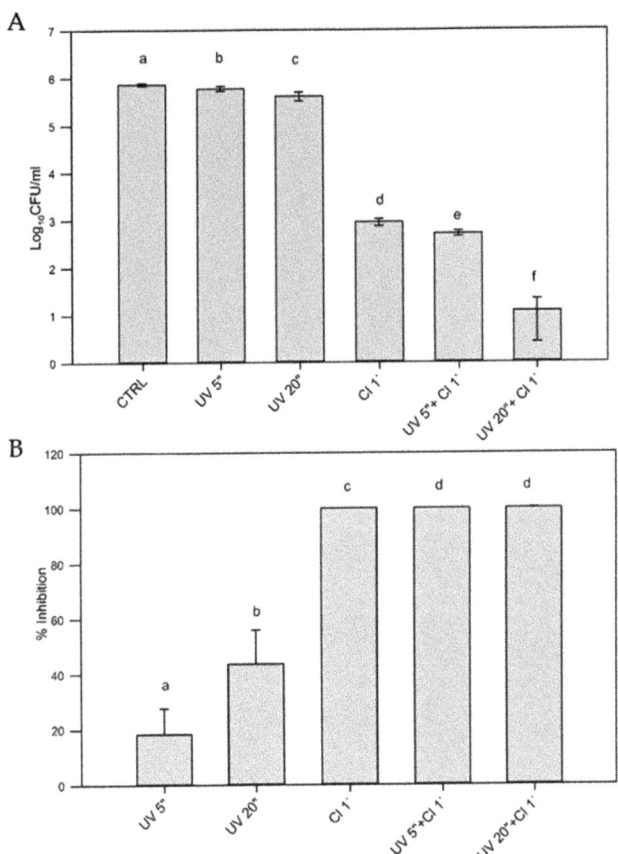

Figure 1. Effect of biofilm creation after pre-treatment of planktonic bacteria with UV 5 s (UV5″), UV 20 s (UV 20″), Cl for 1 min (Cl 1′), combination of UV 5 s and Cl for 1 min (UV5″ + Cl 1′), and UV for 20 s and Cl for 1 min (UV20″ + Cl 1′) and afterward incubation for 5 days ($\log_{10}$CFU/mL) (**A**). (The control is a biofilm created from untreated planktonic bacteria. The mean values are shown along with the standard deviations. (**B**)) % of inhibition of biofilm formation after the above treatments. Lowercase letters above the results indicate the statistical significance. Different letters indicate statistically significant differences tested by Students t-test and Mann–Whitney U test for UV 20″ + Cl 1′.

The results show that the applied treatments significantly reduced the number of bacteria in the biofilm compared to the untreated biofilm as follows: UV for 5 and 20 s ($p = 0.0012$), 1 min Cl ($p = 0.0001$), UV 5 s and 1 min Cl ($p = 0.00018$), UV for 20 s and 1 min Cl ($p < 0.0001$). A significant difference was also found between the effect of individual treatments, from the least effective UV to the most effective treatment, which was achieved by combining UV for 20 s with 1 min Cl. The destruction of a mature biofilm with different treatments shows results ranging from 66.67% to 99.99%. The effects of UV 5 s with reduction of 74.34% and UV 20 s with reduction of 80.19% are less successful in mature biofilm destruction then Cl alone or combined with UV. Cl 1 min treatment achieved biofilm reduction of 97.82%. With UV 5 s and UV 20 s combined with Cl for 1 min treatment, over 99% reduction was observed.

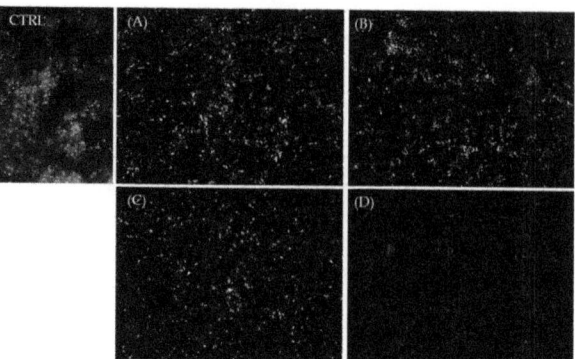

Figure 2. Representative images of dead/live staining of planktonic bacteria after treatment with: (**A**) UV 20 s, (**B**) Cl for 1 min, (**C**) combination of UV 5 s and Cl for 1 min, and (**D**) UV for 20 s and Cl for 1 min. CTRL represent control (untreated bacteria). Green fluorescence represents viable cells while red fluorescence indicates dead cells. Magnification 1000×.

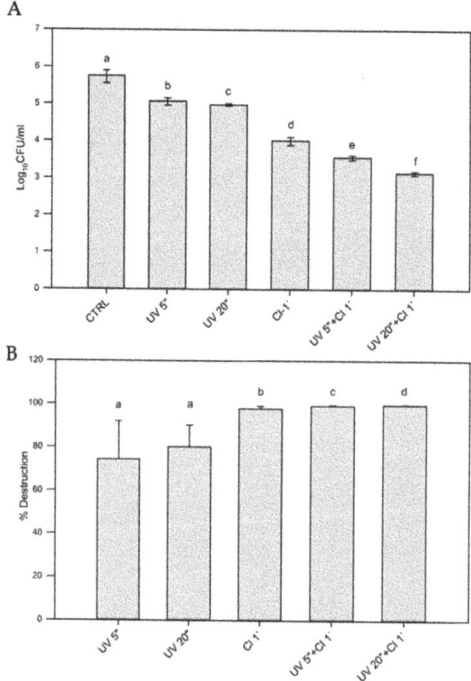

Figure 3. Destruction of a 5-day-old biofilm ($\log_{10}$CFU/mL) (**A**) after treatment with UV 5 (UV 5″) and 20 s (UV 20″), 0.4 mg/L of Cl for 1 min (Cl 1′), combination of UV 5 s and Cl for 1 min (UV 5″ + Cl 1′), and UV for 20 s and Cl for 1 min. The control is represented by an untreated biofilm. The mean values are shown along with the standard deviations. (**B**) % of destruction of a mature biofilm after the above treatments. Lowercase letters above the results indicate the statistical significance. The same letters indicate that there is no statistically significant difference between groups while different letters indicate a statistically significant difference tested by Students t-test for UV 20″ + Cl 1′ vs. UV 5″ + Cl 1′ and UV 5″ + Cl 1′ vs. Cl 1′ and Mann–Whitney U test for other samples.

3.3. The Effect of UV Light and Hyperchlorination on Mature Biofilm Destruction

The effect of a five-time higher concentration of sodium hypochlorite of 2.0 mg/L (Cl-H) was tested on a 5-day old biofilm. Its combined effect with UV for 5 and 20 s was also examined. Afterwards, dependence of the treatment efficiency with hyperchlorination on the exposure was assayed (Figure 4).

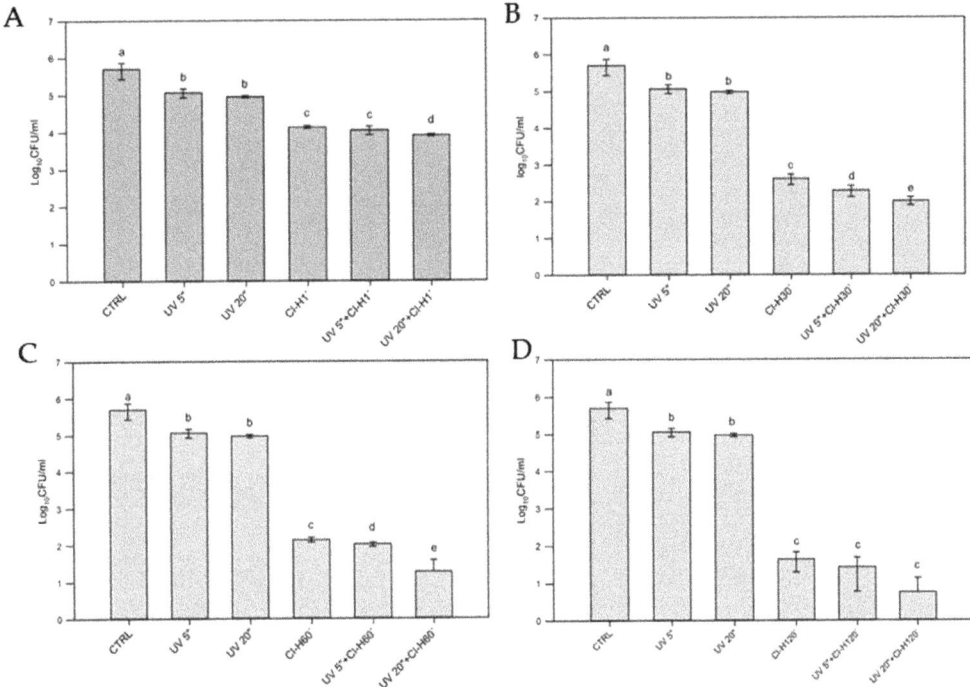

Figure 4. Destruction of a 5-day-old biofilm ($\log_{10}$ CFU/mL) after treatment with UV 5 (UV 5″) and 20 s (UV 20″), and hyperchlorination (Cl-H) for (**A**) 1 min, (**B**) 30 min, (**C**) 60 min and (**D**) 120 min and their combinations. The control is represented by an untreated biofilm. The mean values are shown along with the standard deviations. Lowercase letters above the results indicate the statistical significance. The same letters indicate that there is no statistically significant difference between groups while different letters indicate a statistically significant difference tested by Students t-test and by Mann–Whitney U test for UV 20″ vs. UV 5″; Cl-H120′ vs. UV 20″ and UV 20″ + Cl-H120′ vs. UV 5″ + Cl-H 120′.

All treatments, UV ($p = 0.0012$), hyperchlorination (Cl-H) lasting from 1 to 120 min ($p = 0.01$) and the combination of UV and Cl-H ($p < 0.001$) significantly reduced the number of bacteria in the biofilm compared to the untreated biofilm. As expected, hyperchlorination is significantly more effective than UV light alone. Combined exposure of the biofilm to UV for 5 s and Cl-H did not increase the effectiveness of the hyperchlorination itself, regardless of its duration. On the contrary, the duration of UV radiation had an impact on the effectiveness of the combined treatment. Exposure to UV for 20 s in combination with hyperchlorination for 1, 30, 60 or 120 min led to a significant reduction in the number of bacteria compared to almost all other treatments. Only hyperchlorination for 120 min combined with UV for 5 and 20 s did not differ significantly.

The percentage of mature biofilm destruction was also determined and results are presented in Table 1.

Table 1. Destruction of mature biofilm after different hyperchlorination treatments. Results are presented as a percentage (%). Small letters above the results indicate a statistically significant difference (a according to UV 5″; b according to UV 20″; c according to Cl ($p < 0.05$), non-parametric Mann–Whitney U test).

	Destruction of Mature Biofilm				
	UV 5″	UV 20″	Cl-H 1′	UV 5″ + Cl-H 1′	UV 20″ + Cl-H 1′
Hyperchlorination of mature biofilm 1 min	69.66% (±0.20)	77.73% (±0.12)	96.57% [ab] (±0.02)	97.06% [ab] (±0.02)	97.98% [ab] (±0.01)
	UV 5″	UV 20″	Cl-H 30′	UV 5″ + Cl-H 30′	UV 20″ + Cl-H 30′
Hyperchlorination of mature biofilm 30 min	66.67% (±0.20)	75.74% [a] (±0.11)	=99.90% [ab] (±0.002)	99.94% [ab] (±0.001)	99.97% [abc] (±0.007)
	UV 5″	UV 20″	Cl-H 60′	UV 5″ + Cl-H 60′	UV 20″ + Cl-H 60′
Hyperchlorination of mature biofilm 60 min	69.66% (±0.10)	76.96% (±0.12)	=99.96% [ab] (±0.02)	99.97% [ab] (±0.09)	99.99% [ab] (±0.01)
	UV 5″	UV 20″	Cl-H 120′	UV 5″ + Cl-H 120′	UV 20″ + Cl-H 120′
Hyperchlorination of mature biofilm 120 min	69.66% (±0.10)	76.96% (±0.12)	=99.99% [ab] (±0.01)	99.99% [ab] (±0.01)	99.99% [ab] (±0.001)

Hyperchlorination treatments of the mature biofilm for 1, 30, 60 and 120 min have shown most efficiency combined with UV and results range from 97.06% to 99.99%.

Hyperchlorination, Cl-H of mature biofilm for 1 min was significantly different from UV for 20 s ($p = 0.034$). No other statistical significance was noted in the 1-min treatment. Hyperchlorination for 30 min and UV for 20 s was different from UV for 5 s ($p = 0.02$). Cl-H for 30 min was significantly different from UV for 20 s ($p = 0.004$); a combination of UV for 20 s and Cl-H for 30 min was different from only Cl-H for 30 min ($p = 0.02$). Hyperchlorination for 60 min was significantly different from UV for 20 s ($p < 0.001$). Hyperchlorination for 120 min was significantly different from UV for 20 s ($p < 0.001$). No other statistical significance was noted in the 60- and 120-min treatment.

3.4. Scanning Electron Microscopy (SEM) Analysis

SEM analysis allowed a qualitative presentation of the effect of the combined treatment with UV light and chlorination with sodium hypochlorite on the mature biofilm. Representative images are shown. A dense 5-day-old biofilm with EPS is shown in pictures (Figure 5a). After UV treatments, a cluster of bacteria on the surface of the tile can be seen and they were located inside the tick EPS layer. We noticed the visible difference after Cl 1 min and fewer bacteria that are widespread on the tile surface in smaller clusters or individually can be seen without the presence of EPS. The most significant difference was seen after the combination of UV for 20 s and Cl for 1 min, where individual adhered cells or minor cell clumps can be seen on the tile surface. We did not notice the EPS layer. The figures are consistent with the result of 99% effectiveness of the study treatment described in the section (Figure 1).

Figure 6a showed the biomass with bacteria incorporated into the thick layer of EPS. After treatment of UV for 20 s, the clusters of the cells are fitted with the EPS layer and no significant changes can be seen. After 0.4 mg/L of Cl for 1-min, significant biomass destruction is visible, and fewer bacteria as well as a thinner EPS layer and EPS remains alone, were visible on the tile damage. On smooth parts of the tile, individual bacteria or cluster with fewer bacteria cells and remains of EPS can be seen. In addition to chlorination, it would be necessary to apply regular cleaning for better results. The picture (d) showed individual bacteria or small cluster of cells within a thin layer of EPS and the remains of EPS without bacteria. By combining both methods, fewer bacteria can be seen on the tiles, although EPS remains are still visible.

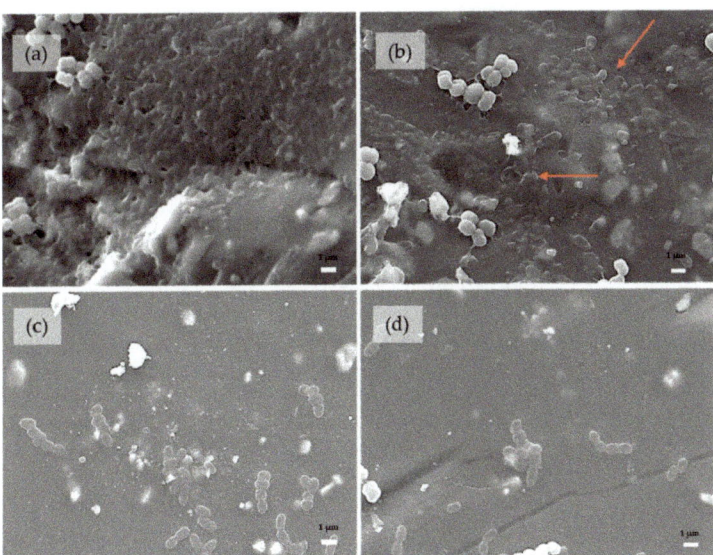

Figure 5. Representative scanning electron microscopy (SEM) micrographs of biofilm inhibition after treatment with UV 20 s (**b**), 0.4 mg/L of Cl for 1 min (**c**), combination of UV for 20 s and Cl for 1 min (**d**); (**a**) represented untreated control of 5-day-old biofilm. Magnifications 5000×. Red arrows point out bacteria embedded in EPS.

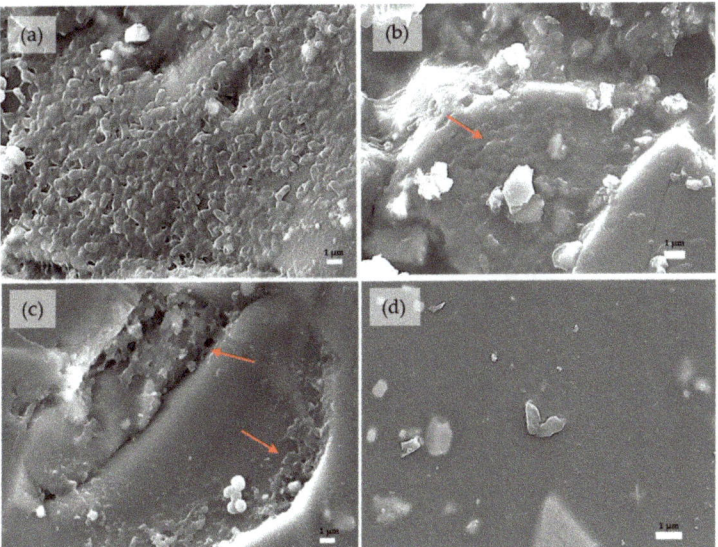

Figure 6. Representative scanning electron microscopy (SEM) micrographs of 5-day-old biofilm destruction after treatment with UV 20 s (**b**), 0.4 mg/L of Cl for 1 min (**c**), combination of UV for 20 s and Cl for 1 min (**d**); (**a**) represented untreated control biofilm. Magnifications (**a**,**c**) 5000×, (**b**) 1000× and (**d**) 2000×. Red arrows point out bacteria embedded in EPS.

4. Discussion

The object of this study was to examine the effect of UV light and sodium hypochlorite on formation, as the pre-treatment and destruction of mature *P. fluorescens* biofilm on ceramic tiles. Our results show that different individual treatments or their combination have diverse effects on planktonic bacteria and their ability to form biofilms, as well as on the destruction of a matured, 5-day-old biofilm.

The effect of different treatments on planktonic bacterial cells has significantly affected the ability of the cells to form a biofilm.

This is consistent with studies stating that planktonic cells are considered more sensitive to external influences such as disinfectants, than those in biofilms [35–37]. In our study, plankton bacteria were treated with individual treatments as well as with their combinations. After the treatment, the planktonic bacteria were incubated for 5 days and their ability to create a biofilm was determined. Immediately after the treatment, we also followed the viability of the cells. Interestingly, a combined treatment with UV for 20 s and Cl for 1 min showed 99.99% inhibition of biofilm formation, but we have proven that some of the bacteria possessed an ability to form the biofilm. It seems that a small number of viable bacteria that survived the combined treatment (Figure 2D) were obviously capable of creating a biofilm, but we did not see the EPS layer present (Figure 5D). In the swimming pools, this type of disinfection of water is used and the pool water repeatedly passes through the UV lamp and is constantly exposed to chlorination. This repeated exposure would certainly be more effective than a onetime exposure. This fact should be investigated further. The mechanism of an individual effect of UV radiation and chlorination is known from earlier studies. Extended exposure to UV radiation alters the genetic material of a bacterial cell. UV affects nucleic acid molecules with wavelengths ranging from 200 to 300 nm, specifically at ~260 nm [38]. This leads to genetic mutations which cause the impossibility of DNA to replicate, and further to cell inactivation. Some bacteria can repair from UV damage and some of them enter a non-cultivable state as a response to this environmental stress [39–42]. Hijnen et al. found that UV can be effectively used for inactivation of suspended, free planktonic cells, without forming harmful disinfection by-products (DBPs) [43]. In a study conducted by Lakretz et al. [44] on *Pseudomonas aeruginosa*, the effectiveness of different UV wavelengths (220–280 nm) on bacterial inactivation and biofilm control was tested. The most effective ones were 254, 260 and 270 nm, because they inactivated more suspended cells, which can contribute to better biofilm control.

The effect of chlorination on the ability of planktonic bacteria to form a biofilm and results then showed that chlorination with sodium hypochlorite leads to a significant inhibition compared to UV radiation treatment or control. Chlorine, in the form of sodium hypochlorite [NaOCl], is a widely used, low-cost disinfectant with effective antimicrobial performance [45]. Chlorine is a very strong oxidant which can cause permeabilization of bacterial membranes causing leakage of protein, nucleic acid, and even lethal DNA damage [46]. Using chlorine alone cannot inactivate species such as *Pseudomonas*, *Sphingomonas* or *Acinetobacter* because they are known for developing resistance to chlorine-based disinfectants [47]. Studies on *P. aeruginosa* or *Escherichia coli* have shown that chlorination, as well as UV irradiation by itself, can induce cells to enter a non-cultivable state [48,49]. We accomplished damaged planktonic cells with chlorine more effectively than with UV light, but even so they can form a biofilm.

Wang et al. studied the effect of UV irradiation or chlorination alone, as well as their combined effect on the model microorganism, *P. aeruginosa*. They found that the number of cultivable cells was effectively reduced by using UV, chlorine, and combined UV/chlorine. This is consistent with our findings, but they also found that non-cultivable cells were present after UV and chlorination but were undetectable after UV/chlorine treatment. Bacterial reactivation was completely suppressed as bacteria were completely damaged by the combined effect of UV and chlorine. This study suggests that the UV/chlorine treatment can completely damage bacteria and is promising for opportunistic pathogen inactivation [50]. In accordance with their findings, that the combined treatment can effectively destroy bacteria or introduce them into a non-cultivable state, we can note that the combined approach to water disinfection contributes to a better reduction of chlorine-resistant opportunistic pathogens and looks promising in sustaining their presence at a barely detectable level. Joint treatments can work more effectively, and the residual effect of chlorine in their combination contributes to avoiding microbial regrowth. Biofilms differ in many ways from planktonic cells. In these complex communities, the EPS composed of extracellular DNA, proteins, and polysaccharides gives microorganisms protection from disinfectants [51,52]. Cells in biofilms may exhibit changes in their characteristics, such as reduced growth rates, because of reduced oxygen levels and lack of nutrient penetration. In addition, the frequency of physiologically resistant cells, by that chlorine resistant cells, is higher in biofilm populations [36].

Due to the above and the assumption that bacteria exhibit different characteristics in biofilms, we exposed the mature 5-day old, single species biofilm of *P. fluorescens* to the effect of UV light and chlorine separately and to their combination. We also examined the separate and combined effects with fivefold increased chlorine levels with prolonged exposure time in a process we labeled as hyperchlorination.

Results showed that UV did significantly affect the mature biofilm compared to control. But despite this, the impact of UV can be described as weaker compared to chlorine or the combination. Data about UV-related technologies for already formed biofilms are limited and often incoherent compared to those related to planktonic bacteria. Despite that, the effect of UV on mature biofilms is desirable and UV technologies and devices are being further developed. Sources of UV radiation that are used or examined in studies are often mercury vapor lamps emitting only 254 nm or a cluster of wavelengths. Some of the other sources that are being used, such as excimer lamps, xenon pulse lamps and light-emitting diodes (LEDs) are even showing enhanced bactericidal effects on biofilms [38,53].

So far it is known that UV minimally affects the EPS of established biofilm [54]. EPS adheres firmly to surfaces, with electrostatic forces, van der Waals forces and chemical bonding with other polymers, which are not easily interrupted with UV [55,56]. Bacteria that are good producers of EPS may have developed a protection mechanism to UV such as increasing the path length of the incident irradiation, emission of free radicals that intercept UV, usage of motility to avoid UV phototaxis, scavenging photogenic reactive oxygen species and protecting the cell structure and components from oxidative damage, light scattering caused by inorganic particles, producing UV-absorbing protective factors such as pigments [38,56,57]. Furthermore, multiple-species biofilms with different microorganisms and their protective mechanisms are less sensitive than single-species biofilms. This was demonstrated in a study conducted on natural biofilms formed on catheters and single *P. aeruginosa* biofilm culture which showed that multiple-species biofilms were much more tolerant of the UV effect than the single-species [58,59]. It is proven that biofilms can repair or recover themselves after irradiation has ended [56,57]. This means that the UV effect is temporary, and bacteria can regrow [44,56,57,60,61].

Formed, matured biofilm is known to be a resistant reservoir of pathogens, which can be spread in bulk water. Biofilms of water distribution systems, or generally other controlled water systems are recognized as areas of concern to be maintained safe [62]. EPS is considered as an adaptation of microorganisms to protect against disinfectants such as chlorine [61,63]. Disinfectants containing halogen species such as chlorine, with their high reactivity, are even neutralized through reaction with EPS, so have an impaired efficiency in reducing biofilm cell density [64]. The presence of EPS is not the only factor that provides biofilm resistance. Cells in biofilms can phenotypically differ from planktonic cells and develop different adaptive responses to sublethal concentrations of the disinfectant [65].

In order to effect even more efficiently on the mature biofilm, in our research we also combined the action of chlorine and prolonged hyperchlorination with UV radiation, which was proved to be the most effective method. Although we did not eradicate the biofilm completely, the synergistic action of hyperchlorination for 120 min and UV radiation for 20 s reduced the biofilm the most. Synergistic actions have been reported in various studies. A combination of UV light with chlorine dioxide was shown to be more effective in eradicating drinking water biofilms than the two treatments applied separately according to Rand et al. [66]. UV treatment systems in combination with chlorine or chlorine dioxide and monochloramine achieved greater log reductions of suspended *E. coli* and its biofilm, than chlorine-based disinfectants alone [67].

By using chlorine-based agents in water, such as sodium hypochlorite, relatively good disinfection results can be achieved as well as residual chlorine. Sodium hypochlorite is added to water as an oxidant that acts on organic and inorganic substances [68]. This results in creating disinfection by-products (DBPs), significantly trihalomethanes (THMs) that are becoming a serious health concern. Due to the genotoxic and carcinogenic effect of THMs, and other DBPs which have not yet been sufficiently investigated, it is preferable to use lower doses of chlorine, and one of the possible solutions is the application of combined disinfection methods, UV radiation and chlorination [68,69]. Complete eradication of biofilm was not achieved with any treatment, so it is necessary to investigate more methods, and their combination, to keep the biofilms of water systems under control. Finally, we want to emphasize that the cleaning and sanitation processes are important as well, so that disinfection methods can be more effective, and their by-products maintained at a safe level.

5. Conclusions

Our study indicates that both chlorine and UV light are effective agents in the inhibition of formation as well as in the treatment of the mature biofilm of *P. fluorescens*. Exposure of plankton bacteria to combined disinfection significantly affects the ability of these bacteria to create a biofilm and, by constantly repeating the procedure, with regular sanitation the formation of bacterial biofilm could be kept under control.

The application of combined methods has proven to be effective on a mature biofilm even though it has led only to its reduction. Therefore, the application of combined disinfection methods should go in the direction of treatment of planktonic bacteria with regular cleaning and sanitation. An additional application of UV radiations directly to the tiles would further facilitate maintaining the biofilm under control. Hyperchlorination has proven to be effective in destroying the biofilm, but due to the creation of by-products it should be used under defined conditions.

Author Contributions: Conceptualization, M.S.Z. and I.G.; methodology, M.S.Z., G.B., I.J.B. and R.K.; investigation, G.B. and M.S.Z.; resources, I.G.; data curation, S.M.; writing—original draft preparation, M.S.Z., G.B., D.T.L. and S.M.; writing—review and editing, I.G., R.K. and D.T.L.; visualization, I.J.B.; funding acquisition, I.G. All authors have read and agreed to the published version of the manuscript.

Funding: This research was funded by the University of Rijeka, grant number UNIRI-biomed 18-171.

Data Availability Statement: Not applicable.

Conflicts of Interest: The authors declare no conflict of interest.

References

1. Falkinham, J.O., III. Common Features of Opportunistic Premise Plumbing Pathogens. *Int. J. Environ. Res. Public Health* **2015**, *12*, 4533–4545. [CrossRef] [PubMed]
2. Moore, M.R.; Pryor, M.; Fields, B.; Lucas, C.; Phelan, M.; Besser, R.E. Introduction of Monochloramine into a Municipal Water System: Impact on Colonization of Buildings by *Legionella* spp. *Appl. Environ. Microbiol.* **2006**, *72*, 378–383. [CrossRef] [PubMed]
3. Hayward, C.; Ross, K.E.; Brown, M.H.; Bentham, R.; Whiley, H. The Presence of Opportunistic Premise Plumbing Pathogens in Residential Buildings: A Literature Review. *Water* **2022**, *14*, 1129. [CrossRef]
4. Vaz-Moreira, I.; Nunes, O.C.; Manaia, C.M. Diversity and antibiotic resistance in Pseudomonas spp. from drinking water. *Sci. Total Environ.* **2012**, *426*, 366–374. [CrossRef]
5. CDC. Implications of Waterborne Disease Estimates. Available online: https://www.cdc.gov/healthywater/surveillance/burden/implications.html (accessed on 10 August 2022).

6. Collier, S.A.; Deng, L.; Adam, E.A.; Benedict, K.M.; Beshearse, E.M.; Blackstock, A.J.; Bruce, B.B.; Derado, G.; Edens, C.; Fullerton, K.E.; et al. Estimate of Burden and Direct Healthcare Cost of Infectious Waterborne Disease in the United States. *Emerg. Infect. Dis.* **2021**, *27*, 140–149. [CrossRef]
7. Soto-Giron, M.J.; Rodriguez-R, L.M.; Luo, C.; Elk, M.; Ryu, H.; Hoelle, J.; Santo Domingo, J.W.; Konstantinidis, K.T. Biofilms on Hospital Shower Hoses: Characterization and Implications for Nosocomial Infections. *Appl. Environ. Microbiol.* **2016**, *82*, 2872–2883. [CrossRef]
8. Scales, B.S.; Dickson, R.P.; LiPuma, J.J.; Huffnagle, G.B. Microbiology, Genomics, and Clinical Significance of the Pseudomonas fluorescens Species Complex, an Unappreciated Colonizer of Humans. *Clin. Microbiol. Rev.* **2014**, *27*, 927–948. [CrossRef]
9. Wong, V.; Levi, K.; Baddal, B.; Turton, J.; Boswell, T.C. Spread of Pseudomonas fluorescens Due to Contaminated Drinking Water in a Bone Marrow Transplant Unit: Table 1. *J. Clin. Microbiol.* **2011**, *49*, 2093–2096. [CrossRef]
10. Sun, Y.-Y.; Chi, H.; Sun, L. Pseudomonas fluorescens Filamentous Hemagglutinin, an Iron-Regulated Protein, Is an Important Virulence Factor that Modulates Bacterial Pathogenicity. *Front. Microbiol.* **2016**, *7*, 1320. [CrossRef]
11. Gershman, M.D.; Kennedy, D.J.; Noble-Wang, J.; Kim, C.; Gullion, J.; Kacica, M.; Jensen, B.; Pascoe, N.; Saiman, L.; McHale, J.; et al. Multistate Outbreak of *Pseudomonas fluorescens* Bloodstream Infection after Exposure to Contaminated Heparinized Saline Flush Prepared by a Compounding Pharmacy. *Clin. Infect. Dis.* **2008**, *47*, 1372–1379. [CrossRef]
12. Anaissie, E.J.; Penzak, S.R.; Dignani, M.C. The hospital water supply as a source of nosocomial infections: A plea for action. *Arch. Intern. Med.* **2002**, *162*, 1483–1492. [CrossRef] [PubMed]
13. Wilkinson, F.H.; Kerr, K.G. Bottled water as a source of multi-resistant *Stenotrophomonas* and *Pseudomonas* species for neutropenic patients. *Eur. J. Cancer Care* **1998**, *7*, 12–14. [CrossRef] [PubMed]
14. Juyal, A.; Otten, W.; Baveye, P.C.; Eickhorst, T. Influence of soil structure on the spread of *Pseudomonas fluorescens* in soil at microscale. *Eur. J. Soil Sci.* **2021**, *72*, 141–153. [CrossRef]
15. Benito, N.; Mirelis, B.; Luz Gálvez, M.; Vila, M.; López-Contreras, J.; Cotura, A.; Pomar, V.; March, F.; Navarro, F.; Coll, P.; et al. Outbreak of Pseudomonas fluorescens bloodstream infection in a coronary care unit. *J. Hosp. Infect.* **2012**, *82*, 286–289. [CrossRef]
16. Daneshvar, A.H.E.; Truelstrup, H.L. Kinetics of biofilm formation and desiccation survival of *Listeria monocytogenes* in single and dual species biofilms with *Pseudomonas fluorescens, Serratia proteamaculans* or *Shewanella baltica* on food-grade stainless steel surfaces. *Biofouling* **2013**, *29*, 1253–1268. [CrossRef]
17. Feazel, L.M.; Baumgartner, L.K.; Peterson, K.L.; Frank, D.N.; Harris, J.K.; Pace, N.R. Opportunistic pathogens enriched in showerhead biofilms. *Proc. Natl. Acad. Sci. USA* **2009**, *106*, 16393–16399. [CrossRef]
18. Masak, J.; Cejkova, A.; Schreiberova, O.; Rezanka, T. Pseudomonas biofilms: Possibilities of their control. *FEMS Microbiol.* **2014**, *89*, 1–14. [CrossRef]
19. Hinsa, S.M.; O'Toole, G.A. Biofilm formation by Pseudomonas fluorescens WCS365: A role for LapD. *Microbiology* **2006**, *152*, 1375–1383. [CrossRef]
20. Puga, C.H.; Dahdouh, E.; Sanjose, C.; Orgaz, B. Listeria monocytogenes Colonizes Pseudomonas fluorescens Biofilms and Induces Matrix Over-Production. *Front. Microbiol.* **2018**, *9*, 1706. [CrossRef]
21. Wang, H.; Cai, L.; Li, Y.; Xu, X.; Zhou, G. Biofilm formation by meat-borne Pseudomonas fluorescens on stainless steel and its resistance to disinfectants. *Food Control* **2018**, *91*, 397–403. [CrossRef]
22. Rossi, C.; Serio, A.; Chaves-López, C.; Anniballi, F.; Auricchio, B.; Goffredo, E.; Cenci-Goga, B.T.; Lista, F.; Fillo, S.; Paparella, A. Biofilm formation, pigment production and motility in Pseudomonas spp. isolated from the dairy industry. *Food Control* **2018**, *86*, 241–248. [CrossRef]
23. Bertelli, C.; Courtois, S.; Rosikiewicz, M.; Piriou, P.; Aeby, S.; Robert, S.; Loret, J.-F.; Greub, G. Reduced Chlorine in Drinking Water Distribution Systems Impacts Bacterial Biodiversity in Biofilms. *Front. Microbiol.* **2018**, *9*, 2520. [CrossRef] [PubMed]
24. Rice, S.A.; Van Den Akker, B.; Pomati, F.; Roser, D. A risk assessment of Pseudomonas aeruginosa in swimming pools: A review. *J. Water Health* **2012**, *10*, 181–196. [CrossRef]
25. Fish, K.E.; Reeves-McLaren, N.; Husband, S.; Boxall, J. Uncharted waters: The unintended impacts of residual chlorine on water quality and biofilms. *NPJ Biofilms Microbiomes* **2022**, *12*, 55. [CrossRef] [PubMed]
26. Lee, J.; Ha, K.-T.; Zoh, K.-D. Characteristics of trihalomethane (THM) production and associated health risk assessment in swimming pool waters treated with different disinfection methods. *Sci. Total Environ.* **2009**, *407*, 1990–1997. [CrossRef] [PubMed]
27. Villanueva, C.M.; Font-Ribera, L. Health impact of disinfection by-products in swimming pools. *Annali dell'Istituto superiore di sanita* **2012**, *48*, 387–396. [CrossRef] [PubMed]
28. van Veldhoven, K.; Keski-Rahkonen, P.; Barupal, D.K.; Villanueva, C.M.; Font-Ribera, L.; Scalbert, A.; Bodinier, B.; Grimalt, J.O.; Zwiener, C.; Vlaanderen, J.; et al. Effects of exposure to water disinfection by-products in a swimming pool: A metabolome-wide association study. *Environ. Int.* **2018**, *111*, 60–70. [CrossRef]
29. Haibo, W.; Chun, H.; Suona, Z.; Liu, L.; Xueci, X. Effects of O3/Cl2 disinfection on corrosion and opportunistic pathogens growth in drinking water distribution systems. *J. Environ. Sci.* **2018**, *73*, 38–46.
30. Hongna, L.; Xiuping, Z.; Jinren, N. Comparison of electrochemical method with ozonation, chlorination and monochloramination in drinking water disinfection. *Electrochim. Acta* **2011**, *27*, 9789–9796.
31. Karimi, B. Formation of disinfection by-products in the swimming pool water treated with different disinfection types. *Desalination Water Treat.* **2020**, *175*, 174–181. [CrossRef]

32. Beyer, A.; Worner, H.; van Lierop, R. *The Use of UV for Destruction of Combined Chlorine*; Version 1.0; Wallace & Tiernan: Tonbridge, UK, 2004. Available online: https://www.pwtag.org.uk/reference/ (accessed on 15 August 2022).
33. Cassan, D.; Mercier, B.; Castex, F.; Rambaud, A. Effects of medium-pressure UV lamps radiation on water quality in a chlorinated indoor swimming pool. *Chemosphere* **2006**, *62*, 1507–1513. [CrossRef] [PubMed]
34. Ivanković, T.; Goić-Barišić, I.; Hrenović, J. Reduced susceptibility to disinfectants of Acinetobacter baumannii biofilms on glass and ceramic. *Arch. Ind. Hyg. Toxicol.* **2017**, *68*, 99–108. [CrossRef] [PubMed]
35. Argyraki, A.; Markvart, M.; Stavnsbjerg, C.; Kragh, K.N.; Ou, Y.; Bjørndal, L.; Bjarnsholt, T.; Petersen, P.M. UV light assisted antibiotics for eradication of in vitro biofilms. *Sci. Rep.* **2018**, *8*, 16360. [CrossRef] [PubMed]
36. Steed, K.A.; Falkinham, J.O., 3rd. Effect of Growth in Biofilms on Chlorine Susceptibility of *Mycobacterium avium* and *Mycobacterium intracellulare*. *Appl. Environ. Microbiol.* **2006**, *72*, 4007–4011. [CrossRef]
37. Davies, D. Understanding biofilm resistance to antibacterial agents. *Nat. Rev. Drug Discov.* **2003**, *2*, 114–122. [CrossRef]
38. Varna, K.; Jones, M. The Effects of Ultraviolet Light on Escherichia coli. *J. Emerg. Investigat.* **2015**, *102*, 23–28.
39. Pullerits, K.; Ahlinder, J.; Holmer, L.; Salomonsson, E.; Öhrman, C.; Jacobsson, K.; Dryselius, R.; Forsman, M.; Paul, C.J.; Rådström, P. Impact of UV irradiation at full scale on bacterial communities in drinking water. *NPJ Clean Water* **2020**, *3*, 11. [CrossRef]
40. Ben Said, M.; Masahiro, O.; Hassen, A. Detection of viable but non cultivable Escherichia coli after UV irradiation using a lytic Qβ phage. *Ann. Microbiol.* **2010**, *60*, 121–127. [CrossRef]
41. Guo, L.; Ye, C.; Cui, L.; Wan, K.; Chen, S.; Zhang, S.; Yu, X. Population and single cell metabolic activity of UV-induced VBNC bacteria determined by CTC-FCM and D2O-labeled Raman spectroscopy. *Environ. Int.* **2019**, *130*, 104883. [CrossRef]
42. Guo, M.; Huang, J.; Hu, H.; Liu, W.; Yang, J. UV inactivation and characteristics after photoreactivation of Escherichia coli with plasmid: Health safety concern about UV disinfection. *Water Res.* **2012**, *46*, 4031–4036. [CrossRef]
43. Hijnen, W.A.M.; Beerendonk, E.F.; Medema, G.J. Inactivation credit of UV radiation for viruses, bacteria and protozoan (oo)cysts in water: A review. *Water Res.* **2006**, *40*, 3–22. [CrossRef] [PubMed]
44. Lakretz, A.; Ron, E.Z.; Mamane, H. Biofouling control in water by various UVC wavelengths and doses. *Biofouling* **2010**, *26*, 257–267. [CrossRef] [PubMed]
45. Gil, M.I.; Gómez-López, V.M.; Hung, Y.-C.; Allende, A. Potential of Electrolyzed Water as an Alternative Disinfectant Agent in the Fresh-Cut Industry. *Food Bioprocess Technol.* **2015**, *8*, 1336–1348. [CrossRef]
46. Virto, R.; Manas, P.; Alvarez, I.; Condon, S.; Raso, J. Membrane Damage and Microbial Inactivation by Chlorine in the Absence and Presence of a Chlorine-Demanding Substrate. *Appl. Environ. Microbiol.* **2005**, *71*, 5022–5028. [CrossRef]
47. Shrivastava, R.; Upreti, R.K.; Jain, S.R.; Prasad, K.N.; Seth, P.K.; Chaturvedi, U.C. Suboptimal chlorine treatment of drinking water leads to selection of multidrug-resistant Pseudomonas aeruginosa. *Ecotoxicol. Environ. Saf.* **2004**, *58*, 277–283. [CrossRef]
48. Guo, M.-T.; Kong, C. Antibiotic resistant bacteria survived from UV disinfection: Safety concerns on genes dissemination. *Chemosphere* **2019**, *224*, 827–832. [CrossRef]
49. Chen, S.; Li, X.; Wang, Y.; Zeng, J.; Ye, C.; Li, X.; Guo, L.; Zhang, S.; Yu, X. Induction of Escherichia coli into a VBNC state through chlorination/chloramination and differences in characteristics of the bacterium between states. *Water Res.* **2018**, *142*, 279–288. [CrossRef]
50. Wang, L.; Ye, C.; Guo, L.; Chen, C.; Kong, X.; Chen, Y.; Shu, L.; Wang, P.; Yu, X.; Fang, J. Assessment of the UV/Chlorine Process in the Disinfection of *Pseudomonas aeruginosa*: Efficiency and Mechanism. *Environ. Sci. Technol.* **2021**, *55*, 9221–9230. [CrossRef]
51. Lopes, F.A.; Morin, P.; Oliveira, R.; Melo, L. Impact of biofilms in simulated drinking water and urban heat supply systems. *Int. J. Environ. Eng.* **2009**, *1*, 276–294. [CrossRef]
52. Flemming, H.-C.; Wingender, J. The biofilm matrix. *Nat. Rev. Microbiol.* **2010**, *8*, 623–633. [CrossRef]
53. Garvey, M.; Rabbitt, D.; Stocca, A.; Rowan, N. Pulsed ultraviolet light inactivation of Pseudomonas aeruginosa and Staphylococcus aureus biofilms. *Water Environ.* **2015**, *29*, 36–42. [CrossRef]
54. Elasri, M.O.; Miller, R.V. Study of the Response of a Biofilm Bacterial Community to UV Radiation. *Appl. Environ. Microbiol.* **1999**, *65*, 2025–2031. [CrossRef] [PubMed]
55. Nguyen, T.; Roddick, F.A.; Fam, L. Biofouling of Water Treatment Membranes: A Review of Underlying Causes, Monitoring Techniques and Control Measures. *Membranes* **2012**, *2*, 804–840. [CrossRef]
56. Song, W.; Zhao, C.; Zhang, D.; Mu, S.; Pan, X. Different Resistance to UV-B Radiation of Extracellular Polymeric Substances of Two Cyanobacteria from Contrasting Habitats. *Front. Microbiol.* **2016**, *7*, 1208. [CrossRef]
57. Luo, X.; Zhang, B.; Lu, Y.; Mei, Y.; Shen, L. Advances in application of ultraviolet irradiation for biofilm control in water and wastewater infrastructure. *J. Hazard. Mater.* **2022**, *421*, 126682. [CrossRef] [PubMed]
58. Yuan, L.; Sadiq, F.A.; Wang, N.; Yang, Z.; He, G. Recent advances in understanding the control of disinfectant-resistant biofilms by hurdle technology in the food industry. *Crit. Rev. Food Sci. Nutr.* **2021**, *61*, 3876–3891. [CrossRef] [PubMed]
59. Bak, J.; Ladefoged, S.D.; Tvede, M.; Begovic, T.; Gregersen, A. Disinfection of Pseudomonas aeruginosa biofilm contaminated tube lumens with ultraviolet C light emitting diodes. *Biofouling* **2010**, *26*, 31–38. [CrossRef] [PubMed]
60. Lakretz, A.; Ron, E.Z.; Harif, T.; Mamane, H. Biofilm control in water by advanced oxidation process (AOP) pre-treatment: Effect of natural organic matter (NOM). *Water Sci. Technol.* **2011**, *64*, 1876–1884. [CrossRef]
61. Lakretz, A.; Ron, E.Z.; Mamane, H. Biofilm control in water by a UV-based advanced oxidation process. *Biofouling* **2011**, *27*, 295–307. [CrossRef]

62. Clayton, G.E.; Thorn, R.M.S.; Reynolds, D.M. The efficacy of chlorine-based disinfectants against planktonic and biofilm bacteria for decentralised point-of-use drinking water. *NPJ Clean Water* **2021**, *4*, 48. [CrossRef]
63. De Beer, D.; Srinivasan, R.; Stewart, P.S. Direct measurement of chlorine penetration into biofilms during disinfection. *Appl. Environ. Microbiol.* **1994**, *60*, 4339–4344. [CrossRef] [PubMed]
64. Stewart, P.S.; Rayner, J.; Roe, F.; Rees, W.M. Biofilm penetration and disinfection efficacy of alkaline hypochlorite and chlorosulfamates. *J. Appl. Microbiol.* **2001**, *91*, 525–532. [CrossRef] [PubMed]
65. Bridier, A.; Briandet, R.; Thomas, V.; Dubois-Brissonnet, F. Resistance of bacterial biofilms to disinfectants: A review. *Biofouling* **2011**, *27*, 1017–1032. [CrossRef] [PubMed]
66. Rand, J.L.; Hofmann, R.; Alam, M.Z.B.; Chauret, C.; Cantwell, R.; Andrews, R.C.; Gagnon, G.A. A field study evaluation for mitigating biofouling with chlorine dioxide or chlorine integrated with UV disinfection. *Water Res.* **2007**, *41*, 1939–1948. [CrossRef] [PubMed]
67. Murphy, H.M.; Payne, S.J.; Gagnon, G.A. Sequential UV- and chlorine-based disinfection to mitigate Escherichia coli in drinking water biofilms. *Water Res.* **2008**, *42*, 2083–2092. [CrossRef]
68. Ekowati, Y.; Ferrero, G.; Farré, M.J.; Kennedy, M.D.; Buttiglieri, G. Application of UVOX Redox®for swimming pool water treatment: Microbial inactivation, disinfection byproduct formation and micropollutant removal. *Chemosphere* **2019**, *220*, 176–184. [CrossRef]
69. Manasfi, T.; Temime-Roussel, B.; Coulomb, B.; Vassalo, L.; Boudenne, J.-L. Occurrence of brominated disinfection byproducts in the air and water of chlorinated seawater swimming pools. *Int. J. Hyg. Environ. Health* **2017**, *220*, 583–590. [CrossRef]

Article

Combined Biocidal Effect of Gaseous Ozone and Citric Acid on *Acinetobacter baumannii* Biofilm Formed on Ceramic Tiles and Polystyrene as a Novel Approach for Infection Prevention and Control

Kaća Piletić [1], Bruno Kovač [1], Matej Planinić [1], Vanja Vasiljev [2], Irena Brčić Karačonji [3,4], Jure Žigon [5], Ivana Gobin [1,6,*] and Martina Oder [7]

1. Department of Microbiology and Parasitology, Faculty of Medicine, University of Rijeka, 51000 Rijeka, Croatia
2. Department of Social Medicine and Epidemiology, Faculty of Medicine, University of Rijeka, 51000 Rijeka, Croatia
3. Toxicology Unit, Institute for Medical Research and Occupational Health, 10000 Zagreb, Croatia
4. Department of Basic Medical Sciences, Faculty of Health Studies, University of Rijeka, 51000 Rijeka, Croatia
5. Department of Wood Science and Technology, Biotechnical Faculty, University of Ljubljana, 1000 Ljubljana, Slovenia
6. Faculty of Health Studies, University of Mostar, 88000 Mostar, Bosnia and Herzegovina
7. Department of Sanitary Engineering, Faculty of Health Sciences, University of Ljubljana, 1000 Ljubljana, Slovenia
* Correspondence: ivana.gobin@medri.uniri.hr

Abstract: *Acinetobacter baumannii* is a prominent emerging pathogen responsible for a variety of hospital-acquired infections. It can contaminate inanimate surfaces and survive in harsh environmental conditions for prolonged periods of time in the form of biofilm. Biofilm is difficult to remove with only one method of disinfection, so combined disinfection methods and biocidal active substances are needed for biofilm eradication. Additionally, having in mind ecological demands, legislators are more prone using fewer toxic substances for disinfection that produce less solid waste and hazardous disinfection byproducts. Gaseous ozone and citric acid are natural biocidal compounds, and the purpose of this study was to determine their combined biocidal effects on *A. baumannii* biofilm formed on ceramics and polystyrene. Twenty-four-hour *A. baumannii* biofilm formed on ceramic tiles and polystyrene was exposed to different combinations of disinfection protocols with 25 ppm of gaseous ozone for 1 h exposure time and 15% citric acid for 10 min exposure. The total number of bacteria was counted afterwards and expressed as CFU/cm^2. The determined disinfection protocols of *A. baumannii* biofilm with combined citric acid and gaseous ozone caused reduction of 2.8 to 5.89 log_{10} CFU (99.99% inhibition rate) of total viable bacteria for each method, with the citric acid–ozone–citric acid disinfection protocol being most successful in eradication of viable bacteria on both ceramics and polystyrene. In conclusion, gaseous ozone and citric acid showed good combined biocidal effects on *A. baumannii* biofilm and successfully reduced early *A. baumannii* biofilm from ceramic and polystyrene surfaces. The given combination of active substances can be a good option for eco-friendly disinfection of hospital inanimate surfaces from *A. baumannii* biofilm contamination with prior mechanical cleaning.

Keywords: *Acinetobacter baumannii*; biofilm; citric acid; combined disinfection; infection prevention; infection control; ozone

1. Introduction

Amongst the many virulence factors that make *Acinetobacter baumannii* interesting for hospital infection control and prevention is its ability to form biofilm on abiotic and biotic surfaces [1–4]. This Gram-negative opportunistic pathogen, during its evolution, acquired characteristics such as flagella and pili, adhesins on bacterial surface) and certain genes that allow it to successfully adhere to surfaces and then form biofilm [3–6]. Because of biofilm formation, *A. baumannii* can survive long stretches of time in harsh environments such as hospital inanimate surfaces [4,5,7–9]. Biofilm represents bacterial congregation embedded in a self-produced extracellular polymeric substance (EPS) that serves as a shield and protects bacteria within from environmental influences [5,10–13]. *A. baumannii* in biofilm form can withstand prolonged and frequent use of antibiotics and prolonged and frequent disinfection and expresses a high survival rate in environments without nutrients or water availability [2–5,9,14]. It is hypothesized that capability of biofilm formation of *A. baumannii* is one of the factors responsible for the remarkable ability of *A. baumannii* to acquire multidrug resistance [15]. *A. baumannii* is one of the nosocomial pathogens that has rapidly developed resistance to multiple available antimicrobial agents and poses great challenge for therapy and outcome of hospital acquired infections [6,16,17]. Even though *A. baumannii* is considered to be a low-virulent bacteria, its ability to rapidly form resistance factors has made it endemic to many hospitals, especially intensive care units, despite implemented infection control strategies [15,18]. The main sources of *A. baumannii* in hospital environment are infected patients and staff, contaminated surfaces, and previous room occupancy by colonized patients [19,20]. Key strategies to stop the spreading of *A. baumannii* contamination through hospital environment are staff hand hygiene and frequent mechanical cleaning and surface disinfection [15,21–23]. These infection control measures can only be achieved by frequent use of antiseptics and disinfectants [15,23], but sometimes frequent or incorrect use of the same available disinfectants can result in development of bacterial resistance towards it [8,24–28]. Additionally, the ability of *A. baumannii* to form biofilm on abiotic hospital surfaces can be related to greater resistance to available disinfectants [9,29]. Numerous studies highlight the fact that bacteria in biofilm are more resistant to disinfectants, potentially due to EPS production that limits disinfectant penetration into biofilm [30–35]. Some authors reported that in Gram-negative bacteria, concomitant antibiotic and antiseptic/disinfectant resistance can occur, and that high multidrug resistance can also result in higher resistance towards disinfectants [8,19,36]. Usually, the introduction of novel disinfection methods to hospital environments can be a potential solution to this challenge [30,37,38], so the occurrence of resistant *A. baumannii* towards standardly used disinfectants in hospitals can possibly be mitigated with the introduction of innovative technologies to fight *A. baumannii* biofilm in hospitals. Such innovative strategies can involve application of gaseous disinfectants, hot vapor, and combinations of the effects of two biocidal active substances trying to evade *A. baumannii* resistance mechanism [22,23,30,39]. Ozone gas is the strongest known oxidizing agent and has proven antimicrobial properties against planktonic bacterial forms and certain biofilms [40,41]. Even though ozone is toxic to humans, it rapidly dissociates into oxygen and is considered environmentally friendly [40]. It achieves its oxidizing action through molecular ozone or free oxygen radicals. An antimicrobial effect is expressed by the oxidation of glycolipids and glycoproteins, and by oxidizing sulfhydryl groups and amino acids of enzymes and oxidizing peptides and proteins. It is also toxic to nucleic acids [42–45]. Due to modern legislators' strategic goals of uses of efficient but less environmentally toxic biocidal substances producing less solid waste, ozone can be considered as a potential good novel disinfectant in *A. baumannii* infection prevention and control [46]. Citric acid is a weak organic acid and a natural compound widely distributed in plant and animal material. It is considered safe to humans and the environment with no toxic residues and has good antimicrobial properties [47,48]. Citric acid achieves its antimicrobial effect by lowering intracellular pH and subsequently damaging proteins, DNA and membranes, leading to cell death [13,49]. It also exhibits chelating activity sequestering metal ions such as calcium, iron and magnesium ions which are (e.g., Ca^{2+}, Mg^{2+}, Fe^{3+}) essential for bacterial homeostasis [50,51]. The antibiofilm action of citric acid has been studied against, Gram negative bacteria like *Pseudomonas aeruginosa*, *Klebsiella pneumoniae*, *Escherichia coli* and Gram positive bacteria such as *Staphylococcus aureus*, mostly in food processing industry [35,49,51,52], but less frequently in hospital acquired infection prevention and control or wound treatments [47,48,53,54]. The combination of two different biocidal substances, as compared with a single biocidal substance, may result in more efficient antibacterial activity that can allow the use of lower doses of each biocidal substance [13,49]. The combined effect of gaseous ozone and citric acid on *A. baumannii* biofilm has not been previously described, so the main objective of this study was to investigate the combined biocidal effect of gaseous ozone and citric acid on *A. baumannii* biofilm formed on ceramics and polystyrene, which are relatively frequently used materials in healthcare settings, as a potential novel environmentally friendly strategy for infection prevention and control.

2. Materials and Methods

2.1. Bacterial Strains and Biofilm Formation on Ceramic Tile and Polystyrene

Two standard strains of *A. baumannii* obtained from culture collection of the Department of Microbiology, University of Rijeka used in this study were *A. baumannii* ATCC BAA-1605 and *A. baumannii* ATCC 19606. Materials used for biofilm formation were upper smooth surface mosaic ceramic tile (2.5 cm × 2.5 cm) and standard 96-well microtiter plates for polystyrene (Pierce™ 96-well polystyrene plates, Thermofisher Scientific, Whaltmann, MA, USA). Prior to the biofilm formation on ceramic tiles, tiles were washed and sterilized, and then a modified method previously described by Ivanković et al. [29] was used. Briefly, 2% agar was melted in autoclave and when cooled, poured aside three mosaic tiles in petri dish, leaving upper surface of the tile's agar free. Then, around 10^5 CFU/mL of diluted overnight bacterial suspension was poured over upper ceramic tiles side and incubated for 24 h at 25 ± 2 °C. Ninety-six-well microtiter plates were used for biofilm formation on polystyrene. In sterile microplates, around 10^5 CFU/mL of diluted overnight bacterial suspension was poured and incubated for 24 h at 25 ± 2 °C.

2.2. Ozone Treatment Test Protocol (Protocol A)

A sealed off experimental chamber with volume of 125 L was used for ozone treatment [55]. Ozone was generated using a mobile ozone generator, model Mozon GPF 8008 (Mozon d.o.o., Sisak, Croatia), and insufflated into the chamber via 6 mm silicone tube. Before the ozone treatment, both ceramic tiles and microtiters plates were rinsed off with saline and dried out for 1 min in a sterile chamber before the ozonation. 24-hour old biofilm on ceramic tiles and microtiters plates re e exposed to ozone action with following parameters: 25 ppm ozone, 1 h exposure time, relative humidity 55–57% and room temperature of 23 ± 5 °C. During the experiment, ozone concentration was monitored with mobile detector model Keernuo GT901 (Shanghai, China), relative humidity and temperature was monitored with an Auriol 4-LD5531 (Berlin, Germany). After the treatment, ceramic tiles were aseptically removed from agar, rinsed off with saline and placed in 50 mL tube with 10 mL saline (1 tile per 1 tube). Tubes containing tiles were then sonicated at 40 kHz/1 min to detach leftover biofilm from the tiles. Afterwards, tiles were once again homogenized using vortex and ten-fold serial dilutions were prepared. Process was similar with microtiter plates. After ozone treatment, saline was added in microplates, then microplates were sonicated at 40 kHz/1 min. After homogenization, bottom of the microplates was scraped off with sterile pipette tip to enhance biofilm detachment. Afterwards, ten-fold serial dilutions were made. When samples were prepared, the number of bacteria was determined, and results were expressed as CFU/cm^2. Non treated biofilm on ceramic tiles and microtiter plates within the same environmental parameters (temperature and relative humidity) served as control. The experiment were done in triplicate.

2.3. Citric Acid Treatment Test Protocol (Protocol B)

Twenty-four-old biofilm of two standard *A. baumannii* strains (ATCC BAA-1605 and ATCC 19606) formed on three ceramic tiles and polystyrene microtiter plates were treated with previously prepared 15% citric acid solution for 10 min exposure time, according to the manufacturer's instructions regarding the usual concentration and exposure time that exhibits adverse biocidal effect. Ceramic tiles were then further processed according to Section 2.2.

2.4. Combined Ozone–Citric Acid Test Protocols (Protocols C–E)

Different combinations of ozone -citric acid disinfection protocols were performed to determine biocidal effect of both active substances. Twenty-four-hour-old biofilms of *A. baumannii* ATCC BAA-1605 and *A. baumannii* ATCC 19606 formed on ceramics and polystyrene were exposed to the following treatments: citric acid–ozone (Protocol C), ozone–citric acid (Protocol D), and citric acid–ozone–citric acid (Protocol E). For Protocol C, biofilm was firstly exposed to 15% of citric acid as described in Section 2.3. After the treatment, ceramic tiles and polystyrene were rinsed off with sterile saline, dried off for 1 min in a sterile environment, and exposed to gaseous ozone as described in Section 2.2. Afterwards, ten-fold serial dilutions were made and inoculated on MH agar and then incubated for 24–48 h at 35 ± 2 °C. For Protocol D treatment, 24 h-old biofilm of *A. baumannii* formed on ceramic tiles and polystyrene was first exposed to gaseous ozone action as described in Section 2.2. Ozone treated biofilm on both materials was removed from the chamber and then exposed to citric acid treatment as described in Section 2.3. In Protocol E, biofilm of *A. baumannii* was first exposed to citric acid as described in Section 2.3, then to gaseous ozone as described in Section 2.2, and then again to citric acid. After all combinations used in this study and after the incubation period, the number of cultivable bacteria was expressed as CFU/cm^2.

2.5. Cell Viability Using Propidium Iodide Dye

Propidium iodide (PI) dye (Molecular Probes, Eugene, OR, USA) was used to determine cell viability and to detect dead bacterial cells. Briefly, following the treatment with ozone gas and citric acid, ceramic tiles and microtiter plates were rinsed off with sterile saline solution and fluorescent dye PI was applied to biofilm on both materials and incubated in the dark for 15 min. After the incubation, to remove the excess dye, both materials were rinsed off with sterile saline. For fluorescence observation, an inverted microscope at 20× magnification (Olympus IX51, Tokyo, Japan) was used. The obtained images were analyzed in ImageJ 1.47 (National Institute for Health, Bethesda, MD, USA). Untreated biofilm represented control samples.

2.6. Crystal Violet Staining and Digital Microscopy

A. baumannii biofilm formed on polystyrene and ceramic tiles was stained with crystal-violet (CV) dye to perform digital microscope images. Treated biofilm from ceramic tiles was rinsed off with sterile saline and then fixated in a dry heat sterilizer (ST-01/02, Instrumentaria, Zagreb, Croatia) at 80 °C for 30 min, while on polystyrene, a blow dryer was used for fixation. Following fixation, biofilm was stained with 0.1% CV for 30 min.

Ceramic surfaces were microscopically examined with a DSX 1000 digital microscope (Olympus, Tokyo, Japan) at 20× magnification with 2-dimensional and 3-dimensional images with the digital microscope. Polystyrene surfaces were examined with an inverted microscope (Olympus, Tokyo, Japan) at magnification 20×.

2.7. Statistical Analyses and Graphing

For evaluation of both combined biocidal effects and solitary effects of gaseous ozone and citric acid, data were analyzed using Wilcoxon signed rank tests ($p < 0.05$), while Microsoft Excel, version 11.00 (Microsoft Home Office, 2021) was used for graphic images. For evaluation of differences between the used material and methods between one strain, Mann-Whitney test was performed ($p < 0.05$), as well as for determination of differences between tested strains and used methods. For determination of differences between the tested methods, Kruskal-Wallis multiple comparison test were performed ($p < 0.05$).

3. Results

To determine the biocidal effects of gaseous ozone and citric acid as solitary disinfectants, and to determine the combined biocidal effects of both disinfectants, a series of experiments with different disinfection protocols with both disinfectants was done, all resulting in significant reductions of viable bacteria in biofilm in comparison to the control (Wilcoxon signed rank test, $p < 0.05$).

3.1. Viable Bacteria Reduction with Gaseous Ozone–Citric Acid Solitary Effect and Combinations on Ceramic Tiles

Tested strains of both *A. baumannii* ATCC BAA-1605 and *A. baumannii* ATCC 19606 showed biofilm reduction on ceramic tiles after the disinfection protocols. The combined biocidal effects of gaseous ozone and citric acid are shown in Figure 1 with the highest $\log_{10}$ CFU reductions of both strains observed with protocol E (combination of pretreatment with citric acid, main treatment with gaseous ozone, and then posttreatment with citric acid). Both citric acid and gaseous ozone in combination, regardless of disinfection protocol used, showed greater biofilm reduction in comparison to solitary gaseous ozone and citric acid treatments. There was a significant difference observed between the two bacterial strains of *A. baumannii* on ceramics and the used disinfection protocols (Mann–Whitney, $p < 0.05$), as well as significant difference between different disinfection protocols on each bacterial strain used on ceramics (Kruskal–Wallis multiple comparison test was performed, $p < 0.05$).

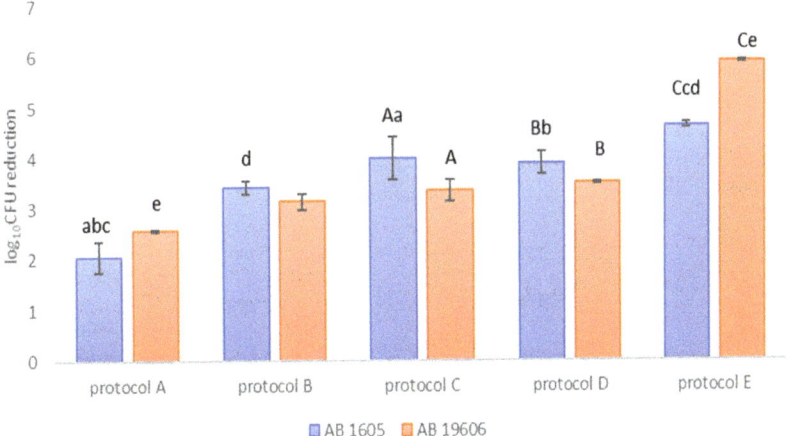

Figure 1. Viable bacteria count expressed as $\log_{10}$ CFU reduction of *Acinetobacter baumannii* ATCC BAA-1605 and *Acinetobacter baumannii* ATCC 19606 with standard deviation. Protocol A marks disinfection with gaseous ozone, Protocol B disinfection with citric acid, Protocol C a combination of citric acid–gaseous ozone, Protocol D a combination of gaseous ozone–citric acid, and Protocol E a combination of citric acid–gaseous ozone–citric acid. Lowercase letters (a–e) express statistically significant differences between disinfection protocols for one bacterial strain (Kruskal–Wallis U, $p < 0.05$). Capital letters (A, B, C) mark statistically significant differences between different bacterial strains per used Protocols C, D, and E.

3.2. Viable Bacteria Reduction with Gaseous Ozone–Citric Acid Solitary and Combination Effects on Polystyrene

The reduction of viable bacteria using different disinfection protocols on biofilm of *A. baumannii* ATCC BAA-1605 and *A. baumannii* ATCC 19606 formed on polystyrene is shown in Figure 2. Protocol E (combination of pretreatment with citric acid, main treatment with gaseous ozone, and then posttreatment with citric acid) caused a reduction greater than 5 $\log_{10}$CFU for both strains. Both strains showed slightly higher bacterial reductions of combined disinfection protocols on polystyrene in comparison to ceramics. There were statistically significant differences between *A. baumannii* ATCC BAA-1605 and *A. baumannii* ATCC 19606 for all protocols (Kruskal–Wallis multiple comparison test was performed ($p < 0.05$). Additionally, there was no statistically significant difference between the used materials and the efficacy of protocols for strain *A. baumannii* ATCC BAA-1605, while for strain *A. baumannii* ATCC 19606, there was a significant difference between the used materials and the efficacy of the tested methods (not shown).

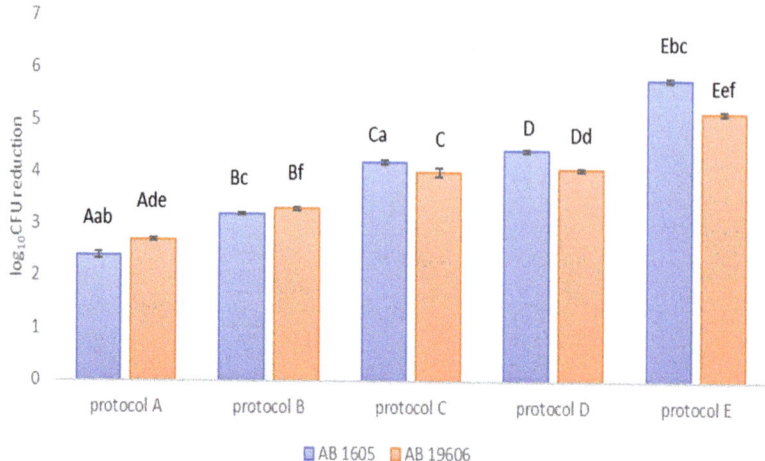

Figure 2. Viable bacteria count expressed as $\log_{10}$ CFU reduction of *Acinetobacter baumannii* ATCC BAA-1605 and *Acinetobacter baumannii* ATCC 19606 formed on polystyrene with standard deviation. Protocol A marks disinfection with gaseous ozone, Protocol B disinfection with citric acid, Protocol C a combination of citric acid–gaseous ozone, Protocol D a combination of gaseous ozone–citric acid, and Protocol E a combination of citric acid–gaseous ozone–citric acid. Lowercase letters (a–f) express statistically significant differences between disinfection protocol and bacterial strain (Kruskal–Wallis U, $p < 0.05$). Capital letters (A, B, C, D, and E) mark statistically significant differences between different used bacterial strain per disinfection protocol.

3.3. Different Disinfection Protocols with Gaseous Ozone and Citric Acid Caused Different Inhibition Rates on Polystyrene and Ceramic Tiles

Gaseous ozone and citric acid used in different combinations of disinfection protocols on *A. baumannii* ATCC BAA-1605 and *A. baumannii* ATCC 19606 biofilms formed on polystyrene and ceramic tiles caused different inhibition rates (Table 1). The inhibition rates varied from 61.63% up to 99.99%, depending on solitary or combined use of biocidal active substances. Biofilm formed on polystyrene showed slightly higher inhibition rates for both strains than biofilm formed on ceramic tiles.

Table 1. Percentages of inhibition of both *A. baumannii* strains of biofilm formed on polystyrene and ceramics after disinfection protocols. Protocol A marks disinfection with gaseous ozone, Protocol B disinfection with citric acid, Protocol C a combination of citric acid–gaseous ozone, Protocol D a combination of gaseous ozone–citric acid, and Protocol E a combination of citric acid–gaseous ozone–citric acid.

Surfaces	*A. baumannii* ATCC BAA1605					*A. baumannii* ATCC 19606				
	Treatments (% Biofilm Destruction)									
	Protocol					Protocol				
	A	B	C	D	E	A	B	C	D	E
Polystyrene	61.6	94.06	99.4	99.33	99.98	80.32	97.35	99.02	99.13	99.93
Ceramic tiles	89.9	82.7	98.29	98.53	99.77	73.3	93.77	96.16	97.4	99.99

3.4. Combined Biocidal Effect of Gaseous Ozone and Citric Acid on Cell Viability

A representative strain of *A. baumannii* ATCC 19606 treated with different disinfection protocols (Protocol A (solitary ozone), Protocol B (solitary citric acid), Protocol C (citric acid–ozone), Protocol D (ozone–citric acid), and Protocol E (citric acid–ozone–citric acid)) is shown in Figure 3. Biofilm not exposed to disinfection with ozone gas and citric acid did not show dead bacterial cells (Figure 3CN), while clustered dead bacterial cells (red) could be seen in the treated biofilm (Figure 3A–E). The absence of dead bacterial cells marked the destruction of bacterial cells and biofilm detachment from the material.

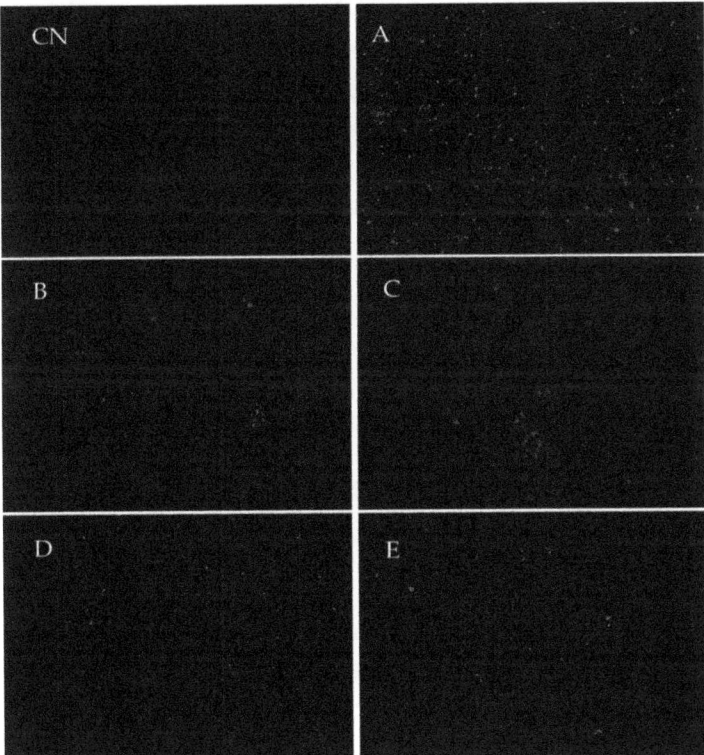

Figure 3. Viability of *A. baumannii* ATCC 19606 biofilm treated with different disinfection protocols ((**A**) solitary ozone, (**B**) solitary citric acid, (**C**) citric acid–ozone, (**D**) ozone–citric acid, (**E**) citric acid–ozone–citric acid) using propidium iodide staining. The control group was non-treated biofilm (**CN**). Red fluorescence indicates dead cells with permeable membranes. Magnification 20×.

3.5. Crystal Violet Microscopy

To determine changes in biofilm morphology after disinfection protocols (Protocol A—solitary gaseous ozone, Protocol B—solitary citric acid, Protocol C—citric acid–ozone, Protocol D—ozone–citric acid, and Protocol E–citric acid–gaseous ozone–citric acid), light microscopy was performed. Morphological changes in biofilm of representative strain *A. baumannii* ATCC 19606 formed on ceramics were found, where 3-dimensional images of Protocols A–D and E can be seen in Figure 4A–E. The distribution of crystal violet dye marked bacterial cell presence. The highest 3-dimensional peaks of *A. baumannii* biofilm were the first exposed to biocidal action and the first to deteriorate after the disinfection. Combined biocidal effects can be clearly shown in Figure 4E, where the absence of crystal violet dye and cells marked the disinfection effects of combined biocides and biofilm destruction and detachment from ceramics and polystyrene.

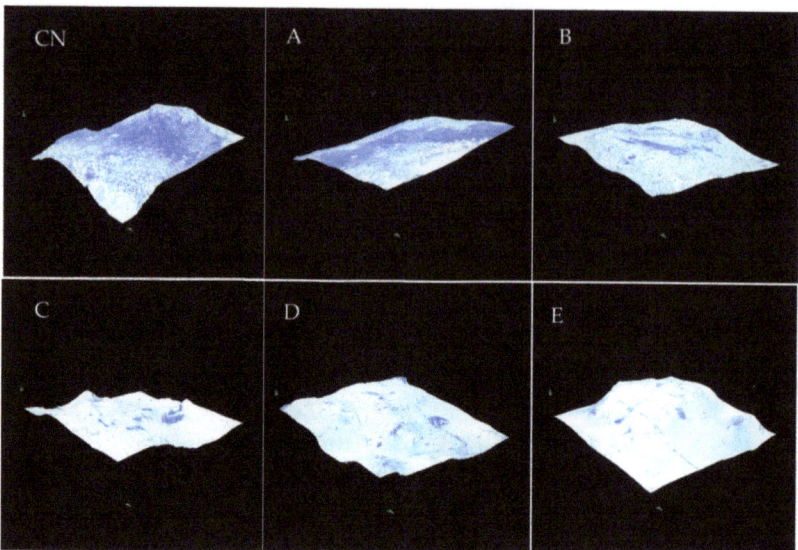

Figure 4. The 3-dimensional images of ceramic tile surface with formed 24 h *A. baumannii* ATCC 19606 biofilm treated with different disinfection protocols (Protocol (**A**)—solitary ozone gas, Protocol (**B**)—solitary citric acid, Protocol (**C**)—citric acid–ozone, Protocol (**D**)—ozone–citric acid, Protocol (**E**)—citric acid–ozone–citric acid) and non-treated control (**CN**). Magnification 20×.

Figure 5 shows 2-dimensional images of representative *A. baumannii* ATCC 19606 biofilm on ceramics after disinfection protocols (Protocol A—solitary ozone, Protocol B—solitary citric acid, Protocol C—citric acid–ozone, Protocol D—ozone–citric acid, and Protocol E—citric acid–gaseous ozone–citric acid). The presented images show that the material surface of tile if rough or uneven can influence the distribution of bacterial cells. Cells were growing more easily in depressed areas or small cavities (crystal violet-stained parts).

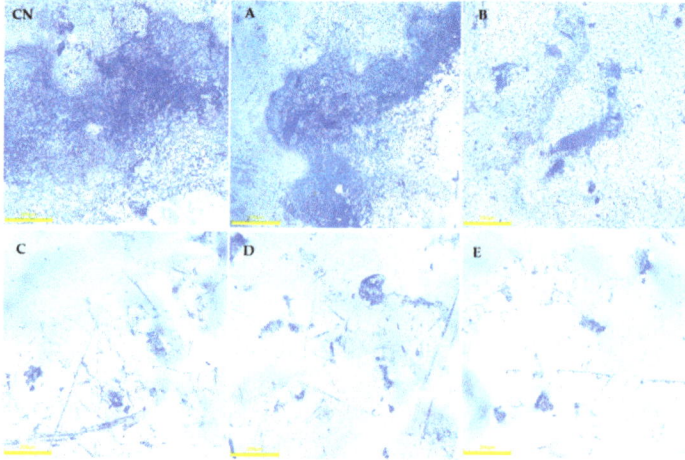

Figure 5. Images of ceramic tile surface with formed 24 h *A. baumannii* ATCC 19606 biofilm treated with different disinfection protocols (**A**–**E**). The control was provided with non-treated biofilm (**CN**). Magnification 20×.

Different combinations and application orders of gaseous ozone and citric acid on representative *A. baumannii* ATCC 19606 biofilm on polystyrene caused morphological changes in biofilm density (Figure 6). The best antibiofilm effect for both materials was observed for Protocol E.

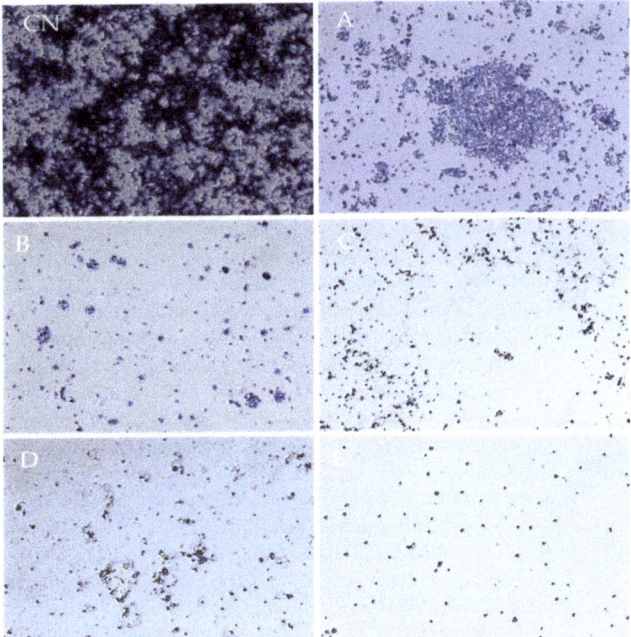

Figure 6. The 2-dimensional images of 24 h representative strain *A. baumannii* ATCC 19606 biofilm formed on polystyrene treated with different disinfection protocols (**A–E**). (**CN**) marks control group. The dark blue stains present the bacteria stained with crystal violet. The control was provided with *A. baumannii* ATCC 19606 biofilm not exposed to combined or solitary ozone gas and citric acid effects. Magnification 20×.

4. Discussion

Contamination of hospital environments with *A. baumannii* biofilm is a potential source of infections, especially in hospital wards with immunocompromised patients, so one way of infection prevention and control is keeping the wards free of biofilm [3,11,14,18]. Once formed on surfaces, *A. baumannii* biofilm is challenging to remove because of biofilm characteristics such as resistance to disinfectants, desiccation, long survival in nutrient free environments, and resistance to antibiotics [3,4,14]. Additionally, the survival of *A. baumannii* in hospital wards where high levels of conventional disinfectants are used on a daily basis can lead to acquired resistance of *A. baumannii* towards them, especially if disinfectants are used contrary to manufacturer's instructions [1,15,16,29]. Thus, one of the main goals of infection prevention teams in hospitals is to maintain high levels of hand and environmental hygiene, choosing the correct disinfectant, and use the optimal concentration to fight biofilm contamination [23,38,56,57]. One of the novel trends in surface disinfection of both environment and foods is the use of environmentally friendly disinfectants such as ozone gas and organic acids such as citric acid [37,40,47,48,52,58–60]. When used in combination, two biocidal active substances can achieve stronger antimicrobial effects with smaller dosages of both disinfectants, which can also have better effects on chemical waste management, less toxicity for staff and the environment, and lower costs of disinfection [35,61]. The aim of this study was to investigate antibiofilm effects of combined disinfection with gaseous ozone and citric acid on early *A. baumannii* biofilm formed on ceramics and polystyrene, two relatively frequent materials in hospitals.

In trying to determine the optimal disinfection protocol for *A. baumannii* biofilm removal, different ozone gas–citric acid combinations were investigated (pretreatment with citric acid then treatment with gaseous ozone, pretreatment with gaseous ozone then citric acid, pretreatment with citric acid then gaseous ozone and posttreatment with citric acid, solitary citric acid treatment and solitary gaseous ozone treatment) using gaseous ozone in effective concentrations determined in a previous study done by authors and citric acid in concentrations according to the manufacturer's instructions. Both ozone gas and citric acid when used in combination, showed good antibiofilm effects and caused significant reduction in viable bacteria count. Additionally, the combination of ozone gas and citric acid resulted in greater reduction of viable bacteria when used in combination in comparison to their effect as solitary disinfectants. These results were similar to the results of Britton et al., Vankerckhoven et al., Cho et al. and Jung et al., where greater antibiofilm effect were achieved when two biocidal active substances were used in combination [37,61–63]. Interestingly, there was no significant difference for both strains and used materials between Protocol C and Protocol D combined disinfection on the viable bacteria count, indicating that in achieving its antimicrobial effect, there was no difference in order of application of these disinfectants. Only the combination of citric acid–gaseous ozone–citric acid showed the highest reduction rates in elimination above 5 $\log_{10}$ CFU reduction of both materials, so only this disinfection protocol can be regarded as efficient according to the *European Chemical Agency Guidance on the Biocidal product Regulation, Volume II*—efficacy [64]. Additionally, this combined disinfection protocol showed a statistically significant difference in comparison to other protocols on both tested strains and materials.

Regarding differences between combined disinfection protocols and the tested materials for each tested bacterial strain (results not shown), there were no statistically significant differences between polystyrene and ceramics on *A. baumannii* ATCC BAA-1605 biofilm, while there were significant differences between the used combined disinfection protocols and *A. baumannii* ATCC 19606 biofilm grown on polystyrene and ceramic tiles, indicating that numerous factors, such as strain sensitivity, material selection, and sanitation protocol, can influence the success of sanitation and disinfection on formed biofilm, as previously emphasized by Gaddy et al., Qi et al., and Rodriguez-Bano et al. [2,3,65].

There is a lack of data on the combined effect of gaseous ozone and citric acid on *A. baumannii* formed on polystyrene and ceramic tiles. Some studies, such as Jung et. al. [61], explored the synergistic effects of sequential or combined uses of ozone and UV radiation on *B. subtilis* spores, and studies such as Cho et al. [63] explored the synergistic effects of citric acid and xenon light on the inactivation of food pathogens. Other studies such as Ha et al. [66] explored the synergistic effects of combined disinfection using sodium hypochlorite and ethanol with UV light to reduce *Staphylococcus aureus*, while Vankerckhoven et al. [61] studied the potential synergistic effects of chemical disinfectants and UV light on biofilm [62]. All these studies have similar conclusions, namely, when used in combination, two biocidal active substances yield better antimicrobial effects than when used alone.

Ozone gas achieves its antimicrobial action through oxidation, while citric acid achieves its action by lowering the intracellular pH and acting as a metal chelator, leading to membrane instability and cell death [35,43,47,48], as shown in Figure 7. Both ozone gas and citric acid achieve their biocidal effects with different mechanisms of actions, so it can be expected that this combination can have good antimicrobial effects on *A. baumannii* biofilm. Additionally, another element of good combined action of ozone and citric acid is emphasized in studies such as Hirahara et al. [67], where the authors underlined the fact that when used in aqueous form, citric acid enables ozone to have a longer half-life in water, which certainly enhances its antimicrobial action.

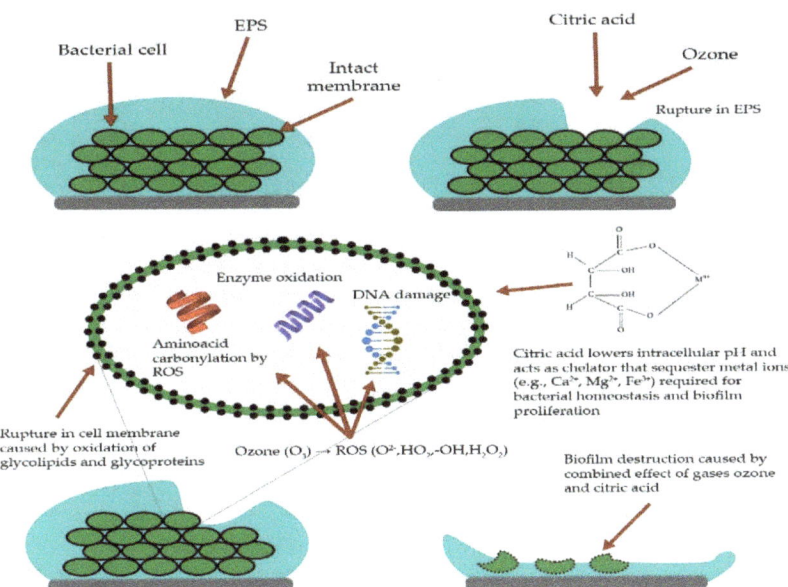

Figure 7. Schematic representation of combined effect of gaseous ozone and citric acid on *A. baumannii* biofilm formed on ceramic tiles.

To determine the effect of ozone and citric acid combination on cell membrane permeability, propidium iodide staining was performed. The combined effect of ozone gas and citric acid led to a greater number of dead bacterial cells as a result of disturbed membrane permeability, which was also previously confirmed by studies such as Piletić et al. and Nagayoshi et al. [67,68]. Additionally, this combination of biocides, in combination citric acid-ozone gas-citric acid, caused total destruction and biofilm detachment from the material, which indicated good practical potential for eradication of biofilm from inanimate surfaces.

To determine how the combined biocidal effect of gaseous ozone and citric acid influenced *A. baumannii* biofilm morphology, light microscopy of all sanitation protocols was performed. All treated biofilms showed reductions in numbers of viable bacteria, clearly visible as blank areas in biofilm surfaces, and the combination of citric acid-ozone gas-citric acid caused total biofilm destruction and detachment from the surface. Additionally, using 3D imagery of treated biofilm, it was clearly shown that both ozone gas and citric acid attacked the topologically highest peaks of biofilm, starting to degrade it from the top, possibly because the highest parts are the first contact points for both biocides. These findings are in line with a previous study done by the authors on gaseous ozone efficacy on *K. pneumoniae* biofilm formed on ceramics, where most morphological changes were observed at the highest topological points of 3D biofilm structures [55].

Regarding the cost effectiveness of using this combination for disinfection protocols in hospitals or other healthcare facilities, there are some issues to address. Ozone gas is relatively cheap to produce with an ozone generator, and it rapidly dissociates to oxygen, therefore leaving no solid waste. In gaseous form it can reach all surfaces in hospital wards, and it is considered to be environmentally friendly [40,58,59]. Additionally, it can be used for air disinfection, which is especially important during hospital-acquired infection outbreaks or COVID-19 outbreaks [69]. Negative side effects are that ozone gas is toxic and must be administered with qualified personnel and can leave an odor, but this can be mitigated with ozone quench gas [55]. Citric acid has numerous advantages; it is not toxic to humans and can be used without the usual precautions, and it is also considered to be environmentally friendly [48]. Both biocides can be favorable according to new policies regarding the usage of chemicals and chemical waste of the European Commission Chemicals strategy for sustainability, which is part of the European Union's zero pollution ambition [46].

Although ozone gas is a strong oxidative agent, and citric acid is known to be a good food disinfectant and to successfully reduce the number of viable bacteria, they failed to completely eradicate early *A. baumannii* biofilm from ceramic tiles and polystyrene in the designed concentrations and exposure times for all tested protocol. This issue can potentially be overcome with thorough mechanical cleaning and prior disinfection using stronger detergents, as surfactants can make changes in membrane permeability and make them more susceptible to biocidal effects.

5. Conclusions

Gaseous ozone and citric acid show good antibiofilm effects when used in sequential, combined disinfection and in comparison, to when used as solitary disinfectants.

The best results, achieving almost eradication of *A. baumannii* biofilm, were observed while using the sequential combination protocol of citric acid–gaseous ozone–citric acid, causing almost full destruction and detachment of biofilm from the surfaces. This combination of biocides has the most implications for practical applications of both biocides, especially for infection prevention and control in healthcare settings.

All tested protocols of combined and solitary used gaseous ozone and citric acid caused biofilm reduction and morphological changes in biofilm structure and made changes in the membrane permeability.

Gaseous ozone and citric acid, when used in the proposed combinations, have good potential to be used for combined disinfection as eco-friendly disinfectants to fight *A. baumannii* biofilm formed on polystyrene and ceramics.

Author Contributions: Conceptualization, M.O. and I.G.; methodology, K.P. and I.G.; validation, B.K.; investigation, K.P., B.K., M.P., V.V. and I.B.K.; resources, I.G. and M.O.; writing—original draft preparation, K.P., B.K. and M.P.; writing—review and editing, I.G., M.O. and I.B.K.; visualization, J.Ž. and I.G.; supervision, I.G. and M.O.; project administration, M.O. and I.G. All authors have read and agreed to the published version of the manuscript.

Funding: This research was funded by the University of Rijeka, grant number UNIRI-biomed 18-171.

Data Availability Statement: Not applicable.

Acknowledgments: The authors express gratitude to the company Mozone d.o.o., Sisak, Croatia, for donation of the ozone generator and other equipment for the experiment.

Conflicts of Interest: The authors declare no conflict of interest.

References

1. Liu, W.L.; Liang, H.W.; Lee, M.F.; Lin, H.L.; Lin, Y.H.; Chen, C.C.; Chang, P.C.; Lai, C.C.; Chuang, Y.C.; Tang, H.J. The impact of inadequate terminal disinfection on an outbreak of imipenem-resistant *Acinetobacter Baumanniiin* an intensive care unit. *PLoS ONE* **2014**, *9*, e107975. [CrossRef]
2. Qi, L.; Li, H.; Zhang, C.; Liang, B.; Li, J.; Wang, L.; Du, X.; Liu, X.; Qiu, S.; Song, H. Relationship between antibiotic resistance, biofilm formation, and biofilm-specific resistance in *Acinetobacter baumannii*. *Front. Microbiol.* **2016**, *7*, 483. [CrossRef] [PubMed]
3. Gaddy, A.; Actis, J. A Regulation of *Acinetobacter baumannii* biofilm formation. *Mol. Cell. Biochem.* **2012**, *23*, 273–278. [CrossRef] [PubMed]
4. Espinal, P.; Martí, S.; Vila, J. Effect of biofilm formation on the survival of *Acinetobacter baumannii* on dry surfaces. *J. Hosp. Infect.* **2012**, *80*, 56–60. [CrossRef]
5. Tomaras, A.P.; Dorsey, C.W.; Edelmann, R.E.; Actis, L.A. Attachment to and biofilm formation on abiotic surfaces by *Acinetobacter baumannii*: Involvement of a novel chaperone-usher pili assembly system. *Microbiology* **2003**, *149*, 3473–3484. [CrossRef]
6. Bergogne-Bé, E.; Zin, R.É.; Towner, K.J. Acinetobacter ssp. as nosocomial Pathogens. *Clin. Microbiol. Rev.* **1996**, *9*, 148–165. [CrossRef]
7. Nor A'shimi, M.H.; Alattraqchi, A.G.; Rani, F.M.; Rahman, N.I.A.; Ismail, S.; Abdullah, F.H.; Othman, N.; Cleary, D.W.; Clarke, S.C.; Yeo, C.C. Biocide susceptibilities and biofilm-forming capacities of *Acinetobacter baumannii* clinical isolates from Malaysia. *J. Infect. Dev. Ctries.* **2019**, *13*, 626–633. [CrossRef]
8. Wisplinghoff, H.; Schmitt, R.; Wöhrmann, A.; Stefanik, D.; Seifert, H. Resistance to disinfectants in epidemiologically defined clinical isolates of *Acinetobacter baumannii*. *J. Hosp. Infect.* **2007**, *66*, 174–181. [CrossRef]

9. Rajamohan, G.; Srinivasan, V.B.; Gebreyes, W.A. Biocide-tolerant multidrug-resistant *Acinetobacter baumannii* clinical strains are associated with higher biofilm formation. *J. Hosp. Infect.* 2009, *73*, 287–289. [CrossRef]
10. Donlan, M. Rodney Biofilms: Microbial life on surfaces. *An. Real Acad. Nac. Farm.* 2016, *82*, 108–126.
11. Vickery, K.; Deva, A.; Jacombs, A.; Allan, J.; Valente, P.; Gosbell, I.B. Presence of biofilm containing viable multiresistant organisms despite terminal cleaning on clinical surfaces in an intensive care unit. *J. Hosp. Infect.* 2012, *80*, 52–55. [CrossRef] [PubMed]
12. Vickery, K. Special Issue: Microbial biofilms in healthcare: Formation, prevention and treatment. *Materials* 2019, *12*, 2001. [CrossRef] [PubMed]
13. Kim, H.W.; Lee, N.Y.; Park, S.M.; Rhee, M.S. A fast and effective alternative to a high-ethanol disinfectant: Low concentrations of fermented ethanol, caprylic acid, and citric acid synergistically eradicate biofilm-embedded methicillin-resistant *Staphylococcus aureus*. *Int. J. Hyg. Environ. Health* 2020, *229*, 113586. [CrossRef] [PubMed]
14. Narayanan, A.; Nair, M.S.; Karumathil, D.P.; Baskaran, S.A. Inactivation of *Acinetobacter baumannii* Biofilms on Polystyrene, Stainless Steel, and Urinary Catheters by Octenidine Dihydrochloride. *Front. Microbiol.* 2016, *7*, 847. [CrossRef]
15. Lanjri, S.; Uwingabiye, J.; Frikh, M.; Abdellatifi, L.; Kasouati, J.; Maleb, A.; Bait, A.; Lemnouer, A.; Elouennass, M. In vitro evaluation of the susceptibility of *Acinetobacter baumannii* isolates to antiseptics and disinfectants: Comparison between clinical and environmental isolates. *Antimicrob. Resist. Infect. Control* 2017, *6*, 1–7. [CrossRef]
16. Kawamura-Sato, K.; Wachino, J.I.; Kondo, T.; Ito, H.; Arakawa, Y. Correlation between reduced susceptibility to disinfectants and multidrug resistance among clinical isolates of Acinetobacter species. *J. Antimicrob. Chemother.* 2010, *65*, 1975–1983. [CrossRef]
17. Soares, N.C.; Cabral, M.P.; Gayoso, C.; Mallo, S.; Rodriguez-Velo, P.; Fernández-Moreira, E.; Bou, G. Associating growth-phase-related changes in the proteome of acinetobacter baumannii with increased resistance to oxidative stress. *J. Proteome Res.* 2010, *9*, 1951–1964. [CrossRef]
18. Martró, E.; Hernández, A.; Ariza, J.; Domínguez, M.A.; Matas, L.; Argerich, M.J.; Martin, R.; Ausina, V. Assessment of *Acinetobacter baumannii* susceptibility to antiseptics and disinfectants. *J. Hosp. Infect.* 2003, *55*, 39–46. [CrossRef]
19. Babaei, M.R.; Sulong, A.; Hamat, R.A.; Nordin, S.A.; Neela, V.K. Extremely high prevalence of antiseptic resistant quaternary ammonium compound E gene among clinical isolates of multiple drug resistant acinetobacter baumannii in Malaysia. *Ann. Clin. Microbiol. Antimicrob.* 2015, *14*, 1–5. [CrossRef]
20. Jawad, A.; Seifert, H.; Snelling, A.M.; Heritage, J.; Hawkey, P.M. Survival of *Acinetobacter baumannii* on dry surfaces: Comparison of outbreak and sporadic isolates. *J. Clin. Microbiol.* 1998, *36*, 1938–1941. [CrossRef]
21. Denton, M.; Wilcox, M.H.; Parnell, P.; Green, D.; Keer, V.; Hawkey, P.M.; Evans, I.; Murphy, P. Role of environmental cleaning in controlling an outbreak of *Acinetobacter baumannii* on a neurosurgical intensive care unit. *J. Hosp. Infect.* 2004, *56*, 106–110. [CrossRef]
22. Manian, F.A.; Griesenauer, S.; Senkel, D.; Setzer, J.M.; Doll, S.A.; Perry, A.M.; Wiechens, M. Isolation of *Acinetobacter baumannii* Complex and Methicillin-Resistant *Staphylococcus aureus* from Hospital Rooms Following Terminal Cleaning and Disinfection: Can We Do Better? *Infect. Control Hosp. Epidemiol.* 2011, *32*, 667–672. [CrossRef]
23. Abreu, A.C.; Tavares, R.R.; Borges, A.; Mergulhão, F.; Simões, M. Current and emergent strategies for disinfection of hospital environments. *J. Antimicrob. Chemother.* 2013, *68*, 2718–2732. [CrossRef] [PubMed]
24. Stickler, D.J.; Thomas, B.; Chawla, J.C. Antiseptic and antibiotic resistance in gram-negative bacteria causing urinary tract infection in spinal cord injured patients. *Paraplegia* 1981, *19*, 50–58. [CrossRef] [PubMed]
25. Thomas, L.; Russell, A.D.; Maillard, J.-Y. Antimicrobial activity of chlorhexidine diacetate and benzalkonium chloride against Pseudomonas aeruginosa and its response to biocide residues. *J. Appl. Microbiol.* 2005, *98*, 533–543. [CrossRef] [PubMed]
26. Suller, M.T.E.; Russell, A.D. Antibiotic and biocide resistance in methicillin-resistant *Staphylococcus aureus* and vancomycin-resistant enterococcus. *J. Hosp. Infect.* 1999, *43*, 281–291. [CrossRef]
27. Russell, A.D. Bacterial resistance to disinfectants: Present knowledge and future problems. *J. Hosp. Infect.* 1999, *43*, 57–68. [CrossRef]
28. Bridier, A.; Briandet, R.; Thomas, V.; Dubois-Brissonnet, F. Biofouling: The Journal of Bioadhesion and Biofilm Resistance of bacterial biofilms to disinfectants: A review. *Biofouling J. Bioadhesion Biofilm Res.* 2011, *27*, 1017–1032. [CrossRef]
29. Ivanković, T.; Goić-Barišić, I.; Hrenović, J. Reduced susceptibility to disinfectants of *Acinetobacter baumannii* biofilms on glass and ceramic. *Arh. Hig. Rada Toksikol.* 2017, *68*, 99–108. [CrossRef]
30. Song, L.; Wu, J.; Xi, C. Biofilms on environmental surfaces: Evaluation of the disinfection efficacy of a novel steam vapor system. *Am. J. Infect. Control* 2012, *40*, 926–930. [CrossRef]
31. Sutherland, I.W. Biofilm exopolysaccharides: A strong and sticky framework. *Microbiology* 2001, *147*, 3–9. [CrossRef] [PubMed]
32. Stewart, P.S.; Rayner, J.; Roe, F.; Rees, W.M. Biofilm penetration and disinfection efficacy of alkaline hypochlorite and chlorosulfamates. *J. Appl. Microbiol.* 2001, *91*, 525–532. [CrossRef] [PubMed]
33. Tachikawa, M.; Yamanaka, K.; Nakamuro, K. Studies on the disinfection and removal of biofilms by ozone water using an artificial microbial biofilm system. *Ozone Sci. Eng.* 2009, *31*, 3–9. [CrossRef]
34. Smith, K.; Hunter, I.S. Efficacy of common hospital biocides with biofilms of multi-drug resistant clinical isolates. *J. Med. Microbiol.* 2008, *57*, 966–973. [CrossRef] [PubMed]
35. Park, K.M.; Yoon, S.; Choi, T.; Kim, H.J.; Park, K.J.; Koo, M. The bactericidal effect of a combination of food grade compounds and their application as alternative antibacterial agent for food contact surfaces. *Foods* 2020, *9*, 59. [CrossRef]
36. Russell, A.D. Possible link between bacterial resistance and use of anticiotics and biocides. *Antimicrob. Agents Chemother.* 1998, *42*, 4804. [CrossRef] [PubMed]

37. Britton, H.C.; Draper, M.; Talmadge, J.E. Antimicrobial efficacy of aqueous ozone in combination with short chain fatty acid buffers. *Infect. Prev. Pract.* **2020**, *2*, 100032. [CrossRef]
38. Boyce, J.M. Modern technologies for improving cleaning and disinfection of environmental surfaces in hospitals. *Antimicrob. Resist. Infect. Control* **2016**, *5*, 10. [CrossRef]
39. Bayan, M.A.G.; McGann, P.; Kwak, Y.I.; Summers, A.; Cummings, J.F.; Waterman, P.E.; Lesho, E.P.; Detusheva, E.V.; Ershova, O.N.; Fursova, N.K.; et al. Distribution of antiseptic resistance genes qacA, qacB, and smr in methicillin-resistant *Staphylococcus aureus* isolated in Toronto, Canada, from 2005 to 2009. *J. Hosp. Infect.* **2016**, *66*, 1–9.
40. Sharma, M.; Hudson, J.B. Ozone gas is an effective and practical antibacterial agent. *Am. J. Infect. Control* **2008**, *36*, 559–563. [CrossRef]
41. Boch, T.; Tennert, C.; Vach, K.; Al-Ahmad, A.; Hellwig, E.; Polydorou, O. Effect of gaseous ozone on *Enterococcus faecalis* biofilm—An in vitro study. *Clin. Oral Investig.* **2016**, *20*, 1733–1739. [CrossRef] [PubMed]
42. Boer, H.E.L.d.; van Elzelingen-Dekker, C.M.; van Rheenen-Verberg, C.M.F.; Spanjaard, L. Use of Gaseous Ozone for Eradication of Methicillin-Resistant *Staphylococcus aureus*. From the Home Environment of a Colonized Hospital Employee. *Infect. Control Hosp. Epidemiol.* **2006**, *27*, 1120–1122. [CrossRef] [PubMed]
43. Giuliani, G.; Ricevuti, G.; Galoforo, A.; Franzini, M. Microbiological aspects of ozone: Bactericidal activity and antibiotic/antimicrobial resistance in bacterial strains treated with ozone. *Ozone Ther.* **2018**, *3*, 1–4. [CrossRef]
44. Megahed, A.; Aldridge, B.; Lowe, J. The microbial killing capacity of aqueous and gaseous ozone on different surfaces contaminated with dairy cattle manure. *PLoS ONE* **2018**, *13*, e0196555. [CrossRef] [PubMed]
45. Fontes, B.; Heimbecker, A.M.C.; Brito, G.d.S.; Costa, S.F.; van der Heijden, I.M.; Levin, A.S.; Rasslan, S. Effect of low-dose gaseous ozone on pathogenic bacteria. *BMC Infect. Dis.* **2012**, *12*, 2–7. [CrossRef] [PubMed]
46. Conto, A. The EU chemical strategy for sustainability towards a toxic-free environment. *Chim. Oggi Chem. Today* **2021**, *39*, 40–41.
47. Akbaş, M.Y. Effectiveness of Organic Acid Treatments for Inhibition and Removal of *E. coli* Biofilms. *Hacettepe J. Biol. Chem.* **2016**, *1*, 35. [CrossRef]
48. Akbas, M.Y.; Kokumer, T. The prevention and removal of biofilm formation of *Staphylococcus aureus* strains isolated from raw milk samples by citric acid treatments. *Int. J. Food Sci. Technol.* **2015**, *50*, 1666–1672. [CrossRef]
49. Park, S.H.; Choi, M.R.; Park, J.W.; Park, K.H.; Chung, M.S.; Ryu, S.; Kang, D.H. Use of organic acids to inactivate *Escherichia coli* O157: H7, salmonella typhimurium, and listeria monocytogenes on organic fresh apples and lettuce. *J. Food Sci.* **2011**, *76*, M293–M298. [CrossRef]
50. Cherrington, C.A.; Hinton, M.; Mead, G.C.; Chopra, I. Organic Acids: Chemistry, Antibacterial Activity and Practical Applications. *Adv. Microb. Physiol.* **1991**, *32*, 87–108. [CrossRef]
51. Wang, J.; Tao, D.; Wang, S.; Li, C.; Li, Y.; Zheng, F.; Wu, Z. Disinfection of lettuce using organic acids: An ecological analysis using 16S rRNA sequencing. *RSC Adv.* **2019**, *9*, 17514–17520. [CrossRef] [PubMed]
52. Tsai, Y.P.; Pai, T.Y.; Hsin, J.Y.; Wan, T.J. Biofilm bacteria inactivation by citric acid and resuspension evaluations for drinking water production systems. *Water Sci. Technol.* **2004**, *48*, 463–472. [CrossRef]
53. Hughes, G.; Webber, M.A. Novel approaches to the treatment of bacterial biofilm infections. *Br. J. Pharmacol.* **2017**, *174*, 2237–2246. [CrossRef] [PubMed]
54. Hughes, G.; Lund, P. The Use of Weak Organic Acids as a Novel Antimicrobial and Biofilm Eradication Agent. In Proceedings of the European Congress of Clinical Microbiology and Infectious Diseases, Madrid, Spain, 21–24 April 2018.
55. Piletić, K.; Kovač, B.; Perčić, M.; Žigon, J.; Broznić, D.; Karleuša, L.; Blagojević, S.L.; Oder, M.; Gobin, I. Disinfecting Action of Gaseous Ozone on OXA-48-Producing Klebsiella pneumoniae Biofilm In Vitro. *Int. J. Environ. Res. Public Health* **2022**, *19*, 6177. [CrossRef]
56. Kampf, G.; Kramer, A. Epidemiologic background of hand hygiene and evaluation of the most important agents for scrubs and rubs. *Clin. Microbiol. Rev.* **2004**, *17*, 863–893. [CrossRef]
57. Boyce, J.M. Environmental contamination makes an important contribution to hospital infection. *J. Hosp. Infect.* **2007**, *65*, 50–54. [CrossRef]
58. Davies, A.; Pottage, T.; Bennett, A.; Walker, J. Gaseous and air decontamination technologies for Clostridium difficile in the healthcare environment. *J. Hosp. Infect.* **2011**, *77*, 199–203. [CrossRef]
59. Moat, J.; Cargill, J.; Shone, J.; Upton, M. Application of a novel decontamination process using gaseous ozone. *Can. J. Microbiol.* **2009**, *55*, 928–933. [CrossRef]
60. Kundukad, B.; Udayakumar, G.; Grela, E.; Kaur, D.; Rice, S.A.; Kjelleberg, S.; Doyle, P.S. Weak acids as an alternative anti-microbial therapy. *Biofilm* **2020**, *2*, 100019. [CrossRef]
61. Jung, Y.J.; Oh, B.S.; Kang, J.W. Synergistic effect of sequential or combined use of ozone and UV radiation for the disinfection of Bacillus subtilis spores. *Water Res.* **2008**, *42*, 1613–1621. [CrossRef]
62. Vankerckhoven, E.; Verbessem, B.; Crauwels, S.; Declerck, P.; Muylaert, K.; Willems, K.A.; Rediers, H. Exploring the potential synergistic effects of chemical disinfectants and UV on the inactivation of free-living bacteria and treatment of biofilms in a pilot-scale system. *Water Sci. Technol.* **2011**, *64*, 1247–1253. [CrossRef]
63. Cho, G.L.; Ha, J.W. Synergistic effect of citric acid and xenon light for inactivating foodborne pathogens on spinach leaves. *Food Res. Int.* **2021**, *142*, 110210. [CrossRef]
64. ECHA. *Guidance on the Biocidal Products Regulation: Volume II Parts B+C*; European Chemicals Agency: Helsinki, Finland, 2022; ISBN 9789290205029.

65. Rodríguez-Baño, J.; Martí, S.; Soto, S.; Fernández-Cuenca, F.; Cisneros, J.M.; Pachón, J.; Pascual, A.; Martínez-Martínez, L.; Mcqueary, C.; Actis, L.A.; et al. Biofilm formation in *Acinetobacter baumannii*: Associated features and clinical implications. *Clin. Microbiol. Infect.* **2008**, *14*, 276–278. [CrossRef]
66. Ha, J.H.; Jeong, S.H.; Ha, S.D. Synergistic effects of combined disinfection using sanitizers and uv to reduce the levels of staphylococcus aureus in oyster mushrooms. *J. Appl. Biol. Chem.* **2011**, *54*, 447–453. [CrossRef]
67. Hirahara, Y.; Iwata, K.; Nakamuro, K. Effect of Citric Acid on Prolonging the Half-life of Dissolved Ozone in Water. *Food Saf.* **2019**, *7*, 90–94. [CrossRef] [PubMed]
68. Nagayoshi, M.; Fukuizumi, T.; Kitamura, C.; Yano, J.; Terashita, M.; Nishihara, T. Efficacy of ozone on survival and permeability of oral microorganisms. *Oral Microbiol. Immunol.* **2004**, *19*, 240–246. [CrossRef] [PubMed]
69. Franke, G.; Knobling, B.; Brill, F.H.; Becker, B.; Klupp, E.M.; Campos, C.B.; Pfefferle, S.; Lütgehetmann, M.; Knobloch, J.K. An automated room disinfection system using ozone is highly active against surrogates for SARS-CoV-2. *J. Hosp. Infect.* **2021**, *112*, 108–113. [CrossRef]

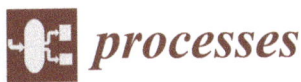

Article

Terpenoids as Natural Agents against Food-Borne Bacteria—Evaluation of Biofilm Biomass versus Viability Reduction

Rok Fink

Faculty of Health Sciences, University of Ljubljana, Zdravstvena Pot 5, 1000 Ljubljana, Slovenia; rok.fink@zf.uni-lj.si; Tel.: +386-13001181

Abstract: This study aimed to analyse the antibacterial potential of limonene, terpineol, and eugenol for the biofilm reduction of food-borne *E. coli*, *S. aureus* and *S. typhimurium*. A microdilution test with resazurin application was used for the minimum inhibitory concentration and a colony plate count was used for the minimum bactericidal concentration. Biofilm biomass was quantified using the crystal violet assay, while biofilm viability was determined using the plate count method. The results show the highest antibacterial potential among terpenoids for eugenol, followed by terpineol and limonene. Both biomass reduction and viability are strongly dependent on the concentration of all terpenoids tested ($p < 0.05$). Moreover, eugenol reduced biofilm biomass most effectively (67% for *E. coli*), while viability was reduced most by terpineol (3.8 log CFU cm^{-2} for *E. coli* and *S. aureus*). The correlation coefficient for the reduction in biomass and viability was highest for eugenol (0.9) and chlorhexidine for all bacteria tested, while the lowest correlation was found for limonene (0.6). Results also demonstrate that tested terpenoids are effective as standard antimicrobial agent chlorhexidine. This suggests that eugenol has potential against food-borne biofilms as it simultaneously reduces both biomass and viability of biofilms.

Keywords: terpenoids; food-borne bacteria; biofilm; minimum inhibitory concentration; viability; biomass

Citation: Fink, R. Terpenoids as Natural Agents against Food-Borne Bacteria—Evaluation of Biofilm Biomass versus Viability Reduction. *Processes* **2023**, *11*, 148. https://doi.org/10.3390/pr11010148

Academic Editor: Shaoan Cheng

Received: 30 November 2022
Revised: 27 December 2022
Accepted: 30 December 2022
Published: 3 January 2023

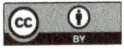

Copyright: © 2023 by the author. Licensee MDPI, Basel, Switzerland. This article is an open access article distributed under the terms and conditions of the Creative Commons Attribution (CC BY) license (https://creativecommons.org/licenses/by/4.0/).

1. Introduction

Managing the bacterial population on the surface plays a crucial role in medicine, technology and in domestic environments, where we try to keep bacteria to a minimum. Under favourable conditions, bacteria attach themselves to the surface of the material and begin to form biofilms in the presence of nutrients, temperature and water. A biofilm is a community of bacterial cells enclosed in exopolysaccharide substances that adheres to the surface of the material and exhibits sophisticated collective behaviour [1]. Bacterial biofilms pose one of the greatest public health problems, as the bacteria within the biofilm are much better protected from chemical and physical stresses than planktonic cells. From a public health perspective, it is estimated that more than 65% of all human microbial infections are related to biofilm exposure [2]. Therefore, the elimination of biofilms on surfaces requires much higher concentrations of chemical compounds compared to planktonic cells [3]. The most common disinfectants on the market contain chlorine-based active ingredients, quaternary ammonium compounds, triclosan, alcohols and aldehydes, which are effective against bacteria and facilitate good hygiene practices. However, the consumption of these chemicals can have worrying effects on humans, animals and the environment as they are washed into the aquatic environment after the cleaning process [4]. In 2020, sales of disinfectants have doubled worldwide, without evidence of their short- and long-term side effects on the environment [5]. Furthermore, experience shows that increased use of disinfectants is associated with increasing resistance, be it from misuse for chronic infections, misuse for viral prophylaxis, or overuse of antibiotic-based disinfectants [6]. A recent report on antibacterial resistance indicates that more than 4.95 million deaths worldwide are associated with antibacterial resistance and that *E. coli* and *S. aureus* are two of the leading pathogens for deaths associated with bacterial resistance [7]. Chlorhexidine, for example, is an antiseptic frequently used in hospitals and industrial environments for disinfection. Moreover, in the last decade, concerns have arisen over the increasing resistance of *E. coli* and *S. aureus* to chlorhexidine [8]. An answer to more sustainable cleaning could be natural agents from plants that are effective against bacteria, are generally recognised as safe (GRAS) and for the environment, and have a low potential for resistance due to their non-targeting effect on bacterial cells [9,10]. Natural antimicrobial agents have attracted much attention among researchers in recent years, and essential oils in particular are considered a source of antimicrobial components. Essential oils are complex mixtures that can contain more than 300 compounds and have antibacterial properties due to bioactive volatile components such as terpenoids, alcohols, esters, thujone, carvone and others. However, the vast majority of active components belong to the class of terpenoids, e.g., terpineol, limonene, eugenol, carvacrol, linalool and others [11,12]. Terpenoids represent one of the largest and structurally diverse groups of naturally-occurring compounds derived from the 5-carbon compound isoprene and its derivatives. Many plants synthesize different kinds of terpenoids that have applications in medicine, pharmacy and technology [13,14]. In recent years it has been found that terpenoids play an increasingly important role in the field of antibacterial activity [15]. Upon contact with bacterial cells, terpenoids disrupt the cell membrane to make it more permeable, disrupt ion transfer, interact with membrane proteins and affect cell enzymes and inhibit DNA synthesis [16]. Limonene is a cyclic monoterpene and is the major component in citrus fruit peel oil. It is commonly used in the pharmaceutical, food and perfumes industry due to its safety [17]. For example, Gupta et al. [18] reported that limonene causes the degradation of proteins at the outer membrane of *E. coli*, leading to increased permeability and formation of hydroxyl radicals by Fenton reaction, which in turn leads to oxidative DNA damage. Moreover, Lee et al. [19] reported limonene is effective against *B. cereus*, *E. coli*, *S. aureus*, and even against methicillin-resistant *S. aureus*. The antibacterial activity of eugenol and limonene also includes the inhibition of *S. aureus* biofilm [20,21]. Terpineol is a monocyclic terpenoid found in many herbs like marjoram, oregano and rosemary and has a wide range of biological properties [22]. Ding et al. [23] reported that the main mechanism of action of terpineol against *E. coli* is to dissolve the outer membrane of the cells by releasing the lipopolysaccharides and increasing the permeability of the cytoplasmic membrane to ATP. Eugenol is a terpenoid derived mainly from clove oil and has attracted scientific interest due to antibacterial, antiviral and antifungal properties [24]. In addition, eugenol is considered a membrane inhibitor, protease inhibitor and source of reactive oxygen species [24]. Yamaguchi [14] tested different terpenoids and found significant bacteriostatic and bactericidal activities at low concentrations. Moreover, the author found the most effective bactericidal activity against Gram negative bacteria. There are several research studies on the antibacterial potential of terpenoids against pathogenic bacteria, but less is known how terpenoids interact with bacteria within the biofilm, especially synergistic effects on biomass and biofilm viability. Therefore, this study aims to analyse the antibacterial and antibiofilm potential of the terpenoids limonene, terpineol and eugenol against the hygienically-relevant bacteria *E. coli*, *S. aureus* and *S. typhimurium*, by comparing the effectiveness of selected terpenoids with the standard antibacterial agent chlorhexidine. Furthermore, the removal of biofilm biomass from the polystyrene and the reduction of the viability of the bacteria within the biofilms were analysed. Finally, to evaluate the potential of selected active components for simultaneous removal of biofilm biomass and reduction of cell viability.

2. Materials and Methods

2.1. Bacterial Strains

For the antibacterial and anti-biofilm assay, standard strains of bacteria that represent hygienically-relevant bacteria were used. The standard strains of *Escherichia coli* ATCC

25922 (*E. coli*), *Salmonella enterica* serovar *typhimurium* ATCC 14028 (*S. typhimurium*) and *Staphylococcus aureus* ATCC 25923 (*S. aureus*) were obtained from Sigma Aldrich (Virginia, St. Louis, MO, USA). Bacteria from the collection were transferred on nutrient agar (Biolife, Italy) and incubated at 37 °C for 24 h. After that, a single colony of a strain was transferred from nutrient agar to the Mueller Hinton broth (Merck Millipore, Burlington, MA, USA) and incubated under the same conditions.

2.2. Chemicals

Terpenoids active components (R)-(+)- limonene (1-Methyl-4-(prop-1-en-2-yl) cyclohex-1-ene), α-terpineol (2-(4-Methylcyclohex-3-en-1-yl)propan-2-ol), eugenol (2-Methoxy-4-(prop-2-en-1-yl) phenol), standard antimicrobial chlorhexidine digluconate and solvent Tween-80 (Polyoxyethylene (20) sorbitan monooleate) were purchased at Sigma-Aldrich (St. Louis, MO, USA).

2.3. Minimum Inhibitory and Bactericidal Concentration

The minimum inhibitory and bactericidal concentration of limonene, terpineol and eugenol against selected bacteria was tested using microdilution methods according to the standard ISO 20776-1: 2020. Bacterial cultures of *E. coli*, *S. typhimurium* and *S. aureus* were transferred from nutrient agar to a 0.9% NaCl solution to achieve a concentration of 0.5 McFarland. Into sterile flat-bottomed 96-well microplates (Nunc, Denmark), 100 µL of bacterial cells in Mueller-Hinton broth were added at a final concentration of 1×10^6 CFU mL^{-1}. In the second step, twofold dilutions of terpenoid active components were added at concentrations ranging from 15 mg mL^{-1} to 0.03 mg mL^{-1}. The active components were diluted in 0.002% (v/v) Tween-80 according to the Clinical and Laboratory Standards Institute [25]. The plates were incubated at 37 °C for 24 h. Then, 10 µL of resazurin solution at a concentration of 0.015% was added and incubated again under the same conditions for 4 h. The negative control was 0.9% NaCl with 0.002% Tween-80, while the positive control was chlorhexidine gluconate at a concentration in the range of 0.003 to 0.25 mg mL^{-1}. The minimum inhibitory concentration (MIC) in the resazurin assay was defined according to Sarker et al. [26] as the lowest concentration of the active component that does not convert blue resazurin to pink resorufin. Subsequently, 100 µL of the suspension above the MIC was inoculated onto the nutrient agar and incubated at 37 °C for 24 h. The minimum bactericidal concentration (MBC) was defined as the lowest concentration at which no colonies grew on solid media (Figure 1).

Biofilm Biomass and Viability

A biofilm test was performed following Fink et al. [27] with some modifications as follows. Bacterial cultures of *E. coli*, *S. typhimurium* and *S. aureus* were prepared in a 0.9% NaCl solution to achieve a concentration of 0.5 McFarland. The bacterial cells were added to Mueller-Hinton broth to achieve a final concentration of 5×10^5 CFU mL^{-1}. Then, 100 µL of the bacterial suspension was added to sterile 96-well flat-bottomed microtitre plates (Nunc, Roskilde, Denmark) and incubated at 37 °C for 24 h. After this, the bacterial suspension was removed, and the biofilms formed on the surface of the microtitre plate were rinsed three times with 100 µL PBS. The biofilms were treated for 15 min at room temperature with 1 MIC, 2 MIC and 3 MIC concentrations of the active components. Samples were then washed three times with 100 µL PBS to neutralise the active components and remove any loosely adhering cells. The biofilm biomass was determined using the crystal violet assay. Cells remaining on the surface were stained with 100 µL 2% crystal violet (Merck Millipore, Darmstad, Germany) and the excess dye removed and washed with PBS. The dye from the cells was remobilised with 100 µL 96% ethanol. The optical density of the solution was measured at a wavelength of 620 nm using the Infinite 200 PRO microplate reader (Tecan, Grödig, Austria). The viability of the biofilm was analysed by counting the bacterial colonies. After neutralisation with PBS, 100 µL 0.9% NaCl was added to each microtitre well and sonicated at 37 kHz and 200 W for 3 min to dissolve the cells from the well surface into the liquid. After serial dilutions, samples were inoculated onto solid media and incubated at 37 °C for 24 h. Colonies were counted and results were expressed as log CFU cm^2 (Figure 1).

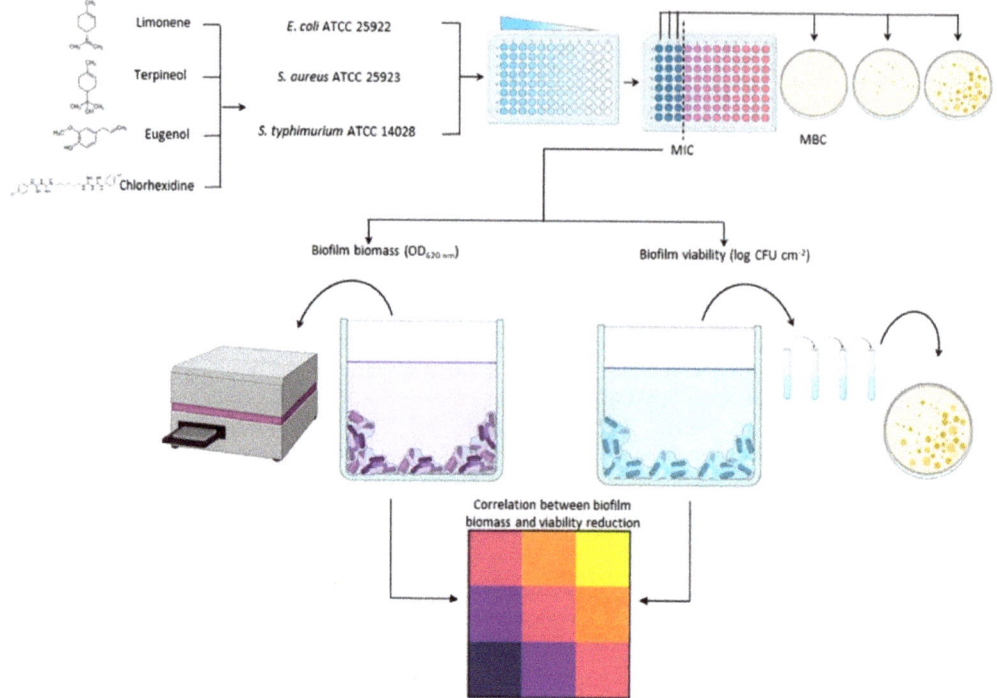

Figure 1. Research design testing antibacterial and antibiofilm potential of limonene, terpineol, eugenol and chlorhexidine against *E. coli*, *S. typhimurium* and *S. aureus* biofilm biomass and viability (Created with BioRender.com).

Statistical analysis was provided using R software version 4.1.1. (Bell Laboratories, Holmdel, NJ, USA). One-way analysis of variance (ANOVA) and the Duncan test were used to determine the significant differences at a significance level of $p < 0.05$. Pearson correlation coefficient (r) was calculated to correlate biofilm biomass and cell viability reduction ($p < 0.05$). The correlation was interpreted as weak (0.1–0.3), moderate (0.4–0.6) or string (0.7–0.9).

Figure 1 was created using BioRender.com (accessed on 25 November 2022).

3. Results and Discussion

One of the principles of green chemistry is to replace classic cleaning and disinfecting agents with less hazardous substances and to offer consumers ingredients that are safer for human health and the environment [28]. Terpenoids have been ported to be GRAS, but to also exert antimicrobial activities against both antibiotic-susceptible and -resistant bacteria at the same time. Notably, carvacrol, eugenol, carvone, geraniol and thymol are among the terpenoids that show antibacterial potential against *S. aureus* [29]. Our study aims to evaluate the potential of the terpenoids limonene, terpineol and eugenol for managing the biomass and viability of biofilms in the food industry. The results show that the lowest MIC for all tested terpenoids and bacteria is 0.1 mg mL^{-1} for eugenol, followed by terpineol (0.1–0.2 mg mL^{-1}) and limonene (0.9–1.9 mg mL^{-1}) (Table 1). In a study by Zhao et al. [30], which investigated the exposure of eugenol to *S. typhimurium*, the MIC was 0.125 mg mL^{-1}, which is consistent with our results. Furthermore, the authors reported that treatment with eugenol deformed the morphology of *S. typhimurium*. As with eugenol, the MIC for terpineol was 0.1 mg mL^{-1} for *E. coli* and *S. aureus*, and 0.2 mg mL^{-1} for *S. typhimurium* (Table 1). Similarly, Huang et al. [31] have shown that *S. typhimurium* and *E. coli* seem to be sensitive to terpineol at a concentration of 0.153 mg mL^{-1}. Limonene appears to be the least antibacterial with an MIC of 0.9 mg mL^{-1} for *E. coli* and 1.9 mg mL^{-1} for *S. typhimurium*. In contrast to our findings, Costa et al. [32] found the MIC of limonene for *S. aureus* at 0.256 mg mL^{-1}, which is lower than the figures reported in our study. One of the reasons for this could be the fact that the researchers used the solvent DMSO. This is particularly important as Van de Vel et al. [33] report that the choice of solvent can have a significant impact on the MIC of essential oils. Meanwhile, the results for chlorhexidine show MIC for *E. coli* and *S. aureus* at 0.02 mg mL^{-1}, which corresponds to Kampf's findings [34] that reported MIC for *E. coli* at 0.0117 mg mL^{-1} and *S. aureus* at 0.02 mg mL^{-1}.

Table 1. MIC and MBC of limonene, terpineol, eugenol and chlorhexidine against *E. coli*, *S. aureus* and *S. typhimurium*.

	Limonene		Terpineol		Eugenol		Chlorhexidine	
	MIC	MBC	MIC	MBC	MIC	MBC	MIC	MBC
E. coli ATCC 25922	0.9	3.7	0.1	0.4	0.1	0.4	0.02	0.03
S. aureus ATCC 25923	1.9	3.7	0.1	0.3	0.1	0.6	0.02	0.06
S. typhimurium ATCC 14028	0.9	2.8	0.2	0.7	0.1	0.6	0.03	0.09

Legend: MIC—minimal inhibitory concentration (mg mL^{-1}); MBC—minimal bactericidal concentration (mg mL^{-1}).

The results of the efficacy of removing biofilm biomass from the polystyrene surface show for all tested bacteria that increasing the concentration of terpenoid agents and chlorhexidine leads to a decrease in biomass ($p < 0.05$) (Figure 2, Table 2). More detailed analysis shows that 2 MIC will significantly decrease the biofilm biomass for all bacteria and all tested compounds, while 3 MIC of limonene will not have a significant effect on *S. typhimurium*, nor will terpineol on *E. coli* and *S. aureus*, or chlorhexidine on *E. coli* (Table 2). We have shown that eugenol can remove up to 67% of *E. coli* biofilm biomass, followed by *S. aureus* (53%) and *S. typhimurium* (46%). A similar trend is observed for limonene (56%, 46% and 27% respectively), while terpineol removes up to 44% of *E. coli* biofilm biomass, followed by *S. typhimurium* (38%) and *S. aureus* (26%) (Figure 2). A study by Yadav et al. [21] investigated the effects of eugenol on *S. aureus* biofilm and found that 0.2 mg mL^{-1} reduced biofilm by 50%, which is comparable to our results. Ding et al. [23] tested 0.3 mg mL^{-1} terpineol against *E. coli* biofilm and found that a 40% reduction was possible with a short exposure time; increasing the exposure time increased the removal of the biofilm. Chlorhexidine can remove up to 57% of *E. coli* biofilm biomass, followed by *S. aureus* (51%) and *S. typhimurium* (37%). Comparable to eugenol, chlorhexidine at 3 MIC removes about 8% less biofilm biomass. Cota et al. [35] tested about ten times higher concentrations of chlorhexidine on wild strains of *S. typhimurium* to demonstrate biofilm eradication.

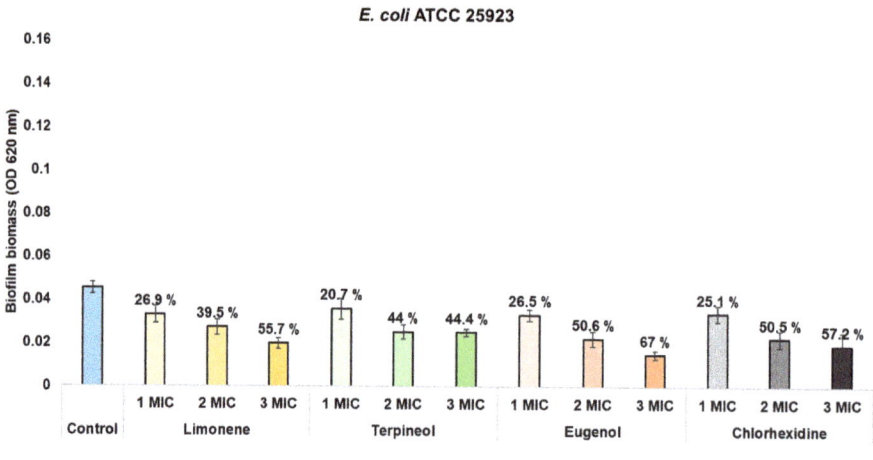
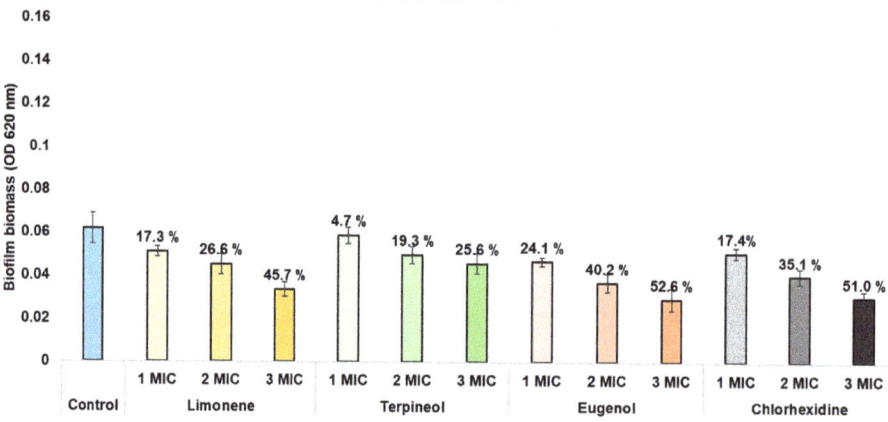
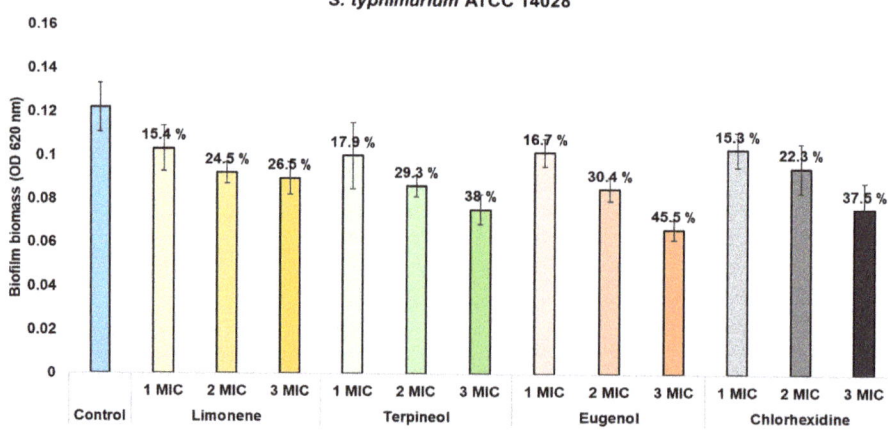

Figure 2. Biofilm biomass (OD620 nm and %) of *E. coli*, *S. aureus* and *S. typhimurium* after exposure to 1 MIC, 2 MIC and 3 MIC limonene, terpineol eugenol and chlorhexidine.

Table 2. Analysis of variance and post hoc Duncan test for biofilm biomass and viability in comparison to limonene, terpineol, eugenol and chlorhexidine concentration.

	Active Component	Concentration	$\bar{x}$	E. coli F-Value	p-Value	Bacteria S. aureus $\bar{x}$	S. aureus F-Value	p-Value	S. typhimurium $\bar{x}$	S. typhimurium F-Value	p-Value
Biofilm biomass (OD 620 nm)	Limonene	Control	0.0454 a	90.28	<0.0000 *	0.0616 a	47.75	<0.0000 *	0.1221 a	22.21	<0.0000 *
		1 MIC	0.0332 b			0.0510 b			0.1033 b		
		2 MIC	0.0275 c			0.0452 c			0.0922 c		
		3 MIC	0.0201 d			0.0335 d			0.0897 c		
	Terpineol	Control	0.0454 a	69.35	<0.0000 *	0.0616 a	16.66	<0.0000 *	0.1221 a	29.73	<0.0000 *
		1 MIC	0.0360 b			0.0587 a			0.1001 b		
		2 MIC	0.0254 c			0.0497 b			0.0863 c		
		3 MIC	0.0252 c			0.0458 b			0.0756 d		
	Eugenol	Control	0.0454 a	190.4	<0.0000 *	0.0616 a	61.3	<0.0000 *	0.1221 a	81.89	<0.0000 *
		1 MIC	0.0334 b			0.0467 b			0.1017 b		
		2 MIC	0.0224 c			0.0368 b			0.0849 c		
		3 MIC	0.0150 d			0.0292 d			0.0665 d		
	Chlorhexidine	Control	0.0421 a	27.75	<0.0000 *	0.0649 a	124.5	<0.0000 *	0.1192 a	17.36	<0.0000 *
		1 MIC	0.0340 b			0.0509 b			0.0103 b		
		2 MIC	0.0225 c			0.0400 c			0.0949 b		
		3 MIC	0.0194 b			0.0301 d			0.0762 c		
Biofilm viability (CFU cm^{-2})	Limonene	Control	8.0261 a	1530	<0.0000 *	8.3507 a	493.5	<0.0000 *	8.5591 a	348.3	<0.0000 *
		1 MIC	5.8995 b			6.4502 b			7.4750 b		
		2 MIC	4.7727 c			5.3065 c			6.5878 c		
		3 MIC	4.5634 d			5.2276 c			5.8535 d		
	Terpineol	Control	8.0261 a	471.6	<0.0000 *	8.3507 a	366.6	<0.0000 *	8.5591 a	869.6	<0.0000 *
		1 MIC	5.9338 b			5.9054 b			6.7936 b		
		2 MIC	5.3726 c			4.6700 c			5.9604 c		
		3 MIC	4.3589 d			4.5578 c			5.6755 d		
	Eugenol	Control	8.0261 a	2073	<0.0000 *	8.3507 a	1,965	<0.0000 *	8.5591 a	470.3	<0.0000 *
		1 MIC	5.9214 b			6.6092 b			6.9335 b		
		2 MIC	4.8198 c			5.7823 c			6.5252 c		
		3 MIC	4.5893 d			5.0638 d			6.3395 d		
	Chlorhexidine	Control	8.1222 a	109.2	<0.0000 *	8.2914 a	475.1	<0.0000 *	8.6001 a	163	<0.0000 *
		1 MIC	3.3453 b			3.8277 b			2.6214 b		
		2 MIC	3.3193 b			3.1963 c			2.3027 c		
		3 MIC	3.2561 c			1.9623 d			1.5898 d		

Legend: $\bar{x}$ mean value; * significant difference at $p < 0.05$; Means (a–d) sharing a common letter are not significantly different at $p < 0.05$.

The viability of the biofilm for all tested bacterial strains and the selected terpenoid agents show an increasing logarithmic decrease with increasing concentration (Figure 3, Table 2). More detailed analysis shows that double concentration will significantly decrease the biofilm viability for all bacteria and for all tested compounds, while for *S. aureus*, 3 MIC of limonene and terpineol will not have a significant effect (Table 2). In contrast to the biomass assessment, biofilm viability shows the highest logarithmic reduction at 3 MIC for terpineol (3.8 log CFU cm^{-2} for *E. coli* and *S. typhimurium* and 2.9 for *S. aureus*). Ulhag et al. [36] tested the extract of *Citrus hystrix* against *S. typhimurium* and found that terpineol was the major antibacterial component acting against bacterial cells. In addition, we found that eugenol and limonene showed similar results against *E. coli*, while limonene reduced more cells at an MIC of 3 (2.9 log CFU cm^{-2}) compared to eugenol (2.2 log CFU cm^{-2}) in the case of *S. aureus* (Figure 3). One study by Umagiliyage et al. [37] tested limonene against *E. coli* and found that 1 mg mL^{-1} limonene can reduce bacterial cells by 1.6 log CFU. Results of chlorhexidine show similar reduction for *E. coli* as for eugenol (3.5 log CFU cm^{-2}) or terpineol for *S. aureus* (3.8 log CFU cm^{-2}), while it was least effective for *S. typhimurium*. Condell et al. [38] reported that *Salmonella* spp., when exposed to sub-lethal concentrations of chlorhexidine, can respond with modification of the cell wall, virulence and a shift in cellular metabolism.

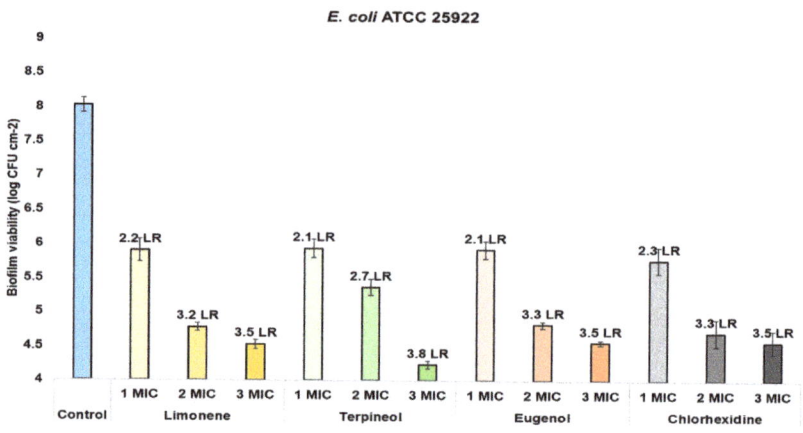

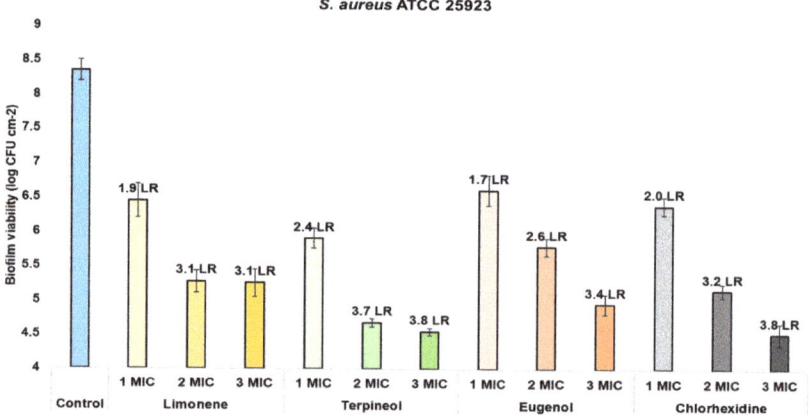

Figure 3. *Cont.*

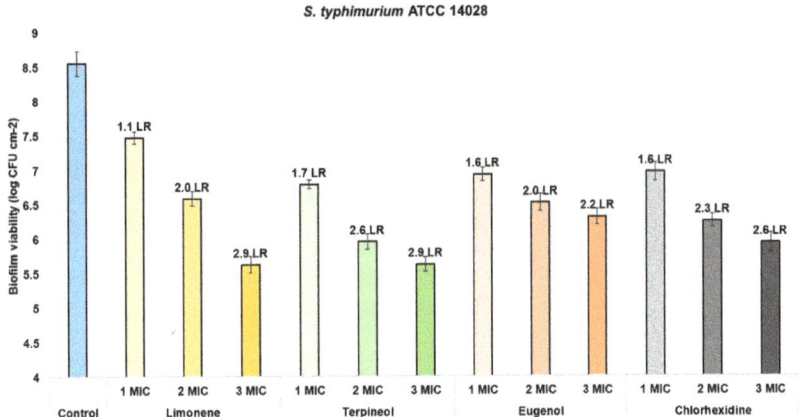

Figure 3. Biofilm viability (log CFU cm^{-2} and LR) of *E. coli*, *S. aureus* and *S. typhimurium* after exposure to 1 MIC, 2 MIC and 3 MIC limonene, terpineol, eugenol and chlorhexidine.

Results of the Pearson correlation coefficient show a strong correlation between the reduction of biofilm biomass and viability for all three tested bacteria against the eugenol (0.835–0.915), while for terpineol, we observed a strong correlation for *S. typhimurium* (0.756) and *S. aureus* (0.790), but moderate (0.612) for *E. coli*. Contrary to those results, limonene shows a moderate correlation between biomass and viability reduction for *S. aureus* and *S. typhimurium*, and only a strong one for *E. coli* (Figure 4). Results for chlorhexidine show a strong correlation for *S. aureus* (0.919) and *E. coli* (0.772), and moderate for *S. typhimurium* (0.643). All this indicates that eugenol is a good antibacterial agent, effectively reducing biofilm biomass and viability, and is comparable to chlorhexidine.

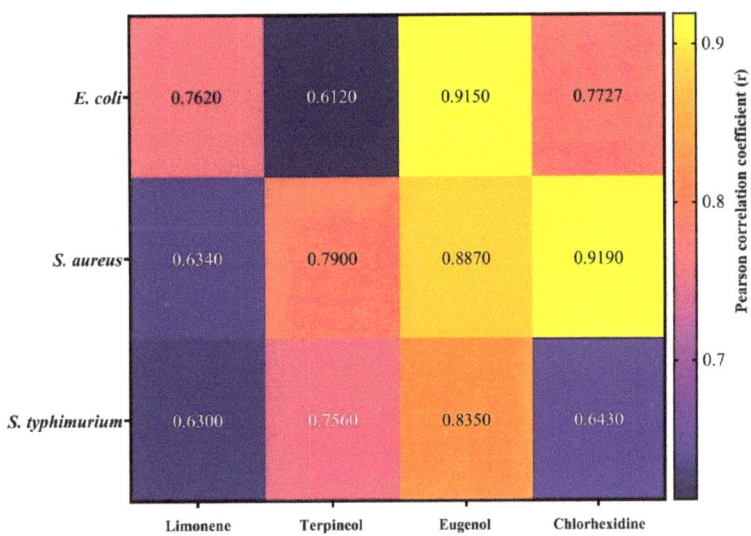

Figure 4. Pearson correlation coefficient between biofilm biomass (OD in %) and biofilm viability (LR in log CFU cm^{-2}) for all three tested bacterial strains and active components.

4. Conclusions

Reducing the environmental impact of cleaning and disinfection products while maintaining their effectiveness is a green chemistry priority. New antibacterial agents must achieve comparable efficiency to classical ones, while reducing the pressure on the environment. Our research has shown that the terpenoids eugenol and terpineol have the strongest antibacterial activity against food-borne *E. coli*, *S. aureus* and *S. typhimurium*, while limonene has less antibacterial potential. Double and triple concentrations of MIC showed significant reductions in both biomass and biofilm viability, with eugenol being most effective in removing biomass, while terpineol was most effective in reducing biofilm viability. We also demonstrated that chlorhexidine is effective against *E. coli* and *S. aureus*, but less so against *S. typhimurium*. A comparison of the correlation of biomass and viability shows that eugenol has the greater potential to simultaneously reduce the biomass and viability of the food-borne biofilms tested. The anti-biofilm properties of terpineol and eugenol are comparable to chlorhexidine and therefore represent a good candidate for substitution in practice.

Funding: This research received no external funding.

Data Availability Statement: https://zenodo.org/record/3543000#.Y7QVpRVBy3A (accessed on 25 November 2022).

Conflicts of Interest: The author declares no conflict of interest.

References

1. Schachter, H.; Kamerling, H. 4.06-Glycobiology of Caenorhabditis elegans. In *Comprehensive Glycoscience*; Elsevier: Oxford, UK, 2007; pp. 81–100.
2. Magalhães, R.P.; Vieira, T.F.; Fernandes, H.S.; Melo, A.; Simões, M.; Sousa, S.F. The biofilms structural database. *Trends Biotechnol.* **2020**, *38*, 937–940. [CrossRef] [PubMed]
3. Abebe, G.M. The role of bacterial biofilm in antibiotic resistance and food contamination. *Int. J. Microbiol.* **2020**, *2020*, 1705814. [CrossRef] [PubMed]
4. Wang, Z.; Wang, Y.Y.L.; Scott, W.C.; Williams, E.S.; Ciarlo, M.; DeLeo, P.; Brooks, B.W. Comparative influences of dermal and inhalational routes of exposure on hazards of cleaning product ingredients among mammalian model organisms. *Environ. Int.* **2021**, *157*, 106777. [CrossRef] [PubMed]
5. Dewey, H.M.; Jones, J.M.; Keating, M.R.; Budhathoki-Uprety, J. Increased use of disinfectants during the COVID-19 pandemic and its potential impacts on health and safety. *ACS Chem. Health Saf.* **2021**, *29*, 27–38. [CrossRef]
6. Lobie, T.A.; Roba, A.A.; Booth, J.A.; Kristiansen, K.I.; Aseffa, A.; Skarstad, K.; Bjørås, M. Antimicrobial resistance: A challenge awaiting the post-COVID-19 era. *Int. J. Infect. Dis.* **2021**, *111*, 322–325. [CrossRef]
7. Murray, C.J.; Ikuta, K.S.; Sharara, F.; Swetschinski, L.; Aguilar, G.R.; Gray, A.; Han, C.; Bisignano, C.; Rao, P.; Wool, E. Global burden of bacterial antimicrobial resistance in 2019: A systematic analysis. *Lancet* **2022**, *399*, 629–655. [CrossRef]
8. Van den Poel, B.; Saegeman, V.; Schuermans, A. Increasing usage of chlorhexidine in health care settings: Blessing or curse? A narrative review of the risk of chlorhexidine resistance and the implications for infection prevention and control. *Eur. J. Clin. Microbiol. Infect. Dis.* **2022**, *41*, 349–362. [CrossRef]
9. Nourbakhsh, F.; Nasrollahzadeh, M.S.; Tajani, A.S.; Soheili, V.; Hadizadeh, F. Bacterial biofilms and their resistance mechanisms: A brief look at treatment with natural agents. *Folia Microbiol.* **2022**, *67*, 535–554. [CrossRef]
10. Saeed, K.; Pasha, I.; Chughtai, M.F.J.; Ali, Z.; Bukhari, H.; Zuhair, M. Application of essential oils in food industry: Challenges and innovation. *J. Essent. Oil Res.* **2022**, *34*, 97–110. [CrossRef]
11. Dhifi, W.; Bellili, S.; Jazi, S.; Bahloul, N.; Mnif, W. Essential oils' chemical characterization and investigation of some biological activities: A critical review. *Medicines* **2016**, *3*, 25. [CrossRef]
12. Nakamura, A.; Kawahara, A.; Takahashi, H.; Kuda, T.; Kimura, B. Comparison between the Antimicrobial Activity of Essential Oils and Their Components in the Vapor Phase against Food-related Bacteria. *J. Oleo Sci.* **2022**, *71*, 411–417. [CrossRef] [PubMed]
13. Kazachenko, A.S.; Vasilieva, N.Y.; Fetisova, O.Y.; Sychev, V.V.; Elsuf'ev, E.V.; Malyar, Y.N.; Issaoui, N.; Miroshnikova, A.V.; Borovkova, V.S.; Kazachenko, A.S. New reactions of betulin with sulfamic acid and ammonium sulfamate in the presence of solid catalysts. *Biomass Convers. Biorefinery* **2022**, 1–12. [CrossRef]
14. Yamaguchi, T. Antibacterial effect of the combination of terpenoids. *Arch. Microbiol.* **2022**, *204*, 520. [CrossRef] [PubMed]
15. Yang, W.; Chen, X.; Li, Y.; Guo, S.; Wang, Z.; Yu, X. Advances in pharmacological activities of terpenoids. *Nat. Prod. Commun.* **2020**, *15*, 1934578X20903555. [CrossRef]
16. Mutlu-Ingok, A.; Devecioglu, D.; Dikmetas, D.N.; Karbancioglu-Guler, F.; Capanoglu, E. Antibacterial, antifungal, antimycotoxigenic, and antioxidant activities of essential oils: An updated review. *Molecules* **2020**, *25*, 4711. [CrossRef] [PubMed]
17. Sun, J. D-Limonene: Safety and clinical applications. *Altern. Med. Rev.* **2007**, *12*, 259–264. [PubMed]
18. Gupta, A.; Jeyakumar, E.; Lawrence, R. Journey of limonene as an antimicrobial agent. *J. Pure Appl. Microbiol.* **2021**, *15*, 1094–1110. [CrossRef]

19. Lee, S.-B.; Cha, K.-H.; Kim, S.-N.; Altantsetseg, S.; Shatar, S.; Sarangerel, O.; Nho, C.-W. The antimicrobial activity of essential oil from Dracocephalum foetidum against pathogenic microorganisms. *J. Microbiol.* **2007**, *45*, 53–57.
20. Subramenium, G.A.; Vijayakumar, K.; Pandian, S.K. Limonene inhibits streptococcal biofilm formation by targeting surface-associated virulence factors. *J. Med. Microbiol.* **2015**, *64*, 879–890. [CrossRef]
21. Yadav, M.K.; Chae, S.-W.; Im, G.J.; Chung, J.-W.; Song, J.-J. Eugenol: A phyto-compound effective against methicillin-resistant and methicillin-sensitive Staphylococcus aureus clinical strain biofilms. *PLoS ONE* **2015**, *10*, e0119564. [CrossRef]
22. Khaleel, C.; Tabanca, N.; Buchbauer, G. α-Terpineol, a natural monoterpene: A review of its biological properties. *Open Chem.* **2018**, *16*, 349–361. [CrossRef]
23. Ding, Q.; Zhuang, T.; Fu, P.; Zhou, Q.; Luo, L.; Dong, Z.; Li, H.; Tang, S. Alpha-terpineol grafted acetylated lentinan as an anti-bacterial adhesion agent. *Carbohydr. Polym.* **2022**, *277*, 118825. [CrossRef] [PubMed]
24. Ulanowska, M.; Olas, B. Biological Properties and prospects for the application of eugenol—A review. *Int. J. Mol. Sci.* **2021**, *22*, 3671. [CrossRef] [PubMed]
25. Weinstein, M.P. *Performance Standards for Antimicrobial Susceptibility Testing*; Clinical and Laboratory Standards Institute: Wayne, PA, USA, 2021.
26. Sarker, S.D.; Nahar, L.; Kumarasamy, Y. Microtitre plate-based antibacterial assay incorporating resazurin as an indicator of cell growth, and its application in the in vitro antibacterial screening of phytochemicals. *Methods* **2007**, *42*, 321–324. [CrossRef] [PubMed]
27. Fink, R.; Potočnik, A.; Oder, M. Plant-based natural saponins for Escherichia coli surface hygiene management. *LWT* **2020**, *122*, 109018. [CrossRef]
28. Babajanian, M.; Marden, M. Safer cleaning products and asthma: Tips and resources for health professionals. *AAP Action* **2021**, 6–10. Available online: https://nysceck.org/wp-content/uploads/2021/11/AAP_-in_Action_November_2021_Newsletter_6-10.pdf (accessed on 25 November 2022).
29. Masyita, A.; Sari, R.M.; Astuti, A.D.; Yasir, B.; Rumata, N.R.; Emran, T.B.; Nainu, F.; Simal-Gandara, J. Terpenes and terpenoids as main bioactive compounds of essential oils, their roles in human health and potential application as natural food preservatives. *Food Chem. X* **2022**, *13*, 100217. [CrossRef]
30. Zhao, X.; Wei, S.; Tian, Q.; Peng, W.; Tao, Y.; Bo, R.; Liu, M.; Li, J. Eugenol exposure in vitro inhibits the expressions of T3SS and TIF virulence genes in Salmonella Typhimurium and reduces its pathogenicity to chickens. *Microb. Pathog.* **2022**, *162*, 105314. [CrossRef]
31. Huang, J.; Yang, L.; Zou, Y.; Luo, S.; Wang, X.; Liang, Y.; Du, Y.; Feng, R.; Wei, Q. Antibacterial activity and mechanism of three isomeric terpineols of Cinnamomum longepaniculatum leaf oil. *Folia Microbiol.* **2021**, *66*, 59–67. [CrossRef]
32. Costa, M.D.S.; Rocha, J.E.; Campina, F.F.; Silva, A.R.; Da Cruz, R.P.; Pereira, R.L.; Quintans-Júnior, L.J.; De Menezes, I.R.; Adriano, A.D.S.; De Freitas, T.S. Comparative analysis of the antibacterial and drug-modulatory effect of d-limonene alone and complexed with β-cyclodextrin. *Eur. J. Pharm. Sci.* **2019**, *128*, 158–161. [CrossRef]
33. Van de Vel, E.; Sampers, I.; Raes, K. A review on influencing factors on the minimum inhibitory concentration of essential oils. *Crit. Rev. Food Sci. Nutr.* **2019**, *59*, 357–378. [CrossRef]
34. Kampf, G. Adaptive bacterial response to low level chlorhexidine exposure and its implications for hand hygiene. *Microb. Cell* **2019**, *6*, 307. [CrossRef] [PubMed]
35. Cota, J.B.; Carvalho, A.C.; Dias, I.; Reisinho, A.; Bernardo, F.; Oliveira, M. Salmonella spp. in pet reptiles in portugal: Prevalence and chlorhexidine gluconate antimicrobial efficacy. *Antibiotics* **2021**, *10*, 324. [CrossRef] [PubMed]
36. Ulhaq, Z.S.; Hendyatama, T.H.; Hameed, F.; Santosaningsih, D. Antibacterial activity of Citrus hystrix toward Salmonella spp. infection. *Enferm. Infecc. Y Microbiol. Clin.* **2021**, *39*, 283–286. [CrossRef]
37. Umagiliyage, A.L.; Becerra-Mora, N.; Kohli, P.; Fisher, D.J.; Choudhary, R. Antimicrobial efficacy of liposomes containing d-limonene and its effect on the storage life of blueberries. *Postharvest Biol. Technol.* **2017**, *128*, 130–137. [CrossRef]
38. Condell, O.; Power, K.A.; Händler, K.; Finn, S.; Sheridan, A.; Sergeant, K.; Renaut, J.; Burgess, C.M.; Hinton, J.C.; Nally, J.E. Comparative analysis of Salmonella susceptibility and tolerance to the biocide chlorhexidine identifies a complex cellular defense network. *Front. Microbiol.* **2014**, *5*, 373. [CrossRef]

Disclaimer/Publisher's Note: The statements, opinions and data contained in all publications are solely those of the individual author(s) and contributor(s) and not of MDPI and/or the editor(s). MDPI and/or the editor(s) disclaim responsibility for any injury to people or property resulting from any ideas, methods, instructions or products referred to in the content.

MDPI
St. Alban-Anlage 66
4052 Basel
Switzerland
Tel. +41 61 683 77 34
Fax +41 61 302 89 18
www.mdpi.com

Processes Editorial Office
E-mail: processes@mdpi.com
www.mdpi.com/journal/processes

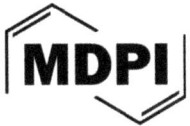

www.ingramcontent.com/pod-product-compliance
Lightning Source LLC
LaVergne TN
LVHW070647100526
838202LV00013B/899